Food:
The Gift of Osiris

VOLUME 2

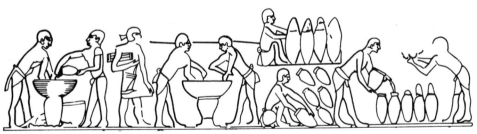

preparation of bread and beer

Frontispiece: The God Osiris. Tomb of Sennutem (number 1) at Thebes. (Deir el Medina); New Kingdom, Ramessid Period, date uncertain. Photographed 1967

Food:
The Gift of Osiris

WILLIAM J. DARBY

*Vanderbilt University, Nashville,
Tennessee, U.S.A. and
The Nutrition Foundation,
New York, U.S.A.*

PAUL GHALIOUNGUI

Cairo, Egypt

LOUIS GRIVETTI

*University of California,
Davis, California, U.S.A.*

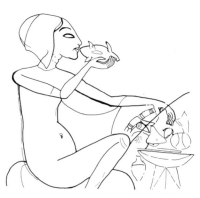

VOLUME 2

ACADEMIC PRESS

1977

London New York San Francisco

A Subsidiary of Harcourt Brace Jovanovich, Publishers

ACADEMIC PRESS INC. (LONDON) LTD.
24/28 Oval Road, London NW1

United States Edition published by
ACADEMIC PRESS INC.
111 Fifth Avenue, New York, New York 10003

Library of Congress Catalog Card Number: 75-19630
ISBN: 0-12-203402-3

Text set in 11/12 pt Monotype Baskerville, printed by photolithography,
and bound in Great Britain at The Pitman Press, Bath

For

Elva Darby
Hugette Ghalioungui
Georgette Grivetti

Preface

The cultural significance of given items of food, in a given society, and at a given time, is widely, though often only subconsciously, recognized. Less generally is it appreciated that the social implications of eating particular foods vary from one period to another or from culture to culture. Conversely, some attitudes persist for exceedingly long periods of time and through diverse social eras, and all the while the current explanations or interpretations of the conditions that gave rise to them may differ considerably from earlier explanations or from their factual origin.

These concepts are particularly well illustrated, retrospectively, by the unparalleled wealth of evidence pertaining to foods over the 7,000 or more years of history recorded in that relatively small geographic area commonly referred to as "the Middle East". Inasmuch as many modern food attitudes are associated with the religious or ethical concepts of the three dominant religions, Christianity, Islam and Judaism, which all originated there, an understanding of the genesis of food habits in this region should be of especial interest to the major cultures of the Western world.

However, these religions and the associated cultural attitudes toward food did not develop *de novo*; they were based upon practices and codes of earlier, highly developed social structures and civilizations, partial records of which are available. These records (or fragments of them) are so scattered through the storehouses of knowledge that they are inaccessible to scholars except within the inventories of their particular scholarly disciplines. We have, therefore, attempted to assemble as much as possible of the evidence that is interpretable in terms of food use and changing attitudes towards foods, as those occurred in courses of the history of the regions studied. Where feasible, we have also tried to relate these concepts to the position of certain foods today.

The constant concern of the ancient physician for diet is a recurrent theme in the writings of the classical physician-scholars Hippocrates, Celsus, Avicenna, and others. The use of foodstuffs in prescriptions from the records of Egyptian physicians from the time of Imhotep onwards, and their instructions, reveal much concerning the "art of food" at a given time, or the availability of food items. Hence, we judge that our account would be incomplete without reference to food in medicine.

The broad understanding thus obtained should provide a useful perspective to our own changing habits and attitudes, as well as to foreign habits that might seem to us strange or incomprehensible. Hopefully, it may afford a greater appreciation of that neglected area of history, namely, the cultural role that food plays in societies. Accordingly, the present work should be of interest to readers of widely diverse backgrounds: agriculturalists, anthropologists, archaeologists, classicists, ecclesiasticists, Egyptologists, food scientists, historians, nutritionists, medical historians, sociologists and others. It should appeal also to that inquisitive general reader who is intrigued with the origin and evolution of his own value judgements and living practices, and who experiences the thrill of romance in the magnificent and colourful fragments of knowledge of earlier civilizations from which the roots of his culture and traditions have been so richly nurtured.

We recognized the enormity of our undertaking and the diversity of sources and disciplines that had to be drawn upon. We have sought, therefore, the counsel and guidance of a wise circle of competent colleagues. We have appreciated the role of food in mythological, mystic, and religious beliefs in determining attitudes and, conversely, the influence of these beliefs upon food acceptability, and have, therefore, sought cues from diverse sources in order that others with deeper knowledge and insight may extend our understanding of food and its cultural significance.

The numerous illustrations have been carefully selected as documentary evidence supplied to allow the reader to appreciate both the wealth and the limitations of this knowledge base. Their inherent beauty may add to the attractiveness of the work, but the reader is urged to study them for their remarkable content.

Due to the richness of the associations, it has been difficult to limit the text, but the focus is on Egypt and the Nile valley, with emphasis on the social and cultural concepts relative to foods through the ages. The diversity of the evidence utilized and the weight given by the thoughtful, critical scholar to particular types of evidence made it desirable to document the sources drawn upon. It is hoped that by so doing others in specialized disciplines may be stimulated to pursue the contribution that their field can offer to improve knowledge of the cultural role and position of foods in society.

Volume 1, after a short survey of the state of nutrition in Ancient Egypt, considers the available information on the major food articles of animal origin—protein rich meats, ranging from the sumptuous beef to the popular and often deprecated fish and seafoods. Reflection on the evidence presented indicates that these food stuffs, then as now, were more accessible to the ruling class, the wealthy, the priesthood, the affluent. Much of the evidence is gleaned from scenes depicting the life-style of the nobility, the leisure class, the pharaohs, or the scholarly traveler. Permanent records of practices by the common man are few, except as seen through the eyes of the élite. Hence, inferences must be drawn from sources of other kinds in order to synthesize a picture of the food culture of the majority of the people of an historical period.

The animal world, however, played more than a nutritive role in Egyptian thought. It did inspire realistic scenes of husbandry and sport, but it was also an inexhaustible source of inspiration that fed the need of symbolic expression, in literature and art, of the powers and virtues of gods and kings who were called bulls or hawks or were given their shape.

A further step was taken when animals were illustrated, not in solemn divine or royal functions, but in plainly human activities. The general tone was humoristic, animals cooking, brewing, plucking the harp or blowing the oboe. More often it was a burlesque caricature of the ceremonious decoration of tombs and temples, a parody that reached at times a philosophy of the absurd, comparable to the contemporary literature of despair: birds using ladders to climb a tree while a hippopotamus is already seated in its foliage and eating its fruits, humans led by goats, cats serving mice, an army of rats storming a fortress manned by surrendering cats, and the like (Curto, no date). It behoves the student, therefore, in examining this symbolic art or the graphic heralds of Aesop, Muqaffah, and other fabulists of old, to bear in mind such artistic motivations.

The items discussed in Volume 2—cereals, vegetables, fruits and alcoholic beverages, especially beer, are better representatives, however, of the staple diet and of the bulk of caloric intake of the majority of the people in antiquity. Rather than the "meat and wine" of the affluent society, "bread and beer" in Ancient Egypt, "bread and salt" in Biblical and Arabian traditions, "bread and butter" in modern Western usage, are the usual synecdoques for daily food.

The East has always been fond of expressing its wisdom in aphoristic metaphores and parables which springing as they do from the common experience of the people, tersely betray the ecological conditions of their birth. A proverb like "What could the Fellah know of apples" expresses better than a lengthy statistical study the relative scarcity of that expensive fruit and its high "social status" in rural Egypt. "Goose chicks can swim", could have been conceived only in a well-watered countryside. Conversely, the ritual use of sand as a cleansing agent, is borne out by the adage "When water comes, cleaning with sand (*tayammum*) is excluded" and the religious injunction to cleanse with sand cooking vessels defiled by dogs could have been born only in a waterless desert: in these two examples, the Arabian peninsula.

Accordingly, since ages immemorial, street-cries and popular maxims express the meaning of food to the Egyptian people. We have tagged some of these to various food items, drawing from our personal experience and from several publications, more especially from the voluminous collection of proverbs by Mrs F. A. Ragheb (1939), many of which re-appear among the over 800 maxims and street-cries that Miss C. Wissa Wassef recorded in her thesis on the rural and alimentary traditions of the Copts (1971). These traditions are mostly general to all ethnic groups in Egypt, underscoring autochthonous practice as distinct from the ostentatious Turkish and Persian Court cuisines imported during the last five centuries. Her work is invaluable to students of food culture and customs in their relation to seasons, fasts, agricultural cycles and milestones of life (birth, baptism, wedding, delivery, mourning).

William J. Darby
Paul E. Ghalioungui
Louis Grivetti

November 1976

Acknowledgements

This investigation was supported in part by Public Health Service Research Grant No. AM 08317 from the National Institute of Arthritis and Metabolic Diseases. Dr Karl Mason of that Institute has been most helpful throughout our researches.

Research facilities and support granted in part by US Naval Medical Research Unit No. 3 (NAMRU-3), Cairo, ARE—supported by Bureau of Medicine and Surgery, United States Navy Work Unit No. MR005.20–0150, and the National Institutes of Health Grant No. 112501.

The opinions and assertions contained herein are private ones of the authors and are not to be construed as official or reflecting the views of the United States Public Health Service, the Navy Department, the Naval Service at large, or the ARE Ministry of Agriculture, Ministry of Culture and National Orientation, or the Ministry of Health.

We wish to thank the several officials of the Arab Republic of Egypt whose skills and assistance, cooperation, and cordial relationships made possible this study.

Our special gratitude is expressed to Dr Gamal Mokhtar, Under Secretary of State, Department of Antiquities, ARE, from whose experience, guidance, and skill we greatly benefited.

Throughout his tenure as Director General of Antiquities, Dr Mokhtar's schedule has been one of accelerated organization, especially during the intense activities of the past few years. He maintains a calm and friendly professional ease, an unhurried cordiality that he extends to all investigators. Dr Mokhtar's field is Egypt, past and present. His goal is to share the accumulated knowledge with all inquiring scholars. For his friendship, hospitality and scholarly assistance, and for the free access he allowed us to the unique collections and holdings of the Department of Antiquities of the ARE, we are most grateful.

The authors acknowledge their special indebtedness to Mrs. Gloria Martin, who skillfully rendered the large number of excellent, accurate, informative pen and ink drawings made from photographs and other documented sources. These add immeasurably to the clarity of the text, the documentation of sources of information and impart a uniformity of illustrative material that could not otherwise have been obtained.

To each of the several hundred persons who helped with this work we are grateful. We wish, however, to recognize especially the interest and assistance of the following persons:

Ministry of Agriculture, ARE:
  Dr Abbas El-Itriby, Under-Secretary of State
  Dr Mahmoud Helmy El-Kawas, Director-General, Agriculture Museum, Dokki
  Mr Edward Riskalla, Deputy Director-General, Agriculture Museum, Dokki
  Mr Hussein Kamel El Monayar, Administrative Assistant, Antiquities Division, Agriculture Museum, Dokki
  Mr William Nazir, Specialist in Ancient Agriculture, Antiquities Division, Agriculture Museum, Dokki
  Mr Hassan Khattab, Specialist in Ancient Agriculture, Antiquities Division, Agriculture Museum, Dokki
  Mr Ramzy Higazi, Director, Training Division, Department of Foreign Relations, Ministry of Agriculture, Dokki
  Mr Medhat Abu Shahba, Engineer, Department of Foreign Relations, Ministry of Agriculture, Dokki

Ministry of Culture and National Orientation, ARE:
  Dr Henri Riad, Director General, Egyptian Museum, Department of Antiquities
  Dr Abdel Hamid Youssef, Director, Centre for Documentation, Department of Antiquities
  Dr Abdel Hamid èl Dahly, Archaeological Inspector, Luxor, Department of Antiquities
  Mrs Zeinab el Dawakhly, Librarian, Centre for Documentation, Department of Antiquities
  Mr Mohamed Salah, Archaeological Inspector, Necropolis of Thebes, Department of Antiquities
  Mr Ramadan Saad, Archaeological Inspector, Karnak, Department of Antiquities
  Mr Ali el-Khouli, Archaeological Inspector, Saqqara, Department of Antiquities
  Mr Magdi Abdel Maboud Abdalla, Chief Guard, Necropolis of Thebes, Department of Antiquities

To Dr Serge Sauneron, Director, Institut Français d'Archéologie Orientale, Cairo, we offer our great appreciation for use of the vast archives and library materials of this unique Egyptological institution, for valuable information on many Egyptological details, and for the hieroglyphs used in the book that were provided by the presses of the Institut.

To Professor Charles Kuentz, the distinguished Egyptologist and former Director of the Institut Français d'Archéologie Orientale in Cairo, we are indebted for highly valuable help and information on historical and philological details.

Members of the Division of Nutrition of Vanderbilt University have long cooperated with the United States Naval Medical Research Unit No. 3 (NAMRU-3) in Cairo, ARE. We particularly wish to acknowledge this support. To both past and present colleagues at NAMRU-3 we are especially grateful,

> Dr John R. Seal, M.C., USN, Director, NAMRU-3 (1958–61)
> Dr James Boyers, M.C., USN, Director, NAMRU-3 (1962–63)
> Dr Lloyd F. Miller, M.C., USN, Director, NAMRU-3 (1964–67)
> Dr Donald C. Kent, M.C., USN, Director, NAMRU-3 (1967–70)
> Dr Henry Sparks, M.C., USN, Director, NAMRU-3 (1970–73)
> Dr Walter Miner, M.C., USN, Director, NAMRU-3 (1973–present)
> Dr Imam Zaghloul El Sayed, Director-General, Ministry of Health Laboratories, ARE.
> Dr Vinayak Narayan Patwardhan, Assistant Director for Nutrition and Biochemistry
> Dr Harry Hoogstraal, Department Head, Department of Medical Zoology
> Dr Dale Osborn, Mammalogist, Department of Medical Zoology
> Mr Kenneth Otto Horner, Ornithologist, Department of Medical Zoology
> Mr Abdel Aziz Salah, Administrative Assistant
> Mr Ibrahim Helmi, Technician, Department of Medical Zoology
> Mr Samir Araman, Technician, Department of Medical Zoology
> Mr Abdalla Diab, Technician, Department of Bacteriology
> Mr Sobhy Gaber, Research Associate, Department of Medical Zoology
> Mr Hassan Touhami, Laboratory Aide, Department of Medical Zoology
> Mr Abdou Hosny Aly, Nurse, Department of Tropical Medicine

With permission of the ARE Department of Antiquities, Mr Ward Patterson has prepared stone rubbings of selected nutrition reliefs from Old Kingdom tombs at Saqqara. Photographs from his unique collection are used with his permission. Mr A. Bergère, Cultural Attaché, French Embassy, formerly in Kuwait, now in Libya, offered friendly assistance and placed at our disposal texts from his fine Egyptological library.

The staff of the library of University of Chicago, particularly Mr Stanley Gwynn, Miss Shirley Lyon, and Mrs Alexandria Denny of the Breasted Library, assisted the authors during early phases of research. Of distinct help in the translation and organization of archaeological texts were Dr Aida Nureddin and Mrs Georgette Stylianos Mayerakis Grivetti.

Miss Juanita Frazor, Executive Secretary, Department of Biochemistry, Vanderbilt School of Medicine, endured our tempers, illegible handwriting and endless revisions. Her tenacity, skill, and cheerfulness are attributes greatly to be admired.

Although the organization and final content are the sole responsibility of the authors, the text benefits from the review by and encouragement and criticism from professional colleagues from several fields:

Dr Paul E. Johnson, Executive Secretary, Committee on Food Protection, National Research Council, National Academy of Sciences, Washington, D.C.

Dr E. Neige Todhunter, Visiting Professor of Nutrition, Department of Biochemistry, Vanderbilt University School of Medicine, Nashville, Tennessee

Dr Dale Osborn, Mammalogist, Department of Medical Zoology, NAMRU-3, Cairo, ARE.

Dr Kent Weeks, Medical Historian/Egyptologist, Metropolitan Museum, New York

Professor V. Täckholm, Faculty of Science, Cairo University

Dr James S. Dinning, Associate Director, Rockefeller Foundation, Bangkok, Thailand

Dr Wallace Aykroyd, Oxford, England

Dr Frederick J. Simoons, Professor of Geography, University of California, Davis

Mr Kenneth Otto Horner, Ornithologist, Department of Medical Zoology, NAMRU-3, Cairo, ARE.

Dr Richard Hall, Vice President, McCormick and Co. Inc., Hunt Valley, Maryland

Dr Maynard Amerine, Professor of Enology, University of California at Davis

To all Egyptologists, from Champollion to present, whose research and insight provided the keys to the mysteries of Egyptian civilization, we are humbly grateful.

Finally, the authors sincerely appreciate the warm understanding, the interest and patience that has characterized our pleasant relationship with the Academic Press Inc. (London) Ltd. during the production of this book. The encouragement, creativity in design and unstinting cooperation of all of the staff, but especially of Jane Duncan, have made this a remarkably happy author–publisher relationship.

William J. Darby   *November 1976*
Paul E. Ghalioungui
Louis Grivetti

Abbreviations

The following abbreviations to references appear throughout the text.

A.R.   *Ancient Records of Egypt*: see Breasted, J. H. (1906).

ASAE   *Annales du Service des Antiquités de l'Egypte*.

Ber.   The Berlin Papyrus: see Wreszinski, W. (1909). *Der grosse medizinische Papyrus des Berliner Museums*, Leipzig: Hinrichs.

B.I.E.   *Bulletin de l'Institut d'Egypte*, Cairo.

B.I.F.A.O.   *Bulletin de l'Institut Français d'Archéologie Orientale*, Cairo.

Carlsb.   *The Carlsberg Papyrus*, Det Kgl. Videnskabernes Selskab histor.-philologische Meddelelser XXVI, E. Iversen, Copenhagen (1939).

Ch.B.   *The Chester Beatty Papyrus*, Hieratic papyri in the British Museum, 3rd series, Translated by Jonckheere, F. (1947). Brussels: Fondation Egyptologique Reine Elisabeth.

Deipnos.   see Athenaeus, *The Deipnosophists*.

Diod.   see Diodorus Siculus.

Eb.   see Ebbell B., *The Papyrus Ebers*, The Ebbell classification is noted in Roman characters; the Wreszinski in Arabic numerals.

F.   Faulkner, R. O. (1962). *A Concise Dictionary of Middle Egyptian*, Oxford University Press.

Fl.   see Loret, V. (1892b). *La Flore Pharaonique*.

G.   Gardiner, A. H. (1950). *Egyptian Grammar*, 2nd Ed. Oxford: Oxford University Press.

Geo.   see Strabo, *Geography*.

Gpfl.   see Keimer (1924a). *Die Gartenpflanze*.

H.   see Wreszinski (1912). *Der Londoner medizinische Papyrus . . . und der Papyrus Hearst . . .* Leipzig: Hinrichs.

Her.   see *Herodotus*.

I. and O.   see Plutarch, *Isis and Osiris*.

J.E.A.   *Journal of Egyptian Archaeology*.

JNEAS   *Journal of Near Eastern Studies*.

K.   *Hieratic Papyri from Kahun and Gurob*, Griffith, F. Ll., London (1898).

L. London Medical Papyrus: see Wreszinski, W. (1912). *Der Londoner medizinische Papyrus . . . und der Papyrus Hearst . . .*, Leipzig: Hinrichs.

MAE see Hayes, W. C. (1964). *Most Ancient Egypt.*

N.H. see Pliny, *Natural History.*

Pyr. *The Pyramid Texts in Translation and Commentary*, by Mercer, S. A. B. (1952). 4 vols. London: Longmans, Green and Co.

Ram III Gardiner, A. H. (1955). *Five Ramasseum Papyri.* Oxford: Oxford University Press; and Barns, J. W. B. (1956). *Five Ramasseum Papyri*, Oxford: Oxford University Press.

S. *The Edwin Smith Surgical Papyrus.* Translated by Breasted, J. H. (1930). Vol. I. Hieroglyphic transliteration, Translatic and Commentary. Vol. II. Facsimile plates and line for line hieroglyphic transliteration. Chicago: The University of Chicago Press.

S.P. *Select Papyri*, see Hunt, A. S. and Edgar, C. C. (1932–34).

Wb. see Erman, A. and Grapow, H. (1957). *Wörterbuch der aegyptischen Sprache.*

Wb.Dr. see von Deines, H. and Grapow, H. (1959). *Wörterbuch der aegyptische Drogennamen*, Berlin: Akademie-Verlag (Grundriss der Medizin der Alten Aegypter, Vol. 6).

Z.A.S. *Zeitschr. für Aegyptische Sprache und Altertumskunde.*

Zaub. Zaubersprüche für Kind und Mutter, Berlin Papyrus 3027 Erman, A. (1901), Abhandlungen der königlichen Preussicher Akademie der Wissenschaften zu Berlin.

T. see Täckholm, V. L. (1941–69). *The Flora of Egypt.*

Note on Vocalization of Symbols used in Transliterating Hieroglyphic Sounds

ʾ the glottal stop heard at the commencement of German words beginning with a vowel, ex. *der Adler* (Arabic *alif hamzatun*)

ỉ Consonantal *Y*

ʿ a guttural sound unknown in English, corresponds to Hebrew *avin*, Arabic *ain*

ḥ emphatic *h*, corresponds to Arabic *ḥa*

ḫ like *ch* in Scottish *loch*

h perhaps like *ch* in German *ich*

š *sh*

ḳ backward *k*; rather like our *q* in *queen*, corresponds to Hebrew *qoph* Arabic *kaf*

ṯ *tsh*

ḏ *dj*

Conventionally an *e* is intercalated between consonants in pronouncing Ancient Egyptian words except when an ʾ or an ʿ which are read *a*, are present.

Adapted from Gardiner (1950), p. 27.

Contents

Contents of Volume 1

List of Illustrations Volume 2

Endpapers:

Front left. Ptahhetep. Saqqara.
Front right. Nefertari. Thebes.
Back left. Mereruka's tomb. Saqqara.
Back right. Tomb of Ptahhetep. Saqqara.

Half-title page. Preparation of bread and beer (Fig. 12.3).
Title page. Youth devouring a duck (Fig. 6.25).
Frontispiece (Colour plate). The god Osiris.

Chapter 11 Grains

All photographs taken by authors except when specifically acknowledged otherwise.

Chapter 12 Bread

Chapter 13 Beer

Chapter 14 Wine (Part I)

Volume 2   Introduction

Agriculture and Irrigation

The inhabitants of the Nile Valley early turned their attention to agriculture, as they outgrew the hunter-gatherer-fisherman stage. Initially, they merely sowed the silt left by the receding flood waters of the Nile god Hapi ("He who overspreadth"); but they soon learned to divide the land into basins, to dig canals and to raise banks. All these arts, they claimed, had been taught to their ancestors by the good god Osiris whose heirs and trustees, the Pharaohs, by faithful performance of the necessary rites assured the perpetuation of these blessings. It is not a coincidence that one of the oldest pictures of pharaohs shows the "Scorpion King", hoe in hand, ceremoniously cutting an irrigation canal (Fig. 11.1), thus ensuring the continued enjoyment of the gifts of agriculture and proclaiming its sanctity. The holiness of grain was further repeatedly stressed in the feasts that were celebrated at fixed times and during the harvest in honour of the serpent-headed harvest goddess Renenet (Fig. 11.2), and in the ritual dances and music that accompanied the various phases of grain gathering (Figs 11.3 and 11.4).

The earliest attempts at bridling the flood of the Nile date to the prehistoric men who raised dykes on its shores to keep the land from periodic devastation. Herodotus exclaimed

"Any one who sees Egypt without having heard a word about it, must perceive. . . that she is an acquired country, the gift of the river. . ." (II, 5)

and Strabo (15, 1, 16) commented that this was the reason why the Nile was called by the same name as the land, Aegyptos, which, in the Odyssey, is the name of the Nile.

There are, indeed, nebulous testimonies to the colossal efforts exerted by Pharaohs to tame this unruly river that ultimately unified its valley. If we are to believe Herodotus, before the founder of the first dynasty, Menes, the Nile

". . . flowed along the sandy range of hills which skirts Egypt on the side of Libya. He [Menes], however, by banking up the river at the bend which

453

it forms about a hundred furlongs south of Memphis, laid the ancient channel dry while he dug a new course for the stream halfway between the two lines of hills. To this day, the elbow which the Nile forms at the point where it is forced aside into the new channel is guarded with the greatest care by the Persians and strengthened every year; for if the river were to burst out at this place and pour over the mound, there would be danger of Memphis being completely overwhelmed by the flood." (II, 99)

There is, unfortunately, no unassailable evidence to support the above statement of Herodotus, but there are solid grounds to credit Amenemhat III of the twelfth dynasty (*c.* 1849–1801 B.C.) with an enormous scheme of irrigation to utilize the flood waters in the intervals between inundations.

In prehistoric times the high Nile ran through a narrow gap in the western high grounds into the low Fayoum basin, creating there a vast lake. Amenemhat and probably other rulers of the same dynasty managed to control the inflow and outflow at the gap, and built in that spot retention walls that enabled them to reclaim for cultivation a total of 27,000 acres (Breasted, 1909, pp. 191–193). In addition, by controlling the flow, enough water was accumulated in the basin to double the volume of the river below the Fayoum during the hundred days of low Nile (Major R. H. Brown, quoted by Breasted, 1909, p. 193). This immense agricultural expansion gained Amenemhat III well deserved praise. It was said of him by the people

"He makes the Two Lands verdant more than a great Nile . . . He is Life . . . The King is food and his mouth is increase." (*A.R.*, I, 747)

When the Greeks visited the area, they were amazed at the size of the works, and they created the legend that the whole basin, which they called "Lake Moeris", was an artificial creation. Says Herodotus (II, 149)

"Wonderful as is the Labyrinth, the work called the Lake Moeris which is close by the Labyrinth is yet more astonishing . . . It is manifestly an artificial excavation, for nearly in the centre there stand two pyramids . . . crowned each of them with a colossal statue sitting upon a throne . . . The water of the lake does not come out of the ground which is here excessively dry, but is introduced by a canal from the Nile. The current sets for six months into the lake from the river and, for the next six months, into the river from the lake. The natives told me that there was a subterranean passage from this lake to Syrtis running westwards into the interior by the hills above Memphis."

It is certainly the silt deposited south of the Illahun dam that is responsible for the exceptional fertility of the land from Beni-Suef down through Asyut, compared with the rest of Upper Egypt. To quote again Herodotus (II, 5)

"The same is true of the land above the lake [Moeris] to the distance of three days voyage [i.e. to about Asyut] . . . which is exactly the same kind of country [as the Delta]."

The statues have disappeared, but on their site were found their bases that Herodotus had taken for pyramids, and some fragments that bear the name of Amenemhat III, who is thus enabled to watch in eternity his gigantic realization.

Watch was kept on the flood far south by nilometers that recorded its vagaries long before they were felt in the north, and such observations, communicated without delay to the officials of Lower Egypt in the vizier's office, enabled them to estimate the crops of the coming season, and, accordingly, to fix the rate of taxation (Breasted, 1909, p. 191). These were the tasks of high ranking officers who appear, from their titles, to have administered an important Department of Irrigation (see Vol. 1, Chapter 2) directly responsible to the Vizier (Petrie, 1925).

Chapter 11   *Grains*

Grain in General

Grain in general, or barley, was depicted by (a) (*F.*, 32) or (b) (*F.*, 428), and later by (c) (*F.*, 270) or (d)[1] (*F.*, 130). An ear of corn (wheat) was depicted by (e) (*F.*, 70), and a seed, or posterity, by (f) and (g).

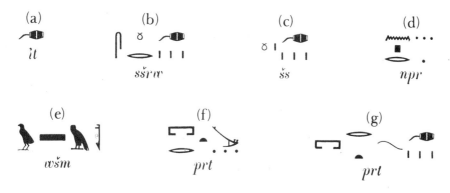

History

Is it wheat or barley?
(Popular saying for "Good or bad news")

The profuse synonymy in ancient writings besets the task of identifying particular grains with great difficulties. It is readily understandable, however, why ancient words for cereals or grains are so confusing, when one considers the number of foreign or national groups that figured importantly throughout Egyptian history. Various travellers identified same grains differently; conquerors added their own appellations, and the resultant confusion is amply documented throughout 12,000 years along the Nile Valley.

In the dawn of Egyptian history, all cereals were termed simply grain, i.e. seeds, and people saw little reason to invent more precise

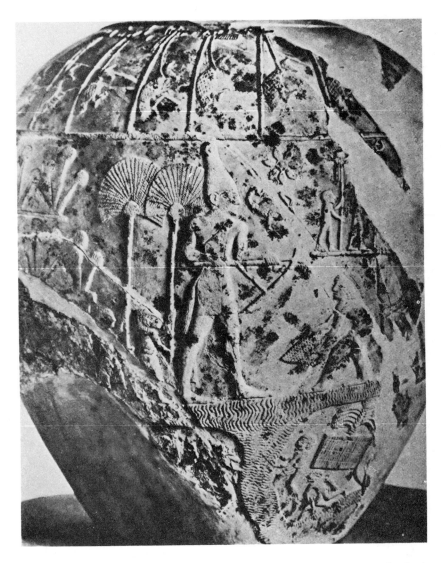

Fig. 11.1. Mace head depicting King Zer opening the irrigation canals at the beginning of the Flood Season. *c.* 2,600 B.C. Ashmolean Museum.

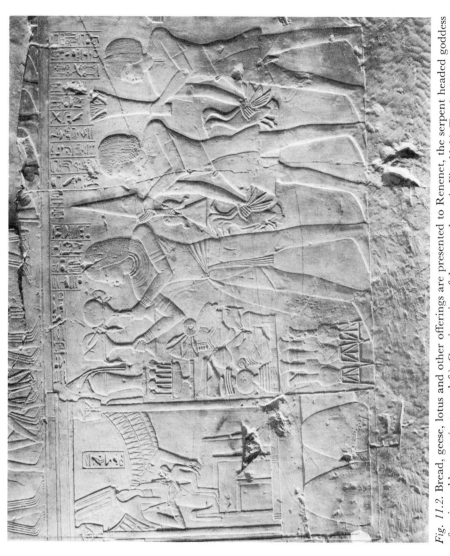

Fig. 11.2. Bread, geese, lotus and other offerings are presented to Renenet, the serpent headed goddess of grain and harvests (extreme left). Continuation of the scene shown in Fig. 11.11. Tomb of Kha-em-hat. Overseer of Granaries of Amenhotep III. Eighteenth dynasty. Luxor West. Centre of Documentation, Cairo.

words dividing the various cereals into categories. Progressively, some distinctions were made; but fuzzy descriptive groupings lingered through the centuries to plague twentieth century botanists and historians. Accurately defined terms, that may be too specific, are products of the modern concern with scientific classification. The Ancients cannot be blamed for a lack of discrimination in respect to grain, that was beyond their interests, and for the resultant confusion of taxonamists.

A word that caused the deepest misunderstanding, both in antiquity and nowadays, is "corn". Today in the United States, this word denotes *Zea mays*, maize; in England it means wheat, and in Scotland, oats (Browning, 1960). Another word, *zea*, as used by Greek authors, denoted five distinct entities, all different from maize, namely: wheat in general, wheat (*Triticum dicoccum*), wheat (*Triticum monococcum*); sorghum and rice.

Corn, in antiquity and the Biblical sense, was the English translation of grain, mostly wheat; but definitely not the American maize that the Spaniards learned from Meso-American Indians only in the fifteenth century A.D. and introduced into Europe, from which it was imported into Egypt via Syria or Morea some time during the eighteenth century A.D. Hence its Egyptian names *dura shami* (Syrian dura), *dura morali* (Morean dura), or *dura Turki* (Turkish dura), *dura* being Arabic for "sorghum".[2]

It is established that grain was harvested in the most remote periods of Egyptian antiquity, although the evidence is indirect and does not stem from finding of grain *per se*. From the Upper Paleolithic, specifically the Sebilian III type horizon, polished grinding stones have been discovered that were used for crushing grain and preparing flour (*MAE*, 60). From the horizon of the oft-debated Mesolithic, between the Paleolithic and Neolithic, small geometric flints, usually rectangular or trapezoidal, have been found in many parts of Egypt adjacent to the Nile and to Lake Fayoum, and in the remote oases of Khargah and Siwa (*MAE*, 70–74). These microliths, when hafted in wooden handles, formed the blades of the sickles used for reaping grains. Continued abrasion from cutting the highly siliceous cereal stems left a worn polished sheen along the cutting edge, further documenting the use of grain at that period (*MAE*, 100). Such polished-microlith sickle blades were found in sites dating throughout the Neolithic Period and far into dynastic times and many are on display at the Cairo Antiquities Museum.

It is speculative as to exactly when man in Egypt ceased his nomadic existence as a hunter-gatherer and started to grow grain, thereby freeing himself from his uncertain dependance for food on migrating herds of meat beasts, and being permitted the settled existence that made possible his cultural and technological developments, but suddenly, at the base occupational levels of the Fayoum "A" type horizon, substantial, even somewhat sophisticated, agricultural techniques appeared. This is, at present, the earliest known site in Egypt where grain has actually been found *in situ*, but the process must have started long before, i.e. during the Upper Paleolithic-Mesolithic Periods.

The ancientness of the use of cereals and of the cultivation of wheat is well documented. Aykroyd and Doughty (1970) state that the Jarmo remains constitute the earliest known archaeological record of the use of wheat as human food but that the process of domestication probably extended much earlier. Both they, and Storcke and Teague (1952) emphasize the evidence from the Natufian culture in Palestine, from sites at Jericho and Mount Carmel, that grains were harvested and perhaps cultivated as early as the ninth millenium B.C. This evidence consists of remains of stone and pottery bowls and flint sickles with bone shafts, the flint possessing the gloss characteristic of used tools.

In addition, wild wheat and barley grow in these regions today, presumably dating from Neolithic times. At any rate, to the Fertile Crescent of Asia may well be ascribed the site of domestication of cultivated wheat at least by 8,000–6,000 B.C., with the simultaneous domestication of sheep and wild goats.

Storcke and Teague depicted the spread of cultivation of wheat in a map reproduced in Fig. 11.5. Their approach, based on genetic and chromosomal studies may be the surest way to trace the avatars of wheat from the earliest days.

Genetically, there are three major groups of wheat.

1. The 14-chromosome group (or Diploid, i.e. containing twice the 7-chromosome grouping called "genome A"). This group includes wild and cultivated Einkorn.

2. The 28-chromosome group (or Tetraploid, i.e. containing twice the two 7-chromosome groupings called "genomes A and B"). This group includes wild and cultivated Emmer and Durum (hard) wheats, used to make pastes and spaghetti.

3. The 42-chromosome group (or Hexaploid, i.e. containing twice the three 7-chromosome groupings, "genomes A, B, and C, or

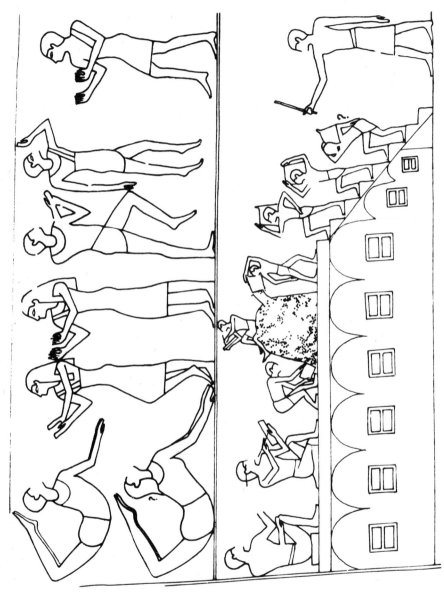

Fig. 11.3. Dances accompanying the harvest. Below, under the supervision of a chief, workmen carry grain into the silos, while scribes register the amounts brought in. Thebes. Middle Kingdom. Tomb of Antefoker. Reproduced from Davies and Gardiner (1920), plate XV.

Fig. 11.4a. (Colour plate, facing page) The harvest packed in basket. Tomb of Nakht. Thebes. New Kingdom. Photographed 1969.

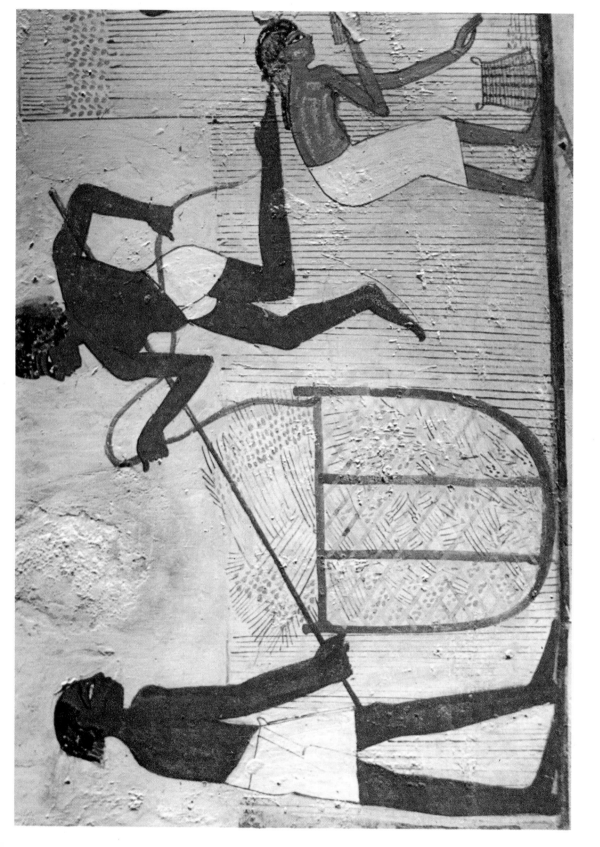

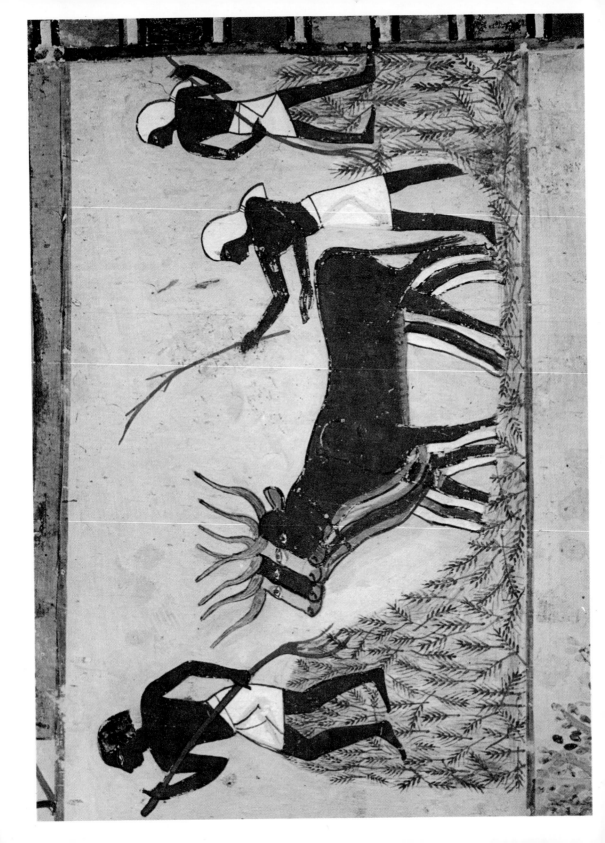

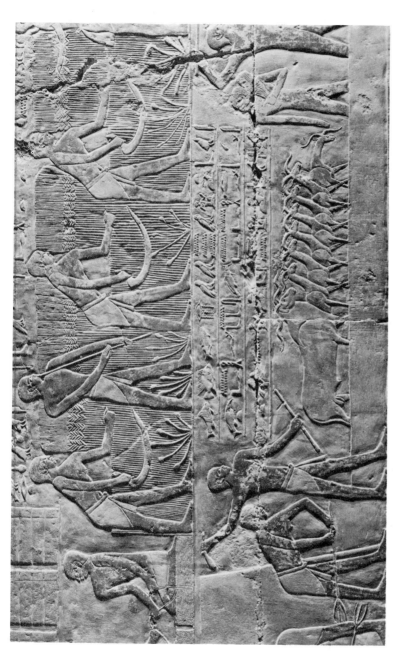

Fig. 11.4b. (Colour plate, facing page) Oxen threshing grain. Tomb of Mena (number 69) at Thebes (Upper Enclosure); New Kingdom, eighteenth dynasty, reign of King Thutmose IV, *c.* 1420 B.C. Photographed 1969.

Fig. 11.4c. (This page) Harvest scenes. Upper: reaping grain and tying the sheaves. Lower: right, rams treading grain in the threshing floor. Tomb of Mereruka. Saqqara. Old Kingdom. Centre of Documentation, Cairo.

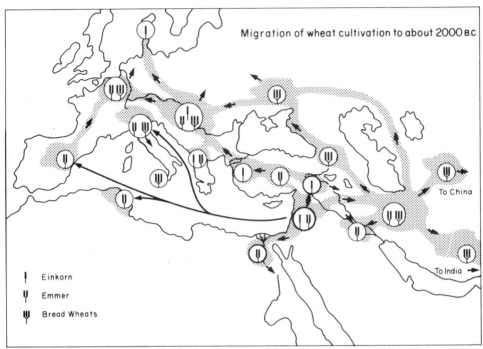

Fig. 11.5. Diagrammatic chart of the spread of the wheats from Syria-Palestine, the place of first cultivation about 7000 B.C. (indicated by the two heavier circles), throughout the Near East and Europe, up to about 2000 B.C. Only the more important paths followed by wheat cultivation in its spread are indicated. Note the central position of Iran in the spread of the bread-wheats, and also the part played by the central Danube Valley as a secondary centre of diffusion. From *A History of Milling, Flour for Man's Bread.* Storcke and Teague (1952), Minneapolis: University of Minnesota Press.

in the case of *Triticum timopheevi*, genomes A, B, and D). To this group belong the bread wheats, including *T. vulgare* the most cultivated wheat and club wheat, *T. compactum.*

Genome A is found in all wheats. It undoubtedly comes from Einkorn. The second group stems from group 1, either through crossing with a new variety, or by doubling and slightly modifying its chromosomes. The third group stems from the second through a similar process.

It is further believed that the three-genome wheat originated in Iran to the northeast of Mesopotamia. Emmer, its parent, was found there at a number of sites; and while actual finds of Emmer wheat have not been reported from Iran, they have been discovered in the surrounding

regions. Storcke and Teague concluded that grain cultivation began
either in Syria-Palestine with Einkorn or Emmer, or that these were
rapidly transferred to Syria after starting somewhere farther north
along the Anatolian foothills. Thence they spread by way of Palestine
to Egypt, and by way of Mesopotamia to Iran where wheat somehow
hybridized.

To state, however, that the initial impetus for grain cultivation, or
any other cultural trait, whether it be social, technical or nutritional,
originated with "X" people at "Y" time is unduly to simplify a highly
complex situation. Man's early movements in and through the Nile
Valley during these formative years in African and Asian history have
to be better understood, and more critical palaeobotanical studies must
be made before the correct understanding of agricultural diffusion is
possible.

It is, therefore, preferable to leave the question open, for there is
indeed evidence that these same early Egyptians were also in contact
with populations further to the south that influenced them (Wendorf
et al., 1970). This latter contact is clear in many legacies, *inter alia* in the
Sed festivals in which the ritual death and rebirth of the Egyptian king
was played out periodically in order to assure the renewed strength and
virility of the monarch. This ritual was not a product of Semite diffusion,
but it represented early Nilotic and East African patterns, like the still
existing "king-must-die" tradition of the Shilluks who presently live
along the Nile in central Sudan, south of Khartoum.

Grain was not only a staple of the diet, but a source of income for
land-owners and for government as well. In times of need Egyptians
sold their grain to less fortunate foreigners

> ". . . and all countries came into Egypt to Joseph for to buy corn [wheat];
> because the famine was so sore in all lands . . ." (Genesis, 41–57)

In the great temple of Abu Simbel, built by King Rameses II (nineteenth dynasty, 1298–1232 B.C.), the King instructed his craftsmen to
carve the words of the God Ptah as they were revealed to him

> ". . . I (the God) give to thee (Rameses II) constant harvests, to feed the
> Two Lands at all times; the sheaves thereof are like the sand of the shore,
> their granaries approach heaven, and their grain-heaps are like mountains
> . . ." (*A.R.*, III, 404)

Later, Egypt, so rich in grain, was considered to be the "breadbasket"
of the Roman world.

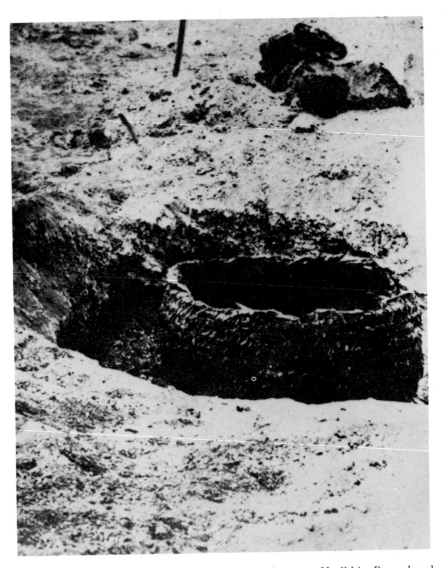

Fig. 11.6. Baskets kept underground, serving as grain stores. Neolithic. Reproduced from *The Desert Fayum*, Caton-Thompson and Gardner (1934), plate XXVII, silo no. 12.

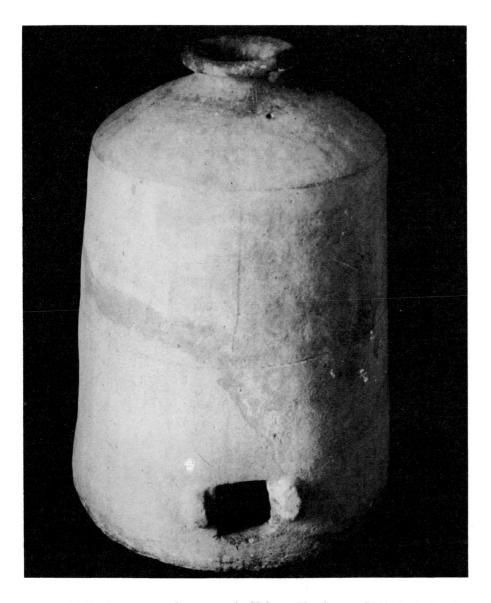

Fig. 11.7. Earthenware vessel to store grain. Helwan. First dynasty. Dokki Agricultural Museum.

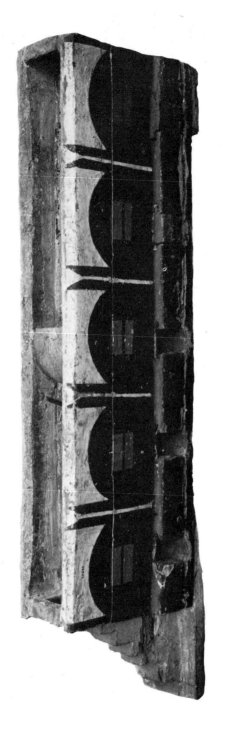

Fig. 11.8. Model of granary. Found in Akhmim, Upper Egypt. Cairo Museum, J. 28839.

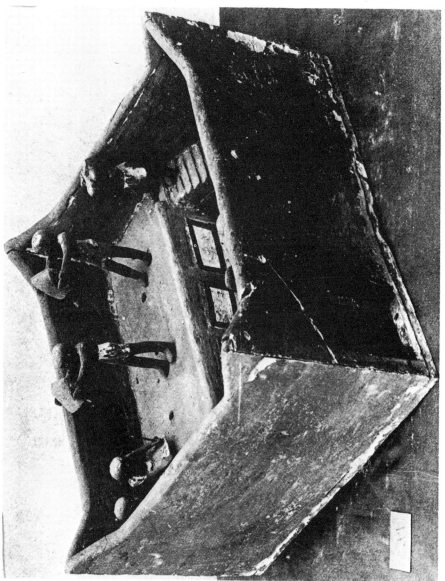

Fig. 11.9. Model of granary with farmers pouring grain from above into the silos, and others withdrawing it from openings below. Right: a supervisor. Upper left: scribes. Saqqara. Middle Kingdom. Cairo Museum.

Famine

Yet, with all this seeming abundance, famine occasionally raged through Egypt creating dietary and economic disasters. Africanus, quoting from the lost texts of Manetho (Waddell, 1940, p. 29) reported the great singular event that, during the rule of King Uenephes,[3] a great famine seized Egypt. There exists a more accurately dated report from the eighteenth year of the reign of King Zoser (third dynasty, *c.* 2750 B.C.) (see Volume 1, Chapter 2).

> ". . . the Nile has not risen in my time for the space of eight years. Corn [wheat] is scarce, there is lack of herbage, and nothing is left to eat . . ."

More than seven hundred years later, during the reign of King Senusret I (second king of the twelfth dynasty, *c.* 1970–1936 B.C.) Prince Amenemhat (or Ameni) recorded his own benevolence in his tomb at Beni Hassan,

> ". . . when the years of famine came, I plowed all the fields of the Oryx nome . . . preserving its people alive and furnishing its food so that there was none hungry therein . . ." (*A.R.*, I, 523)

Kheti, a nomarch of the ninth to tenth dynasty who devoted himself to the improvement of his city said

> "I was rich in grain. When the land was in need, I maintained the city with *Kha* and with *Heket*.[4] I allowed the citizen to carry away for himself grain, and his wife, the widow, and her son." (*A.R.*, I, 408)

Such disasters called for special religious functions that, in Buto, included a personal intervention of the king in the temple of the goddess Wadjet, public supplications and prostrations in the "Castle of Silence", and processions in Min's chapels throughout the territory. Drioton (1943a), who published the stele on which this tradition is preserved, stated that, although it dates to the Roman era, the reference to the king indicates that it stemmed from Pharaonic times.

Overseers of Granaries

To forestall such calamities, grain was stored ever since the Neolithic; at first in baskets buried underground (Fig. 11.6) or in earthenware jars

(Fig. 11.7); later in communal silos and granaries (Figs 2.8, 11.8, 11.9, 11.10) stacked with provisions, that were administered by an "Overseer of Granaries" who ranked next to Pharaoh, although this title appears so exalted that it might have lost its literal meaning and come to be purely honorific.

Thus, Ineni was Hereditary Prince, Count, and Chief of all Works in Karnak; the Double-Silver House was under his charge; the Double-Gold House was on his seal; he was Sealer of contracts in the House of Amon, Excellency, Overseer of the Double Granary of Amon (*A.R.*, II, 43).

Hemi, a minister of Mentuhotep III, arrayed a picturesque list of titles

> "his real favourite servant, Wearer of the Royal Seal, Overseer of that which is and that which is not, Overseer of the Temples, Overseer of the Granary and White House, Overseer of horn and hoof, Chief of the Sixth Courts of Justice, high-voiced in proclaiming the name of the King, who judges the prisoner according to his desert." (*A.R.*, I, 428)

These lofty personages who held in their hands the strings of the most important Ministries were so highly trusted that they were charged with the most delicate missions, like judging the robbers of the Royal Tombs (*A.R.*, IV, 156), or reporting on the activities of other officials

> "Reward of the stewards of the estates of Pharaoh . . . after the statement of the Overseer of the Granary concerning them: they have increased the harvest of the year 30." (*A.R.*, II, 872)

They were even buried close to the kings. Thus, under Rameses IX, robbers broke their way into the burial place of King Sekhem-Re-Shed-Kawy from the outer chamber of the tomb of the Overseer of Granaries of Thutmose III, Nebamon (*A.R.*, IV, 517).

Import and Tribute

Clearly, the Biblical tradition of Joseph and the seven "fat" years and seven "lean" years does not want more documented antecedents. The lessons learned from severe famine were not forgotten and, though Egypt was blessed with abundant harvests, she also imported grain. In Kha-em-hat's tomb at Thebes, large ships are seen unloading bags of cereals (Fig. 11.11) that are offered to the goddess of grain and

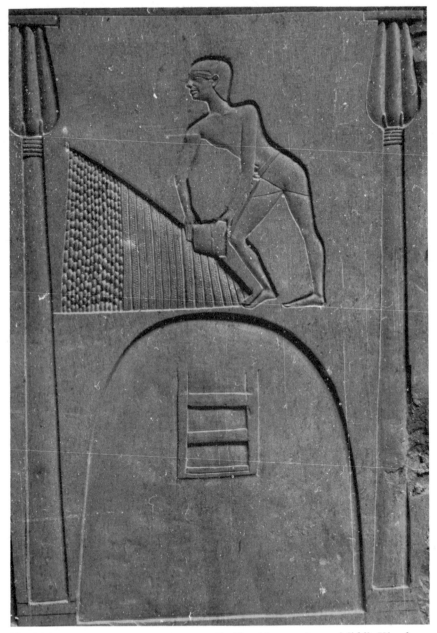

Fig. 11.10. A peasant pouring grain into a silo. Kawit's sarcophagus. Middle Kingdom. Cairo Museum.

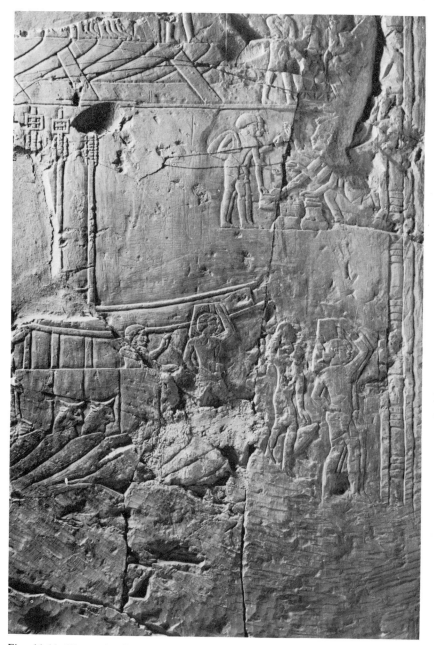

Fig. 11.11. The unloading of grain from merchant ships. Tomb of Kha-em-hat, Overseer of Granaries of Amenhotep III (eighteenth dynasty). Luxor West. Centre of Documentation, Cairo. Continuation of Fig. 11.2.

harvests Renenet (Fig. 11.2). These were imported mainly from Syria from which barley is often mentioned in offerings (*A.R.*, IV, 287, 344, 391). The tribute lists of King Thutmose III (eighteenth dynasty, *c.* 1504–1450 B.C.), give examples of grain exacted from other countries

". . . Behold, the cultivable land was divided into fields which the inspectors of the Royal House calculated in order to reap their harvest; a statement [of the harvest] was brought to his Majesty from the fields of Megiddo . . ." (*A.R.*, II, 437)

". . . list of tribute brought to his Majesty: loaves, various loaves, clean grain in kernel, and ground . . ." (*A.R.*, II, 462)

and

". . . He [Thutmose III] arrived at the city of Kadesh, overthrew it, cut down its groves, harvested its grain . . ." (*A.R.*, II, 465)

He did the same in Tw-nep (*A.R.*, II, 530); took grain as booty from Nahorin (*A.R.*, II, 480); and from Retenu (*A.R.*, II, 473).

Donations

The records are numberless wherein the kings and nobles prided themselves in their largesses to the commoners

". . . I gave bread to the hungry, clothing to the naked, and of grain, and of oxen . . ." (*A.R.*, I, 378)

King Amenemhat I (first king of the twelfth dynasty, *c.* 2000–1970 B.C.), narrated

". . . I was one who cultivated grain and loved the harvest god . . ." (*A.R.*, I, 483)

The edict of Horemheb (nineteenth dynasty) enumerated, likewise, his lavish distributions (*A.R.*, III, 66).

Donations to temples were, naturally, larger. The papyrus Harris records the huge quantities given by King Rameses III (*c.* 1198–1166 B.C.) to the gods and temples of Egypt

". . . I gave to thee ten-thousand measures of grain to provision thy divine offerings of every day . . ." (*A.R.*, IV, 206)

and the same king described his generosity and berated the "stinginess" of his predecessors

". . . I made for thee [the God] granaries filled with grain which had begun to fall waste, and they became millions . . ." (*A.R.*, IV, 267)

A most unusual account recorded during the reign of King Rameses IX (twentieth dynasty, *c.* 1100 B.C.), tells of grave robbers captured by officials in the act of looting a tomb and of their subsequent interrogation

". . . the thief (though caught 'red-handed' the speaker denied his involvement in the crime and blamed his accomplice), *he* made me take some grain, I seized a sack of grain and when I began to go down [*flee*] . . ." (*A.R.*, IV, 550)

The human trait of blaming others for one's crime seems to be an ancient one.

Taxation

On the other hand, cultivators were expected to contribute part of their harvests to the treasury, though, in what proportion, we do not know. "Barley of the impost of the peasants" is thus recorded in a document of the time of Rameses III (*A.R.*, IV, 229).

Inscriptions from the tomb of Rekhmire, the prestigious vizier of Thutmose III, list grain in several places and record three unidentified grains, *yhe, sh,* and *tb,* as partial payment for governmental taxes in the districts of Coptos and Diospolis Parva (*A.R.*, II, 733–737).

Grain in Graeco-Roman Times

During the Graeco-Roman period, travellers to Egypt repeatedly mentioned the profusion of grain in that country, but Strabo (17, 1, 35) generally failed to comment on the vast amounts produced in Egypt. He simply stated that grain was harvested in the Arsinoite nome (near Fayoum), and mentioned the feeding of grain to the sacred crocodiles at Fayoum (17, 1, 38), a food probably not especially suitable to reptilian fancy! Diodorus (1, 36, 5) was amazed at the "ease" of Egyptian agriculture, especially the methods of planting and harvesting

". . . and they gather great heaps of grain without exertion or much expense . . .".

He also recorded a food taboo connected with the death of dogs

". . . if any wine or grain or any other [food] thus necessary for life happens to be stored in the building [private home] when one of these animals expires, they would never think of using it thereafter for any purpose." (1, 84, 2)

Importance of Bread and Cereals as Food

Apart from rice in the Far East and Central Asia, bread, in most areas of the world, constitutes the largest single dietary source of energy and nutrients. It predominates in Europe, America and western Asia. Indeed, wheat, the world's most widely cultivated food plant, makes the greatest contribution of any single foodstuff to man's supply of calories and protein.

In the Arabian Peninsula, its contribution to nutrition is probably equal to or slightly less than that of rice; and this finds expression in the different meanings given to the word ʿaish in different Arab countries (see p. 492). On the world scale, Table 1, taken from Horder *et al.* (1954, p. 14) underlines the preponderance of wheat among world cereals.

Table 1

World production of cereals
(in million metric tons)

	Average, 1934–38	1951	1952
Wheat	152·7	173·6	196·1
Oats	63·5	60·1	59·9
Barley	49·0	55·2	58·9
Maize	112·8	131·2	140·0
Rye	42·4	41·4	39·7
Rice	139·5	150·6	159·2

The role of bread in the fare of the common man is further illustrated in Table 2 which lists its share in the provision of energy and of some essential nutrients to various groups of the population of the United Kingdom, graded downwards from A to D according to their incomes; while Table 3 shows the contribution of wheat and cereals to the nutrition of a number of countries, and underlines its importance to man especially in the Near East and Western Hemisphere.

Table 2

Percentage of total daily intake supplied by flour and bread

		Social Class				
				D		
Nutrient	A	B	C	Excluding old-age pensioners	Old-age pensioners	All Class D
Energy	22·0	23·6	27·7	28·6	28·0	28·4
Protein	23·2	25·6	30·7	30·3	30·6	30·7
Calcium	18·7	21·7	27·0	28·4	26·2	27·9
Iron	23·5	26·0	29·9	31·3	32·5	31·6
B_1	30·9	33·7	37·6	39·5	38·5	39·0
Riboflavin	10·9	11·9	14·7	15·0	14·5	15·0
Nicotinic acid	21·7	23·3	26·9	26·6	27·5	26·8

From a report on Domestic Food Consumption and Expenditure (1950), prepared by the British Ministry of Food (HMSO, 1952), London. (After Horder, Dodds, and Moran, 1954, p. 172.)

To most Mediterraneans, no fare is complete without a large allowance of bread. At sunrise, the Egyptian fellah (peasant) breaks his fast with a loaf, some cheese, an onion, or greens, which he washes down

Table 3

Contribution of wheat and cereals to calories
and protein intake in different countries

Country	Grammes of wheat *per capita* daily	Percentage of total calories from wheat	Percentage of total calories from all cereals and starchy foods	Percentage of protein from animal sources
Romania	340	38	65	29
Israel	301	37	42	43
Spain	286	37	50	30
France	261	30	37	56
United Arab Republic	239	31	73	15
Ireland	279	29	39	60
New Zealand	226	23	28	68
Switzerland	220	24	33	57
United Kingdom	204	22	30	60
Sweden	145	21	29	66
Pakistan	120	20	73	21
Canada	161	19	25	66
United States	149	17	24	70
German Fed. Rep.	148	18	35	61
Peru	99	16	59	25
India	73	13	68	12
Japan	71	10	68	24

Modified from Tables 11, 12, and 13 of Aykroyd and Doughty (1970).

with heavily sugared strong tea and milk. At midday, his young children and wife bring him his meal wrapped in a large, pliable, flat loaf. Urbanites in popular quarters are awakened in the early morning by the squeaking donkey-pulled carts that peddle fresh hot bread. The very poor live largely on bread with beans and a few garnishings. The more wealthy whet their appetites by dipping morsels of white wheaten bread into sesame, chick peas, or egg plant, worked into a paste with oil, garlic and spices; and they accompany their meals with large portions of bread.

Little does anybody, there or elsewhere, ponder over the long human experience and experimentation that preceded the present perfection of their bread.

Barley (Hordeum vulgare)

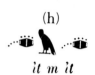

(h)

it m it

'*it*: Barley, also grain in general [see (a) p. 457]
(h): Barley as barley, or barley proper (*F.*, 32)
(i): Barley of Upper Egypt (*F.*, 266)

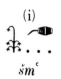

(i)

Our barley rather than another's wheat
(popular saying)

*sm*ꜥ

Whereas it is certain that the major class of food-stuffs utilized by the Ancient Egyptians in the Post-Paleolithic Period was constituted by cereals, which cereal was grown first is debatable. There is evidence, however, that it may have been barley.

One cannot positively date the use of barley prior to the Neolithic, despite the previously presented evidence pointing to a very long history (pp. 460, 461), and to its use in the Late Paleolithic.

Finds of barley ranging from the Neolithic Merimde (over 4000 B.C.) through the Tasian, Fayoum, Badarian, Maadi, Mostagedda, New Kingdom (Fig. 11.12), and Coptic cultures, have been enumerated by Täckholm *et al.* in their encyclopaedic "Flora of Egypt" (*T.*, I, 288–292). According to measurements carried out by Jackson on grains found in Fayoum settlements by Caton-Thompson and Gardner (1934), these did not differ from modern types. The material was examined by Hans Helbaek (personal communication to Dr Täckholm), who identified four species: *Hordeum distichum, H. deficiens, H. vulgare* and *H. hexastichum,* together with Emmer, *Triticum dicoccum.* This is the only time all these *Hordeum* species were found. In finds of the Dynastic Period, only *H. vulgare* occurs, and in a slender strain corresponding to the barley nowadays called "Mansuriya".

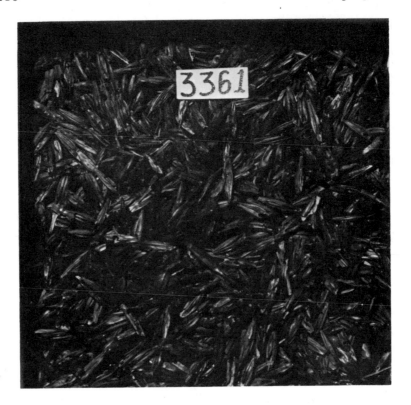

Fig. 11.12. Barley found in Tut-ankh-Amon's tomb. Dokki Museum.

Nevertheless, a somewhat elaborate mathematical analysis of the distribution of straight and twisted grains among the find led Jackson (1934) to identify "two-rowed" grains (*H. vulgare distichum*); but Täckholm prudently warned that the identification must remain doubtful as long as no ear or rachis has been discovered. The varieties that were mainly used, however, were certainly the 4-row (*H. tetrastichum*) (Schulz, 1916, *T.*, I, 287, 292) and the 6-row (*hexastichum*) ones (Brunton and Caton-Thompson, 1928; Brunton, 1937); and, because the 4-row grains found in Ani's tomb (eleventh dynasty) were of different shades, it has been surmised that the "red", "black" and "white" varieties probably belonged to that type (*T.*, I, 287). Specimens of that variety were found in the underground galleries adjacent to the step Pyramid of Zoser (Lauer *et al.*, 1951). Botanists, however, do not agree when it comes to more accurate identification of the finds.

In Egyptian literature, barley (*'it*) is mentioned as early as the first dynasty, and is often qualified: barley of "Upper Egypt", or barley of "Lower Egypt". Inscriptions from the time of King Thutmose III (*c.* 1504–1450 B.C.) tell of the king presenting offerings of barley to the gods

> "My Majesty established for him the god [Ra-Harakhte] a divine offering of barley, in order to perform the ceremonies therewith, at the feast of the new moon, at the feast of the sixth day of the month; and as a daily income of each day, according to that which was done in On [Heliopolis]—Behold, My Majesty found it very good to plow the barley . . ." (*A.R.*, II, 562)

King Horemheb (*c.* 1341–1320 B.C.) showed his generosity by offering gifts of barley to the common people

> ". . . yea, they took grain heaps in the granary, every one of them bore barley and spelt . . ." (*A.R.*, III, 66)

Herodotus (II, 36) referred to barley as being

> ". . . a disgraceful food among the Egyptians . . ."

but Atheneaus (*Deipnos.*, 3, 114, D) some 600 years after Herodotus stated that a special sour bread made from barley, the *Kyllastis* bread, was commonly eaten in Egypt and was greatly esteemed by the people living there (see Chapter 12).

There are subtle indications, though, that the Herodotian viewpoint was at least partially correct. Athenaeus (4, 149, F) reported that in Naucratis, the town of his birth, barley gruel was eaten three times a year during the three major religious festivals. This might suggest that barley was not eaten throughout the rest of the year, at least among the upper-middle class and wealthy Graeco-Egyptians who were primarily wheat consumers; or that it had a special religious significance, like the wheat gruel eaten on the eve of the tenth day of the month of Moharram by Moslems and called *Ashoura*, and on St Barbara's day by Eastern Christians, and called *Burbara*. The extreme view adopted by Herodotus should be seen with caution, however, for when all the evidence is examined, it is difficult to tag barley as "disgraceful" especially seeing that so many Egyptian kings took pride in offering this grain to the most important gods of Egypt. Even today, the popular saying: 'Like barley, eaten but maligned', witnesses to the feeling that barley is not fairly judged.

Despite Egypt's wealth in barley, it often had to be imported. As recorded in the Papyrus Harris, Rameses III, following the example of preceding kings, levied it from conquered lands

". . . 2000 heket[5] of Syrian barley to be offered to the sun god Re at On [Heliopolis] . . ." (*A.R.*, IV, 287)

Funerary texts of the New Kingdom, give additional credit to barley

". . . let my hands lay hold upon the wheat and the barley which shall be given unto me therein in abundant measure." (Budge, 1949, 72, p. 242)

In the Nu papyrus, the deceased had to say

". . . let me live upon bread made of white barley, and let my beer be made from red grain." (Budge, 1949, 52, p. 194)

A papyrus dated to the third to fourth centuries A.D. tells of a man, named Melas, who was forced to pay with barley for a debt incurred by his friends at a funeral (*S.P.*, I, 157).

Barley entered into many of Egypt's legends. Strabo (17, 1, 6) related that when the foundations of fortified Alexandria were being laid out, the workmen exhausted the supply of architectural chalk and substituted barley to mark the outlines of the fort on the earth. But birds soon flocked about and quickly consumed the "grand design". The workers moaned that this indeed was a sorrowful omen. But Alexander the Great consulted his soothsayers who interpreted the sign favourably (they could have scarcely done otherwise, since Alexander himself had chosen the site). Hence, the city of Alexandria was constructed as designed, partially planned by this unique use of barley.

Historically, according to the discovered finds, barley seems to have preceded wheat. Husks of barley have been isolated from almost every sample of intestinal contents of Pre-Dynastic Egyptians both in Egypt and Nubia (Netolitzky, 1911). Precedence of barley is also suggested by linguistic and religious evidence. In the Old and Middle Kingdom texts, when barley and wheat are mentioned, barley always comes first. In accordance with their grammatical genders, barley was said to have grown out of man and wheat out of woman (Sauneron, 1960). The same correlation must also have been the basis of a test to foretell the sex of unborn children by the different effect of pregnancy urine on these cereals (p. 485); and a religious pun was often made on *it*, that meant both barley and father.

Necklaces of barley were commonly placed on mummies to symbolize resurrection. In some finds, the barley was found germinated. While it is possible that malt, which is germinated barley, was used as a food and in the preparation of beer, it is more likely that germination of this cereal represented a funerary rite of resurrection that figured in some Osirian rituals.

On display in the Cairo Museum are several wooden "Osiris beds" constructed of thin strips of wood made in the life-size outline of the god (Carter, 1933, p. 61 and plate 64). These frames were covered with mud, planted with barley, completely wrapped in linen and placed with the deceased inside his tomb to identify him with the god. The sprouted grain that filled in time the frame with yellowish-white shoots symbolized the resurrection and rebirth of the dead. This custom of planting "dead" rapidly growing seeds, which shortly are "reborn", is not unique to Egypt, and is habitual in many folk traditions. In Greece, it is currently observed on Saint Spiridon's day, December 12th; in Russia, the Christians plant seeds in shallow pans just before the Easter season. The Egyptian Greeks and Copts, likewise, observe this custom. While their observance cannot with certainty be traced back to the Ancient Egyptians, the parallel is strongly suggestive.

On the contrary, connections of wheat with gods are less obvious in Egyptian mythology, although this cereal predominated in ritual preparations and on wealthy tables.

Varieties of Barley

There is thus general agreement on the antiquity of the use of barley in Ancient Egypt. Most discussions concerning "varieties" of barley relate to the geographical origin of the harvested grain, rather than to varieties in the botanical sense. Kees (1961, p. 74) referred to these simply as Upper and Lower Egyptian varieties, while Rawlinson (1881, 1, p. 31) classed them as "red" and "white", two varieties mentioned in the *Book of the Dead* (Budge, 1949, 52, p. 194). On the other hand classifying barley by colour may reflect the duality of the land of Egypt, the Red Crown symbolizing Upper Egypt, and the White Crown, Lower Egypt (see Chapter 15, pp. 607–608).

Other Uses of Barley

Hunt (*S.P.*, 1, 93) recorded, from a papyrus dating to 252 B.C., that barley was commonly *fed to animals;* and Rawlinson (1881, 1, pp. 82–83) further elaborated that it was fed to horses and to cattle, the latter for both sacrifice and human consumption. To find that it was given to both man and beast may have been the reason why Herodotus called it a disgraceful food (see p. 481).

Apart from food, barley was used in brewing (see Chapter 13), as a medium of exchange, and in therapeutics.

A papyrus of 256 B.C. (*S.P.*, I, 39) quoted the value of barley at three-fifths that of wheat. Four centuries later, a castanet dancer was hired for an evening's entertainment and paid with barley (*S.P.*, II, 391). The dancer named Isidora (the gift of Isis) was paid, in addition, 36 drachmae and 20 paired (?) loaves of bread. The host guaranteed donkey transportation to and from her home and promised to guard her garments and gold ornaments.

Medically, even more than wheat, barley (*'it*) had wide applications, and was prescribed in different forms: as grain, powder (barley meal), roast grain, fermented grain, groats, or barley water. Even its straw (*rwjw*) was utilized in a fumigation (*L.*, 35).

Against burns it was mixed with manna, rush nut from the field, northern salt, papyrus, burnt leather, grease of ox, oil, wax, and applied every day (*Eb.*, LXVIII, 484). As a purgative, it was toasted and fully dried, shaped into cakes, put in oil, and then eaten (*Eb.*, XII, 37).

Roasted and mixed with frankincense (or terebinth?) and oil, it was applied in bandages (*Eb.*, LXXI, 532). Barley water "whose substance is removed" was drunk with pounded toasted barley, costus? and sycamore (*Eb.*, XLVI, 240).

Barley meal was mixed with dregs of wine, northern salt, dates and honey, and made into suppositories to cool the anus (*Eb.*, XXXIII, 163); and, with cow's milk, it was anointed onto contusions (*Eb.*, LXIX, 512).

But three prescriptions retain one's attention. The first is said to be a "secret remedy for the one who is under the physician except thy own daughter", prescribed for a phlegm (?) obstacle

> "Do not abandon him . . . fresh barley without it having been dried, boiled, and mixed with dates." (*Eb.*, XLII, 206 *b*)

The second was a remedy for the eyes imparted by an Asiatic from Byblos. It was made of fresh barley (?), barley, dates, red ochre, alum, salt, antimony (?) lead (?) a leg marrow, galena, fresh balanites oil, and an unidentified ingredient (*Eb.*, LXIII, 422).

The last is a diagnostic-prognostic test that has excited the curiosity and imagination of physicians and patients for centuries. It was supposed to detect not only pregnancy but, also, the sex of the unborn child. This has always been a major concern of kings and nobility who were anxious to assure their dynastic continuity, for history repeats itself and the worry of Pharaohs over male heirs must have been equal to that of Henry VIII or Napoleon in more recent times. This no doubt explains the importance of such practices as the following, which was copied by Hippocrates, the Arabs and European mediaeval physicians, and is said to be still current in some parts of the Near East.

The woman's urine was added to wheat and to barley. If the barley grew first, the woman was pregnant with a boychild. If the wheat grew better, she was expecting a girl. If none grew, she was not pregnant (*Ber.*, 199). A recent trial (Ghalioungui *et al.*, 1963) has shown that urine of non-pregnant women uniformly prevents any growth, while pregnancy urine "permits" growth of both cereals in about 40% of cases. No relation was found, however, between the cereal that grew first, and the sex of the child.

After the Egyptians, the Greeks continued to use barley medically. Pliny (*N.H.*, XXIV, XLII, 71) who visited Egypt in the first century A.D. and recorded some therapeutic methods he observed there, stated that barley mixed with brya (tamarisk bark or berry?) taken internally, heals ulcers. He also recalled the opinion of Hippocrates who commended barley water made from double pointed barley grains, as giving strength and health (*N.H.*, XVIII, XV, 75). It may be significant that barley water is today widely recommended by physicians for infantile diarrhoeas and as a diuretic.

Aelian (3, 17, 5), on the authority of Phylarchus, gave a fanciful explanation why the people of Egypt do not suffer from asp bites. It is, he said, because they mix barley with wine and honey, and set these aside as offerings to the asps that live in the house. When the master of the house claps his hands in a special manner the snakes come and feast while the family retires for the night, apparently respecting the asps' right to roam at will about the house. If one rises during the night, he claps his hands in a manner different than the earlier snake signal, thus commanding the asps to go to their holes and not to bite.

Wheat

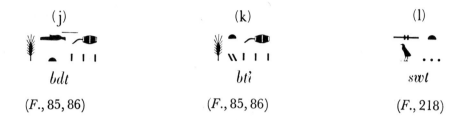

(j)	(k)	(l)
bdt	*bti*	*swt*
(F., 85, 86)	(F., 85, 86)	(F., 218)

The bread is baked and water fills the cups
(popular saying for: "we are ready")

Wheat, like many food items utilized by the inhabitants of Ancient Egypt, is surrounded by the most confusing terms, synonyms, and spelling variants. Transliteration of the hieroglyphics into English is now conventionalized; but the exact vocalization of Egyptian words is not known, owing to the omission of vowels in that writing. The early Egyptologists tried to overcome this by inserting tentative vowels, each in his own way. Thus, *sout, sou, suut, sw,* and *swt* became variants of the same word! The Classical Greek authors, often merely borrowing from each other terms and descriptions, added their own interpretations of the equivalence of various grains. Thus, the *zea* of Herodotus probably equals sorghum while the same word, as used by Theophrastus, could be equated with no less than five distinct entities. At the same time another term, *olyra,* may or may not be equated with *zea,* depending on the author.

Wheat, usually only generally identified, has been obtained from numerous tombs[6] (Fig. 11.13) throughout the Dynastic Period (Engelbach, 1961, 265); and the Papyrus Harris, dating from the reign of King Rameses III, tells of the great offerings of wheat (wheat in general) given by the king to the temples and gods of Egypt (*A.R.,* IV, 206, 244, 259).

Kees (1961, p. 74) stated that wheat was not in common usage or of major importance as an edible grain until the New Kingdom when it

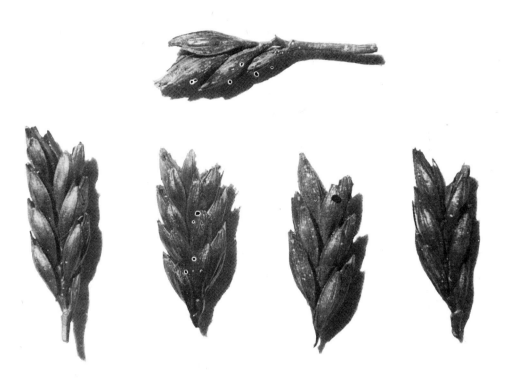

Fig. 11.13. Heads of wheat from Saqqara. Dokki Agricultural Museum no. 1430.

supplanted barley as the chief grain of the land. This seems to be a gross generalization, especially when one considers the evidence for consumption given above and in the section on barley. It is usually assumed, though, that wheat was not commonly utilized by the poor, possibly because it was expensive. As noted on p. 484, Hunt (*S.P.*, I, 39) reported that wheat cost more than barley; yet it is likely that the poor ate wheat at least part of the time, perhaps as they do today.

It is difficult to determine which breads were made from wheat and which from barley. Kyllistis[7] bread, already mentioned in the section on barley, illustrates this point. Herodotus (II, 36) stated that it was not made from wheat, but from spelt, which is the Roman term for wheat (*Triticum spelta*), while others wrote that barley was the base flour (*Deipnos.*, III, 114, D), and Gulick, who translated Athenaeus (*Deipnos.*, X, 418, translatory note), stated that it was probably from rye!

Additional dishes made from prepared wheat were also popular. Groats, the general term applied to preparations made from "cracked" wheat, were often served. From Athenaeus (*Deipnos.*, IV, 131, D), we may infer that they were of the best quality since he reports that groats made in the "Egyptian" manner, were served at Greek wedding feasts.

There were certain times, however, when people avoided wheat and wheat products. Diodorus (1, 72, 2) describing the days of mourning following the death of an Egyptian king, when men and women formed into groups of two or three hundred to recite dirges, chant the praises and recall the virtues of the deceased said

> "nor would they eat of the flesh of any living thing, or food prepared from wheat."

In the minds of the populace wheat symbolized vast richness, a viewpoint that Athenaeus (*Deipnos.*, II, 39, F) described in the spinning daydream of a man intoxicated with wine

> ". . . and every man dreams of being a monarch, with gold, yes, and with ivory, his house glitters; wheat-laden ships carry over the shining sea mighty wealth from Egypt . . ."

But as grain grew and ripened, this richness was obvious for all to see, especially to the keen eye of the tax assessor (Montet, 1958, p. 113). For wheat was as heavily taxed in Egypt throughout antiquity as hard earned income is today, and the Egyptian monarchs, like the "powers-that-be" in the twentieth century, took out their generous share of it.

As with barley, the classical travellers were astounded that wheat was harvested so often in Egypt, sometimes three times a year, Pliny (*N.H.*, XVIII XLV, 161, 162) related that, at Babylon,[8] wheat was cut twice, and the third extravagantly wasted, left for the cattle to eat! He pondered over this and believed that the great abundance of Egyptian wheat had to be due to the heat (*N.H.*, XVII, III, 31).

Like barley too, wheat was a standard barterable commodity, being traded either alone, or mixed in various proportions with grain of lesser value (*S.P.*, II, 391). It could be used in payment for rent (*S.P.*, I, 39) or taxes (*S.P.*, II, 347). When stored in quantity, it represented considerable wealth, and could be left to heirs (*S.P.*, I, 84). This tempted wheat farmers, dealers, and profiteers into illegal transactions that King Ptolemy Auletes (*c.* 70 B.C.) tried to halt by a royal decree

". . . no one purchasing wheat or pulse from the nomes above Memphis, shall carry it down to the low country [the Delta] or carry it up to the Thebaid [Upper Egypt] on any pretext . . . on pain of being liable to death if detected . . ." (*S.P.*, II, 209)

A harsh law, but no doubt, to try to control profiteering from a flourishing black market was the object.

Since a standing crop of wheat was like the proverbial "money tree", any threat of crop damage caused great alarm among landowners; and Aelian (2, 6, 41), in his interesting collection of tales, discussed just this problem

". . . when it rains, mice are born which damage the crops of corn [wheat] by nibbling the stems and attacking the stacked sheaves, causing the Egyptian great concern . . ."

Varieties of Wheat

As discussed on p. 465, Emmer, the three genome *Triticum dicoccum*, seems to have been the main variety grown and consumed in Egypt. It has been found at Merimda—Beni Salama (Junker, 1929) and in granaries in various sites in Fayoum, a fact that indicates, as it does with barley, a long history of prior usage (Caton-Thompson and Gardner, 1934).

The word *bd.t* designating a cereal, is met with as early as the first dynasty, along with *it*, barley, from which it is obviously different (Emery, 1958, III, p. 36); and, as most Egyptian finds consist of Emmer, it probably denotes that variety.

Seven varieties of *bti* have been described in Egyptian texts, a fact that led Gardiner to postulate the existence of seven varieties of wheat, and the possibility of *spelt* having been one of them. However, as four of these varieties are distinguished by their different colours, and as *spelt* has never been found in Egypt, the distinction may have been only a superficially descriptive one, although in the eighteenth dynasty and in Ramessid times, red ink was utilized by scribes to write *bdt*, wheat, and black ink to write *it m it*, barley (Gardiner, 1947, p. 222).

Ciferri, cited by Kees (1961, 74) concluded, though from limited information, that *T. spelta* var. *saharae*, a variety found in the Western Desert oases of Egypt, is the prototype of later varieties cultivated in the Nile Valley. Nevertheless, "spelt" that often appears in translations and discussions of Ancient Egyptian texts, has never been found in Egypt (Dixon, 1969).

Regarding Egyptian wheat, *bdt* or *btt*, Täckholm gave us the following information, based on findings of H. Helbaek personally communicated to her (February 1974).

From Pre-Dynastic times up to the Roman era, Emmer, *Triticum dicoccum* has been continuously cultivated in Egypt. The so-called "naked wheats" of both hexaploid and tetraploid types (*Triticum vulgare, T. durum, T. turgidum*) occur among the old Emmer first in Ptolemaic and Roman times.

Triticum monococcum has erroneously been recorded in the Pre-Dynastic settlements of El Omari (Debono, 1948) and in the Pyramid of Zoser (third dynasty) (Lauer *et al.*, 1951). The material in question was redetermined by Helbaek who found it to represent unripe *T. dicoccum;* and he further states that true *T. monococcum* has never been found in Egypt.

Among carbonized material from Merimde and El Omari, both of Neolithic age, Helbaek identified a small amount of *Triticum aestivum* among the Emmer. He published it earlier as being Club wheat, *Triticum compactum*, but he later changed his opinion and considered it only a strain of *T. aestivum*, different from the true Club wheat of Europe. This wheat was found only in the above-mentioned two Neolithic collections; it is not found in any dynastic material.

swt, sw

The variety called *swt* or *sw*, as distinct from both *it* and *bdt*, was first said to be "naked wheat" (*T.*, I, 253). It was later translated "Einkorn" (Lauer *et al.*, 1951). The following are the conclusions of Helbaek regarding the interpretation of *swt*, kindly communicated to us by V. Täckholm (February, 1974).

Ensete edule, *swt* or *sw*, the Ensete banana, which is an important bread plant in present Ethiopia, is not growing in Egypt nowadays, but it may have been cultivated in the Neolithic, during the so-called

Gerzean or Middle Nagada time. The fruits are inedible, but the plant is cultivated for the starch in the flowery stems. It is a plant of swampy habitats and is pictured on ancient Gerzean pottery, always in connection with boats, waves, flamingos, etc. In ancient pictures, a ring is frequently drawn across the middle of the stem. It is, therefore, interesting that up to the present day, the natives of Ethiopia make a ring-like leaf scar when they want to propagate the plant. At the edge of the incision, buds are then formed that could be used for propagation.

The Ensete motive disappeared during the Later Neolithic Periods. It is probable that the Gerzean Period had a wetter climate (the Neolithic wet phase) when the Nile inundated the shores and made them into swamps unsuitable for cereal cultivation. This may have been the reason for the Ensete cultivation. When the climate dried up, this cultivation must have been abandoned, but *Ensete edule* survived in the hieroglyph of the *sw* plant, that gives a very vivid representation of its shape, and that denoted the South or the plant of the South. During the early dynasties, it became the heraldic plant of Upper Egypt, but it was later replaced by the "Lily of the South".

After the disappearance of the Ensete culture, the ancient name *swt* or *sw* may have been transferred to a cereal. There has been a proposal to the effect that it denoted one of the hard-wheats, *Triticum durum* or *T. turgidum* of late times. But it may have just as well have represented the *Triticum aestivum* found in the Pre-Dynastic settlements of El Omari and Merimde (see above). This is not yet finally settled.

One should add that Keimer (1953) did not agree with these conclusions concerning *Ensete*.

bs ꜣ

A cereal used in the production of beer, *bs ꜣ* was tentatively identified with malt by Nims (1950) (see Chapter 13).

Medical Uses

bdt. The medical papyri mention white, black and a variety (*ankh.t*) translated as either fresh or goat's wheat (*Wb. Dr.*, 184). It was pre-scribed mainly in external applications (*Eb.*, 568, 572, etc.; *Ram.*, III,

1); only once internally (*H.*, 51). It served also in birth prognosis (see p. 485).

swt, untranslated by Ebbell (1937b), was, on the other hand, extensively used, though less frequently than barley; it was given as whole grain, as flour, or as groats; and its applications were mostly internal, rarely external. As grain, we meet it prescribed with honey, boiled and strained, to expel exudation (?) in the belly (*Eb.*, LXXV, 597). Ebers (XI, 31) recommends as a laxative wheat flour, [?], juniper, colocynth, senna, mustard, shaped into *šnš* bread.

As a dressing, groats were mixed with ox-beef, spleen, northern salt, dragon's blood,[8] grease of ibex and brain of ox (*Eb.*, LXXX, 645).

Two recipes are remarkably picturesque. The first was a remedy made by the god Shu for himself: powder of wheat, northern salt, oil, coriander, soot, bean, frankincense [? terebinth], costus, yellow ochre and viscous fluid, mixed together; and the sick places are bandaged therewith (*Eb.*, XLVI, 243).

The second was meant to expel *áaá* caused by a god or a dead man, and to smite all evil things: figs, sebesten, groats of wheat, ochre and water, strained and taken for four days (*Eb.*, XLV, 229).

Medicinal use of wheat persisted in Greek times. Pliny (*N.H.*, XXVII, XLV, 161, 162) related that wheat, aged for three months and mixed with seriphum root, was prescribed to expel intestinal worms.

Rice

Coptic: *pi-arros*
Greek: *oryza*
Arabic: *arozz*

Rice, whether it originated in Asia or Africa, seems to have been first cultivated in Asia, somewhere between southern China and Cochinchina (Mosseri, 1922). It became known early in Babylon, where it was given the Aramaic name *ourouzza*, from which its Arabic and Greek names were derived. Nowadays, its dietary importance equals that of bread in some parts of the Arab world where it is called *aish* (life), a term applied in Egypt only to bread.

Today in Egypt rice is a popular cereal, especially in the North; but it is a comparative newcomer. According to Täckholm (*T.*, I, 411), it was introduced by the Arabs between the Arab conquest (seventh century A.D.) and the Turkish invasion (sixteenth century). In the fourteenth century, An-Nabulsy mentioned it among the products of Fayoum, so that it must have been introduced some time before that period (Salmon, 1901; Shafei, 1939).

No remains of rice were ever identified beyond doubt in Ancient Egyptian remains, except some pieces of rice straw said by Caylus (1752) to be included in the gilded plaster covering of a statuette of Osiris (of which neither the date nor the present location are known) (Daressy, 1922). Daressy thought the identification acceptable; but Täckholm (*T.*, I, 412) does not believe it possible, since even the Coptic name of this plant, Pi-arros, is derived from Arabic *arozz*.

Pliny (*N.H.*, XVIII, XIX, 81) however, stated that rice grew in Egypt

". . . while zea, olyra, and rice or tiphe are found only in Egypt, Syria, Cilicia and Asia and Greece . . ."

Elsewhere, he stated

". . . the same authority [Tarranius] is of the opinion that olyra and oryza are the same plant . . ." (*N.H.*, XVIII, XV, 75)

This author, however, could not have meant the rice we know; and much of the confusion over his discussion of this grain seems to spring from the closeness of the Greek work *olyra*, with its varied usage, to *oryza*, the Roman word for rice. The error possibly started in the Middle Ages or later, in the course of the translation of his writings from various fragments, as a result of misreading, illegibility, or innocent scholarly misidentification.

Millet

Arabic: *dokhn*[9]

Pearl millet, *Pennisetum glaucum*, is now widely cultivated in Sudanic Africa where it probably originated, and where it is of great economic importance. In the Sudan and in the Aswan area, this cereal is made into bread, or ground and made into a kind of dough eaten with milk and molasses. It has not been identified in Ancient Egyptian remains, but many varieties of "millet" are cultivated in Egypt today (*Pennisetum typhoideum, Setaria italica, Panicum miliaceum, Echinochloa frumentacea*). Members of the panicum species have been identified in ancient bricks (Unger, 1862); a specimen of *Setaria verticillata* was found in a garland at El-Lahun (*T.*, I, 460); and grains of *Echinocochloa colonum*, referred to under the old name *Panicum colonum*, were identified by Netolitzky in the intestinal contents of bodies excavated at Naga-el-Deir (1911) in quantities and in a degree of purity that suggest that the plant was cultivated at that time as a cereal (Dixon, 1969, p. 136). As discussed in the preceding sections, durra, sorghum, millet, and maize (corn) have intertwining and confusing synonymies, and Dawson (1930, p. 11) was of the opinion that the millet found in the intestinal contents of mummies was probably sorghum (see under that cereal).

Sorghum

Arabic: *Dura rafi'a, D. 'ewega, D. seify,* or *D. baladi*

Sorghum is widely cultivated at present in Egypt, but mainly in Middle and Upper Egypt where it is mixed with wheat and barley in making bread, and is included in the dough used to make *bouza* (see under Beer) (*T.*, I, 535).

Most recent investigators agree, however, that sorghum was not grown in Ancient Egypt. This was the opinion of Schweinfurth (1891) who stated that the cultivation of this cereal did not start before the Roman-Byzantine Period, the only certain finds being those discovered in the Coptic monastery of St Cyriacus (sixth to seventh century A.D.). Other finds, exhibited in the Berlin-Dahlem and Cairo museums, as well as reports of other archaeological finds are judged doubtful by Täckholm (*T.*, I, 537); and nowhere does Hayes (1964) in his extensive survey of Pre-Dynastic Egypt mention the existence of sorghum in burials or village refuse deposits.

In direct opposition, Engelbach (1961, pp. 354, 355) stated that sorghum was found in Pre-Dynastic Egyptian burials; but he did not admit that it was found in the tombs of the Dynastic Period He denied that reliefs and paintings of Dynastic Egypt illustrate the harvesting of that cereal.

Both Wilkinson (1854, 2, pp. 50, 51) and Rawlinson (1881, I, pp. 34, 83, 84), however, published illustrations from several tombs, that they label the harvesting of *doura*, although omitting accurately to identify these tombs.

Moreover, Rawlinson (1881, I, p. 31) reported five distinct varieties of sorghum existing in modern Egypt, and he made the assumption that these, though possibly not all, were also there in antiquity. He equated the zea and olyra of Herodotus (II, 36) with sorghum, and concluded that this was probably the grain eaten by most Egyptians. In another passage he stated that sorghum is a kind of spelt, thus increasing confusion by identifying sorghum with a variety of wheat, *Triticum spelta* (1881, I, p. 82). On the other hand, Wilkinson (1854, I, p. 179) made no attempt to elaborate on sorghum or to present any solid arguments for its existence for he withdrew from the scholarly arena with the bland remark that sorghum was made into cakes for the poor, and contented himself with an attempt to equate the Egyptian medicinal preparation *athera*, that he thought was very beneficial for babies, with a preparation made from *Holcus sorghum*. Jones, however, in an author's translatory remark, distinctly referred to *athera* as being ground from "two-grained wheat", i.e. *triticum dicoccum* (*N.H.*, XXII, LVII, 121).

Wilkinson and Rawlinson, both agreed that identification presents serious problems, owing to the similarity in appearance of flax and sorghum in illustrations. Even Plutarch seems to have confused these two plants when he remarked

". . . the flax springs from the earth which is immortal; it yields edible seeds and supplies a plain and cleanly clothing . . ." (*I. and O.*, 352, 4)

Dawson (1930, p. 11) presents what appears to be the most convincing evidence concerning sorghum, which he calls millet, noting that on analysis of human intestinal contents, in a number of cases,

"those grain husks of millet were also found . . ."

He added

"The finding of millet is of great interest because its use in Egypt has been denied, and the species found is not now cultivated except in the East Indies."

Unfortunately, he gave no details of the finds.

The classic Greek writers never mentioned sorghum as a product of Egypt. Herodotus does not report having seen it, although he said that it grew in Babylon of Asia into trees of which he knew the height but would not say it, for those who have not visited these countries were already sceptical of what he said of its harvests (I, 193). Nor did Pliny, one of the main sources on the food habits of the Ancient Egyptians, mention it. Nevertheless, relatively recent writers commented on its culture in Egypt, like Abdul Latif al-Baghdady (1965) who saw it cultivated in the southern part of Upper Egypt in the twelfth century A.D., and the scientists of Bonaparte's expedition (Girard, 1813, p. 517).

In an interesting linguistic discussion, Loret (*Fl.*, 26), after mentioning that specimens of *S. vulgare* from Egypt are on exhibit in various museums, notably in Florence, compared the Biblical word *dokhan*[9] for *S. saccharatum* to Arabic *dokhn* for millet and *S. saccharatum*. He added that in a Coptic scala (a Coptic-Arabic lexicon), the Coptic word *boti* that exists also in Ancient Egyptian [see (k), p. 486] is translated as both chick pea and doura (sorghum). On that account, he stated that it might be concluded that the Egyptians knew sorghum, were it not that *boti* in the Coptic Bible translates also *olyra*. He added that one might also be tempted to compare Arabic *doura* to the hieroglyph (m) which possibly designated a reed (*F.*, 295, Lefebvre, 1956, p. 121), and to a possible varient depicted by (n) which he claimed was certainly a cereal.

(m)

twr

(n)

twrwt;

Oats (Avena)

Arabic: *shoufan*

Oats cannot compete in Egypt with wheat or barley because, like rye, they need cooler, harsher climates than obtain in Egypt. Newberry (1889, 1890), however, discovered a few grains of a species of *Avena* in two necropoles, both situated between the Fayoum and the Nile Valley: El-Lahun dating to the twelfth dynasty, and Hawara to the second to third century A.D. This author thought that they were specimens of *A. strigosa* Schroeb; but Täckholm (*T.*, I, 330) was of the opinion that they belong to *A. fatua* or *A. sterilis*. These few grains constitute the only evidence of the existence of oats in Ancient Egypt. In view of their small number, they may well represent insignificant impurities in imported grain.

Rye

". . . and the flax and the barley was smitten: for the barley was in the ear, and the flax was boiled. But the wheat and the rie (sic) were not smitten: for they were not grown up . . ." (Exodus, 9, 31–32)

This Biblical quotation is often marshalled as evidence of the existence of rye in Ancient Egypt, and Gulick (translatory note, *Deipnos.*, X, 418, E) concurred. At present, however, there is neither archaeological nor literary evidence to prove that rye was utilized by the Ancient Egyptians. The "rie" of Exodus appears to be a mistranslation for either barley or spelt (Holy Bible, 1956), for rye has never been known in Egypt; and indeed the grain is a poor substitute for wheat, and needs a much colder climate in order successfully to compete with it.

Sesame (Sesamum orientale)

Ancient Egyptian: *smsm.t* (*Wb. Dr.*, 493?)
Coptic: *oke* (*Fl.*, 57)
Arabic: *smsm*

The sesame plant is probably central African in origin, but it is grown abundantly in Egypt nowadays. As olive oil production in Egypt can scarcely cover the needs of the population, before the advent of arachis, cotton-seed, and corn oils, sesame oil was the staple fat in the diet of those sectors of the population who may not use animal fats consistently, like the Copts during their long fasts, or the Jews in the preparation of animal foods. Ground into a paste now called *tahina*, sesame was known since at least the second century B.C. (see below). It still is a favourite relish and dip and enters into the preparation of many dishes, especially in Syria and the Lebanon.

There are positive records of the existence and use of sesame in Egypt as early as the third century B.C. Of these, Hunt cites several

". . . Kindly buy me, so that I may get them when I arrive, 3 metretae of the best honey and 600 artabae of barley for the animals, and pay the cost of them out of the produce of the sesame and croton [castor oil bean] . . ." [252 B.C.], (*S.P.*, I, 93)

". . . I sent him off telling him to come early next morning in order to get from me in Memphis a quarter of an artaba of sesame and pound me a paste, as I wished to give it to someone to take to the city . . ." [*c.* 160 B.C.], (*S.P.*, I, 98)

". . . they shall sell the oil in the country at the rate of 48 drachmae in copper for a metretae of sesame oil—if anyone is detected manufacturing oil from sesame or croton or cnecus in any manner whatsoever, or buying sesame oil or cnecus oil or castor oil from any quarter except from the contractors, the king shall decide his punishment . . ." [259 B.C.], (*S.P.*, II, 203)

Pliny (*N.H.*, XV, VII, 25) also mentioned wild sesame (*sesamon silvestre*), but though this translation seems to be accepted by Lucas (1962, p. 336), other authors believe that Pliny's sesame was the castor oil plant.

The only remains of sesame ever discovered are a few capsules found by Schiaparelli in a Theban tomb, but which Schweinfurth (1886) hesitated to call pharaonic. Loret commented that bakers in a painting in Rameses III's tomb may be seen mixing aromatic grains to dough; but these could be any grains, not necessarily sesame seeds. He also pointed to a plant of which the grains were edible and were called *shemshem*, a name very close to Arabic *semsem* (*Fl.*, 57). This is at variance with the opinions of Keimer (*Gpfl.*, 135) and of Dawson (1934), who translated *shemshem* "hemp".

On the other hand, Coptic for sesame is *oke*, which is possibly a late form of a still unidentified medicinal plant *ake* (*Fl.*, 57).

Notes: Chapter 11

1. The word *nabary*, used today for grain in some Egyptian districts, is possibly derived from this word. Another non-understood word *noub*, possibly derived from it, is chanted in a harvest song during the thrashing of wheat: "*heb, heb, yazar'el-noub*" (rise, rise, noub plant).

2. As with wheat and barley in the Ancient Middle East and Mediterranean countries, maize was held in godly reverence in Pre-Columbian America, and a host of deities looked after it. Of these, the most important were the two goddesses *Chicomecoatl*, and *Xilomen*, the guardian of immature ears;

and *Kan* who was honoured with corn meal sprinkled on burning incense. The form of worship varied in different Meso- and South-American countries. In some areas, parts or deformities of the plant were shaped into idols. Elsewhere maize bread was prohibited during fasts, or grinding corn was forbidden for five days following the death of kings. Special maize cakes were eaten during cannibalistic ceremonies and, in another equally gruesome rite, maize was eaten sprinkled with genital blood. What seems to the modern mind appallingly cruel is the practice of cutting into pieces the bodies of young girls sacrificed to the spirit of corn, and burying these with the sown corn to promote its growth. These and other habits have been collected by Weatherwax (1954) in *Indian Corn in Old America*.

3. King Uenephes (Africanus version of Manetho) or Vavenephis (Armenian version by Eusebius) has not been identified with certainty with any Egyptian ruler from the other king lists.

4. Two measures of grain.

5. A measure equal to just over a gallon.

6. It has often been stated that grains of wheat recovered from Ancient Egyptian tombs have been made to grow again, and some authorities faithfully perpetuated this myth! What really happened when water was added to these grains, is that they swelled and split, and the already formed germ emerged; but no further development took place.

7. Greek transcription of neo-Egyptian *kršt*.

8. The Egyptian Babylon or *Bab-el-On*, whose etymology is yet to be ascertained, was located at the apex of the Delta, two miles south of Cairo. *On* is derived from *Iwnw* (in Greek, *Heliopolis*), where the worship of the sun god Ra first developed.

9. The name *dokhan* occurs in Ezekiel, IV, 9, as a cereal grown in Babylon, but it is not certain to which plant it refers, since it was formerly applied also to sorghum.

Chapter 12   *Bread*

Bread

(a)

t

> *The hungry dream of a bread market*
> (Popular saying)

History of Bread

It is unlikely that we will ever know when man first learned to prepare flour and bread. Diodorus showed fine historical insight by placing these inventions immediately after the stage of cannibalism and meat-eating

> "After subsisting in this manner over a long period, they finally turned to the edible fruits of the earth, among which may be included the bread from the lotus." (1, 43, 5)

Primitively, a meat-eater with occasional or seasonal additions of seeds or fruits, man could not settle, leave behind his wandering hunting life, plan, legislate and organize a fixed society, until he could depend on a stable supply of storable and satiating food, not the perishable meats and fruits to which he had been used. This he found in cereals and, later, in bread. Since that remote time, he has relied for the greatest part or, in some countries wholly, on vegetable food.

How he upgraded his use of these foods from chewing the raw grain, to breaking, winnowing and sieving it in more and more efficient ways, then making it into gruels, baking it into groats and, finally, preparing bread, is a long story of which Storcke and Teague (1952, p. 5) said

"There is no other single thread of development that can be followed so continuously throughout all our history and none which bears so constant cause-and-effect relation to every phase of our progress in civilization."

In Egypt, the earliest finds of bread date to the Omarian horizon (*MAE*, 119); but this bread was far different from the full, soft, present-day loaves of Western countries. Although early bakers were less sophisticated than their adroit present-day colleagues, one may assume that their products were similar to the thin, pliable loaves of today's fellaheen, or to the sun bread (*'aish shamsy*) of Upper Egypt. The latter is made from a thick batter left to dry and leaven in the sun before being baked, ultimately producing a hard crusted loaf with a sweet, soft interior. In fact, the Neolithic specimens found at El-Badari were sufficiently porous to indicate that leavening was practiced even at that period.

By the Dynastic Period, bread was well established as a food of poor, rich and gods, alike. The fifth dynasty nomarch Henku boasted that he gave bread to all the hungry (*A.R.*, 1, 281). A proud text, attributed to Mentuhotep III (*c.* 2019–2007 B.C.) records his workmen's rations

"I went forth with an army of 3,000 men. I made the road a river and the Red Land [the desert] a stretch of field, for I gave a leathern bottle, a carrying pole, 2 jars of water, and 20 loaves to each one among them every day."

Breasted, commenting on the above text, likened these loaves, in size, to small table rolls. The frequent trips to the quarries of Wadi Hammamat worked by these people were by no means short-term ventures. The daily provision of 20 loaves to each of the 3,000 men represented a total of 1,800,000 rolls a month. Even accounting for some exaggeration in Mentuhotep III's statement, the production, delivery and distribution of such immense numbers of loaves is a logistic feat that staggers the imagination.

Each day priests had bread baked for them out of sacred corn (wheat) (*Her.*, II, 27). Thus Sesostris[1] enjoined that Hepzefi, the

"superior prophet, triumphant, be given in the first months of the first season, on the 18th day, the day of the *Wag*-feast, 400 flat loaves, and 10 white loaves for his own use; and, on behalf of his fellow-priests, 200 flat loaves and 5 white loaves to each of the Announcer, the Master of Secret Things, the Keeper of the Wardrobe, the Overseer of the Storehouse, the Keeper of the Wide Hall, The Overseer of the House of the Ka, the Scribe of the Temple, the Scribe of the Altar, and the Ritual Priest." (*A.R.*, 1, 550)

In another contract, Hepzefi received also a jar of beer, a large *rrt*-loaf, 500 flat loaves and 10 white loaves (*A.R.*, 1, 590).

Bread as Ritual Offering

An impressive list of offerings made by Pharaoh Sahure shows the anthropomorphism of gods in respect of their food

". . . to Nekhbet[2], 800 daily offerings of bread and beer; to Buto[3], 4800 daily offerings of bread and beer; to Re, 138 daily offerings of bread and beer, etc." (*A.R.*, 1, 159)

Under the same king (*c.* 2500 B.C.) the noble Persen made an offering,

"being the payment of *heth* loaves, pesen (*pzn*) loaves, and *sefet*-oil which comes from the temple of Ptah, for the King's mother, every day, as perpetual offering." (*A.R.*, 1, 241)

The variety of words for bread in these lists will remain the bane of scholars until it is possible to determine their distinctive differences in composition, quality, size or shape. Under the New Kingdom, the names multiplied even more profusely. A list presented by Rameses III to Amon-Ra enumerated an amazing array of varieties

"1057 large oblation loaves of *fine bread*; 1277 large *syd*-loaves; 1277 large *bḥ*-loaves; 440 *ddmt-ḥr.t* loaves; *r-'h wsw*-cakes; 62,540 *by*'.t-loaves; 160,992 *prsn*-loaves; 13,020 white loaves of fine bread; 6200 *'k* loaves; 24,800 *s'b*-loaves; 17,340 *pws'-'k*-loaves; 572,000 white *oblation loaves;* 46,500 *pyramidal* loaves; 441,800 *kyllestis* loaves; 127,400 *wdnwnt*-loaves; 116,400 white *t'*-loaves; *kwnk* bread; 262,000 *p't*-loaves of fine bread." (*A.R.*, IV, 238)

Even sacred animals, like the sacred cats and ichneumons, were fed bread and milk (*Diod.*, 1, 83, 2). But mortuary offerings were often replaced by clay or stone models of loaves or cakes, sometimes stamped with the name of the offerer. These could by prayers and magic effectively replace what they imitated, with the advantage of being more durable and less likely to tempt pilferers.

Social usage, too, regulated the use of bread and cakes according to set traditions. Mourners over a dead king avoided wheaten foods (*Diod.*, see p. 488). The Scriptures narrate how, when Joseph's folk ate with the Egyptians, their meal was set apart because

"the Egyptians would not eat bread with them" (Genesis, 43,32),

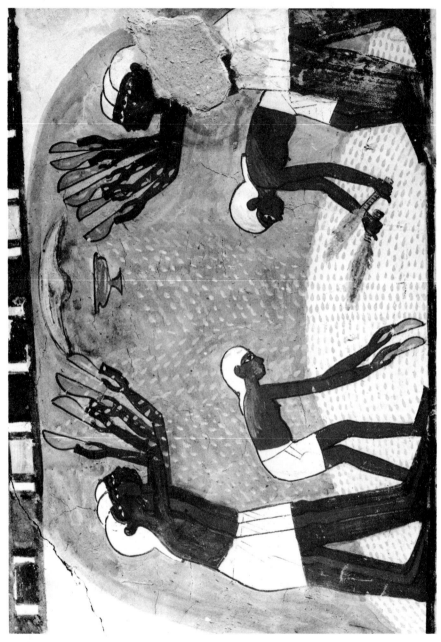

Fig. 12.1. Winnowing grain, The Tomb of Nakht at Thebes. New Kingdom.

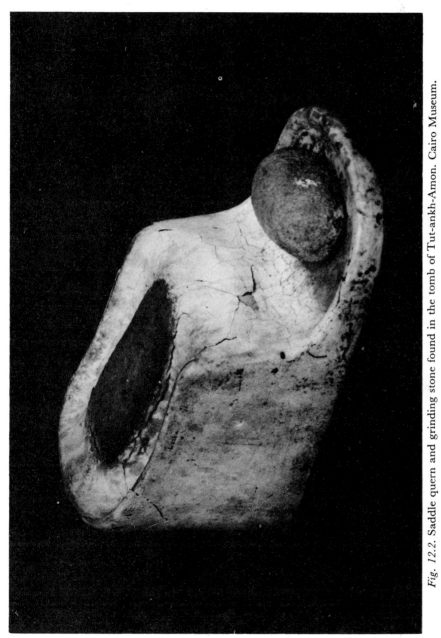

Fig. 12.2. Saddle quern and grinding stone found in the tomb of Tut-ankh-Amon. Cairo Museum.

although the latter expression might have meant merely sharing a meal. Athenaeus, likewise, wrote of the habit of Naucratites never to serve eggs and honey cakes at wedding banquets (*Deipnos.*, 4, 150, A).

Preparation of Bread

"Take thou also unto thee wheat, and barley, and beans, and lentiles, and millet, and fitches, and put them into one vessel, and make thee bread thereof . . ." (Ezekial, IV, 9)

"And thou shalt eat it as barley cake, and thou shalt bake it with dung that cometh out of man, in their sight." (Ezekial, IV, 12)

"Lo, I have given thee cow's dung for man's dung, and thou shalt prepare thy bread therewith." (Ezekial, IV, 15)

Baking appears, at least until the New Kingdom, to have been a task of the housewife or, in large households, of the domestics. In Rome, Pliny said that there were no bakers until the war with Perseus (171–168 B.C.), and that baking was especially the task of women (*N.H.*, XVIII, XXVIII, 107).

At first, grain was used, unmilled, to make gruels and unleavened biscuits and flour that were then baked to be eaten or brewed. The first revolution occurred when it was crushed or ground. The process was made easier by previous parching or roasting (*N.H.*, XVIII, XXII, 97), a measure that facilitated threshing and grinding and, by converting starch into dextrin, sweetened the flour and promoted fermentation.

Another practice that became common around the Mediterranean was to steep grain into water, and then to dry it in the sun before pounding it (*N.H.*, XVIII, XXII, 98). This allowed the skin to resist pulverization, and thus to be easily separated from the powdered flour.

At first, after winnowing (Fig. 12.1) grinding and pounding were performed on a saddle quern by means of a round or roller-shaped stone (Fig. 12.2 and Fig. 12.3, lowest two rows) and it was usually a job left to women. The circular rotary mills of which specimens of about the eighth century B.C. were found in Eastern Anatolia (Storcke and Teague, 1952, p. 77) were invented later, probably in more than one place at the same time. According to Forbes (1955, Vol. 3, p. 58), in Egypt, one hears of a miller only about 1500 B.C., and the rotary quern appeared only shortly before Hellenistic times, probably as an import from

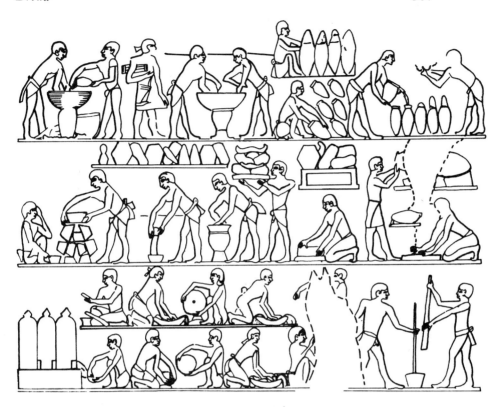

Fig. 12.3. Preparation of bread and beer. Ti's tomb. Saqqara. Old Kingdom. Redrawn from Daumas and Goyon (1939).

Mesopotamia, where animal-driven rotary querns were known since Assyrian times, after 1000 B.C.

The crushed grain was then cribbled and sieved (Fig. 12.3) through sieves made of rush or papyrus (*N.H.*, XVIII, XXVIII, 108). Actually most flour in antiquity was simply whole meal and, calculating from figures given by Pliny (XVIII, 86–89), an 80% extraction was the best that could be achieved. But examination of specimens of bread found in tombs shows that a lot of grit was allowed through. Filce Leek (1972) recently reported on several loaves that were examined microscopically, radiologically and by petrographic techniques. The results showed the presence of husks of grain, and of radio-opaque particles of quartz,

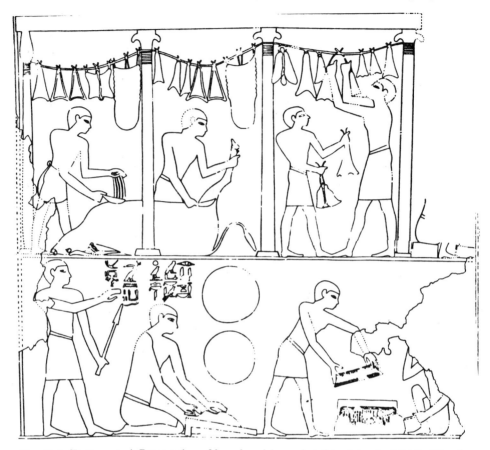

Fig. 12.4. (Bottom row) Preparation of bread and beer. Antefoker's tomb. Middle Kingdom. Thebes. (Davies and Gardiner, plate IX.)

feldspar, mica, ferromagnesium minerals probably hornblende and other rock fragments. He attributed these to a variety of sources, like the soil where the grain had grown, the flint sickles, sand carried with the wind during winnowing or from the silos, the grinding stones, and possibly inorganic material added to hasten the grinding process. He ended by quoting a papyrus of the Greek period substantiating the belief that impurities were sometimes found in grain, but his statement that Pharaoh's chief baker who was imprisoned with the Biblical Joseph for his having offended Pharaoh was punished because he thus adulterated bread, is not substantiated in the Scriptures.

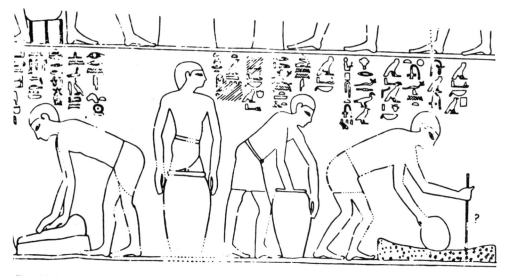

Fig. 12.5. Preparation of bread in Antefoker's tomb. Second figure from left is kneading, with feet in pottery vessel. (Davies and Gardiner, 1920, plate VIII.) Thebes Middle Kingdom.

Kneading and Leavening

Flour being thus obtained, its transformation into bread became possible. Mechanical kneading, invented in Rome to satisfy the huge demands on bread doled to the Romans, does not seem to have been practiced in Egypt. On the other hand, workers are often seen in tomb illustrations kneading dough with their hands (Fig. 12.3, middle register) and, in large households, with their feet (Fig. 12.5), thus confirming the statement of Strabo (17, 2, 5) and the astonished comment of Herodotus (II, 36)

"Dough they knead with their feet, but they mix mud with their hands."

Spices and salt were added, but priests seem to have avoided salted bread (Plutarch, *Table Talk*, 10, 684, 685).

Fermentation was started by adding sour dough, leaven, or yeast. In Greece, leavened bread introduced from the East was still a luxury in the time of Solon, but, in the Egyptian specimens of beer residues he examined, Grüss (1932) found *torula* mixed with organisms resembling

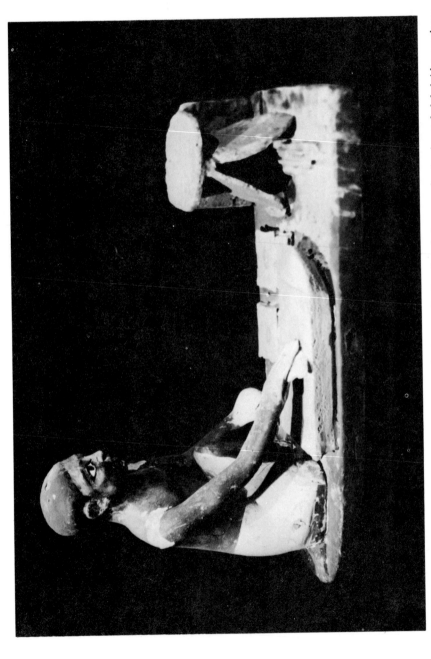

Fig. 12.6. Cooking and baking on an oven made of a few vertically placed stones and a horizontal slab laid over them. Old Kingdom model. Cairo Museum.

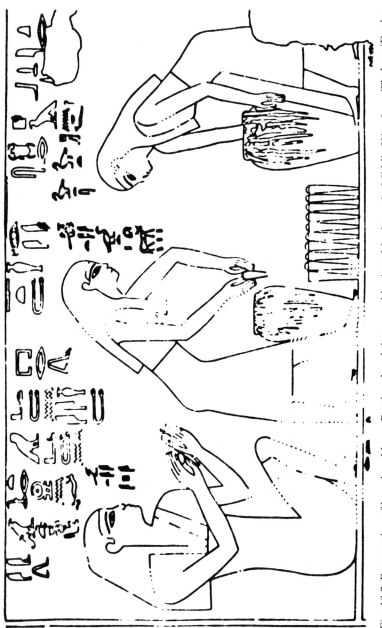

Fig. 12.7. Preparation of bread and beer. Putting dough into moulds. Antefoker's tomb, Middle Kingdom. Thebes. (Davies and Gardiner, 1920, plate XII).

Saccharomyces winlocki. According to this author it is probable that an almost pure yeast was available by 1500 B.C.

By Pliny's time several methods of leavening were known, and the rather lengthy description of leaven by this author may have some bearing on Egyptian practice. He stated that this was made especially of millet or of bran after steeping them in unfermented wine. This of course would assist fermentation. Apart from the vinting season, leaven was made of browned barley cakes shut up in vessels until they went sour, or of wheat dough kept over from the previous day (*N.H.*, XVIII, XXVI, 102–104). Of course, in Alexandrian times, the leaven trade was in the hands of specialized professionals.

If current interpretations of iconographic material be correct, the result was a semi-solid preparation.

Baking

> *Give your bread to the baker even though he eat half of it*
> (popular saying)

The dough so prepared then was baked. At first, baking was on an open fire (Fig. 12.4) or over ashes (Fig. 12.5, extreme right). A rudimentary oven was subsequently contrived by lighting a fire between a few vertically placed stones with an overlaying horizontal slab (Fig. 12.6). Sometimes, as may be seen in Antefoker's tomb, the dough was baked in pre-heated moulds (Fig. 12.7). Later, came cylindrical ovens inside of which a fire was lit (Fig. 12.8). Some of these ovens were open above; when the oven was sufficiently hot, the dough loaf was pressed against the inside of the heated walls (Borchardt, 1932). This gave flat curved loaves. Such ovens are still in use in rural North-Africa (Fig. 12.8b).

The whole process of bread making is profusely illustrated in many tombs of all epochs, in many scenes accompanied by explanatory legends. Despite this, the interpretation of some details is still debated.

In the Ancient Kingdom tomb of Ti, in Saqqara, the wall of the store-room facing the entrance is covered with several horizontal panels illustrating the preparation of bread and beer (Fig. 12.3). On the side walls are shown these being offered to Ti and his family.

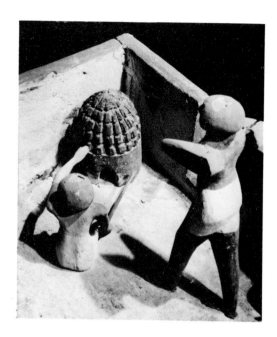

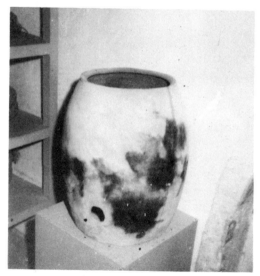

Fig. 12.8a. (Upper) Model of round oven. Middle Kingdom. Cairo Museum.

Fig. 12.8b. (Lower) Traditional bread oven still in use in rural North Africa. A fire is lit inside the oven, and when this is sufficiently hot, the dough loaves are applied through the upper opening on the inside of the walls. Courtesy of the authorities of the Tripoli museum.

The lowest panel in this illustration which, in the tomb, roughly occupies the middle of the wall, illustrates the first steps common to the production of both bread and beer—grain being withdrawn from storage, measured, pounded, cleaned, ground and cribbled.

Upward from this common panel run brewing scenes and downward are bread-making scenes, although the distinction is not absolute between the two. The baking scenes are interpreted thus by Wild (1966).

In the lowest register (Fig. 12.3) the grain, after being withdrawn from its stores (extreme left) and pounded, is being ground on a concave stone by kneeling women. Some grain is spilled onto the floor. Each woman is faced by a squatting companion who cribbles the product on a circular sieve. On a higher register, the grinding operation is repeated, and each group of two or three grinders is faced by a squatting companion who sieves the product through a rectangular sieve into a jar, where it can be seen falling. The operation is repeated by successive teams (lower two panels) until all the grain has attained the desired fineness.

In the third panel from above (the sixth on the wall) conical moulds, called *bedja*, are heated over a fire, stirred by workers who protect their faces from the heat (right and left extremities). In the middle scenes, divided into two horizontal ones, the dough is mixed and poured into the heated moulds in the lower half; in the upper half, its condition is controlled by the woman to the left; the moulds are closed and, finally, emptied.

The middle panel of the same wall depicts in addition the heating and filling of moulds in which dough is then poured to prepare hexagonal loaves called *kmḥw*. These moulds are made of two trapezoidal halves that, after being filled, are placed atop of each other. The dough in the two then sticks together to give the loaf an hexagonal shape. Other loaves in the same picture, shelved or carried on trays, are rounded, oval, conical or crescentic.

The kinds of grain mentioned in these pictures (the names are not reproduced in the figure) are: *zwt*, determined by ovoid cereal grains; and *bš?*, determined by round circles. The latter circles determine also the aromat *sgnn* (see Chapter 3, Beer), green-bread (*t-w?ḏ*), dough (*šdt*), and leaven (*hz?*). The use of a peculiar determinative sign with all of these terms as well as with *bš?* suggested to Wild that *bš?* was a grain specially prepared or set aside for brewing.

Figure 12.4, taken from Antefoker's tomb (Davies and Gardiner, 1920, plate VIII), shows the making of round pancakes. An overseer, armed with a stick, encourages his men; and the baker who works the dough on a sloping block answers "All right! I am hard at work." His fellow carries a disc of dough in a pan to a clay hearth, that a companion is stirring below a griddle. The result must have been very close to the wafer-like bread of the present day fellah.

At the end of the same row (Fig. 12.5), dough is kneaded both by hand and by treading in a jar; a worker is extracting out of the jar some dough that, made into a cake, is placed by the next man on a bed of hot ashes(?) or hot sand(?), that he is raking with a poker.

All these men maintain a lively conversation registered in many rows of hieroglyphs.

Another scene (Fig. 12.9) from the same tomb was described in detail by Davies and Gardiner (1920). It represents both bread making and brewing. The following is a slightly modified account of his description

> On the right we see two men pounding the grain with pestles in a solid cylindrical mortar. The man with uplifted pestle gives the word "Down!" and receives the equally brief assent "Right!" ("I do your pleasure"). A woman passes the coarse flour thus obtained through a sieve into a tray to remove husks, and a companion grinds it still finer between a pestle and a stone slab set on a clay bench within a hollow in which it collects. One woman is piously mindful of the object of her labour, saying, "O all ye gods of this land, bless my powerful master"; but what is left of her companion's reply seems prosaic enough ". . . . This is for food". Three women (named in less prominent script "the handmaid, Apa," "the handmaid, Sitepiḥu" and "her daughter, Sitantef") (Fig. 12.7) make the cakes. One mixes flour with water in a jar with more vigour than deftness, for it slops over the rim at every point. Another rubs each roll of dough that is destined for a loaf with a lump of red material. The third, the middle one, fills a batch of ten conical moulds with dough. All are chattering. The baker (Fig. 12.4 right) then takes the moulds, and stacks them in the flames which issue from the top of a fireplace the fuel of which is introduced and poked from below.

Nature and Varieties of Ancient Egyptian Bread

Brunton and Caton-Thompson (1928) found, at the Neolithic site of El-Badari, pieces of bread of which the porosity indicated that they had

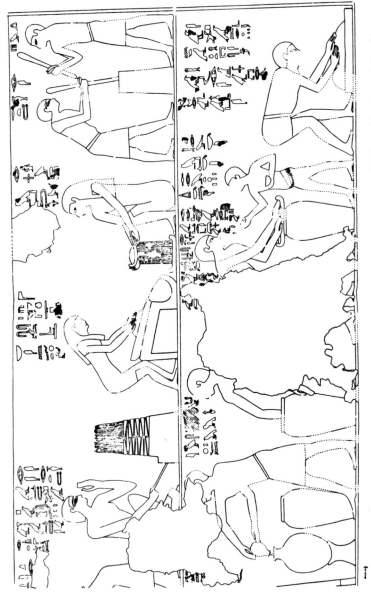

Fig. 12.9. The preparation of bread and beer. Antefoker's tomb. Middle Kingdom. Thebes. (Davies and Gardiner, p. 15 and plate XI.)

been subjected to leavening. At Deir el-Bahari (Schweinfurth, 1883) and elsewhere, masses of lichen similar to varieties nowadays utilized to increase the porosity of cakes (*Evernia furfuracea*, Arabic: *sheba*) have been found; and, on the strength of this finding, it has been suggested that these may have been utilized to the same purpose. In that connection, Filce Leek (1973) stated that

". . . at least in 1930 bread made from lichens was still sold in Teheran. Certain lichens contain highly characteristic proteins detectable by thin-layer chromatography, whilst the proteins of other lichens remain difficult to detect. A positive result would prove definitely that lichens were used in the production of bread, but a negative result would leave the question open."

He further quoted negative experiments carried out by Dr D. L. Hawksworth at the Commonwealth Mycological Institute on three samples of Ancient Egyptian bread.

Herodotus, who observed that Egyptians were bread-eaters said that they ate *kyllestis* and Hecataeus was credited with the same assertion (*Deipnos.*, 3, 114, C–D). This kyllestis, records of which go as far back as Rameses III (*A.R.*, IV, 238) was sourish, according to Athenaeus, who added, on the authority of Nicander, that it was made of barley. Nevertheless, Gulick, in a note to his translation (*D ipnos.*, 10, 418, C–D note *a*) asserted that it was probably made of rye, although this cereal is not known to have been cultivated in Egypt.

In fact, the majority of specimens of bread that were examined were found to be made of Emmer (*T.*, I, 248), as were all the samples in the Berlin Museum (Grüss, 1932). This apparent contradiction between Athenaeus and the laboratory is most probably due to the fact that the specimens that found their way to museums were offering breads that had to be made of this superior cereal, wheat.

A particular kind of bread, attested since the earliest times, had a special significance. This was a conical white bread called *t-ḥd* that was used in offerings (Figs 12.10, 12.11, 12.12). In hieroglyphic writing, it was determined by a pointed pyramidal sign depicted by (b) (*F.*, 292) which represented the loaf and generally bread, and either drawn alone, or on the palm of the hand, as in (c) meant "to give".

Other loaves were roughly circular or ovoid, with slashes to allow the gas formed during fermentation and baking to escape (Figs 12.13, and 1.6, Vol. 1). A triangular loaf was apparently much in favour, for it figures in most illustrations and museums (Figs 12.14 and 12.15).

A semi-circular loaf (Fig. 12.16) must have been very traditional, since

(b)

(c)

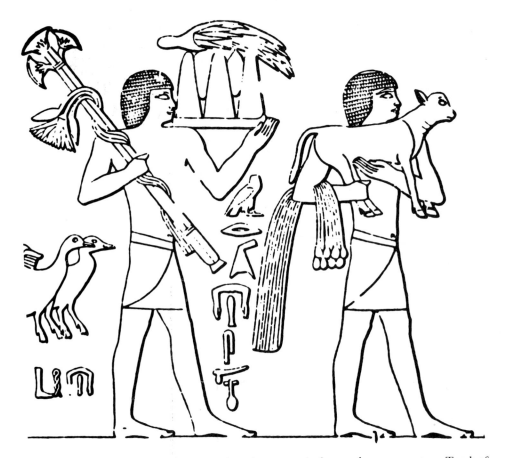

Fig. 12.10. Offerings of loaves, lettuce, onions, lotus wreathed around a papyrus stem. Tomb of
Akhet-hotep. Saqqara. Old Kingdom. (Davies, 1901, part 2 plate XXXII.)

the figure was used ever since writing was invented as a hieroglyph for
bread [see (a) p. 501] and for the sound *t* that designated it. This phonetic
use of semi-circular loaves is clearly seen in Fig. 6.45 (Vol. 1), just
above the royal cartouche.

There was also a flat loaf that was often curved, having taken the
shape of the inner wall of the cylindrical oven where it was baked
(Borchardt, 1932). A variety that had in its centre a crater surrounded
by a raised or everted lip (Fig. 12.13) recalls a present-day custom of

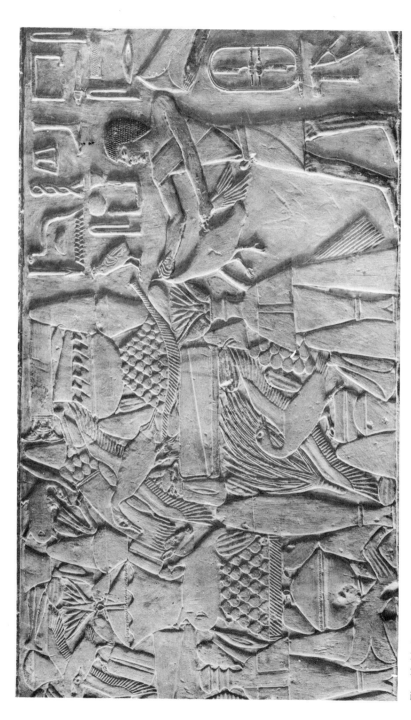

Fig. 12.11. Food offerings: Loaves of various shapes, figs, lotus, lettuce, onions, melons, papyrus, gourds, geese, joints of meat. Tomb of Ptahhetep. Saqqara. Old Kingdom. Centre of Documentation. Cairo.

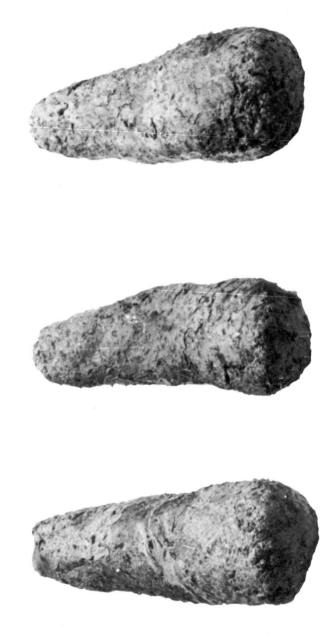

Fig. 12.12. Conical loaves. New Kingdom. Dokki Agricultural Museum, Cairo. No. 4272.

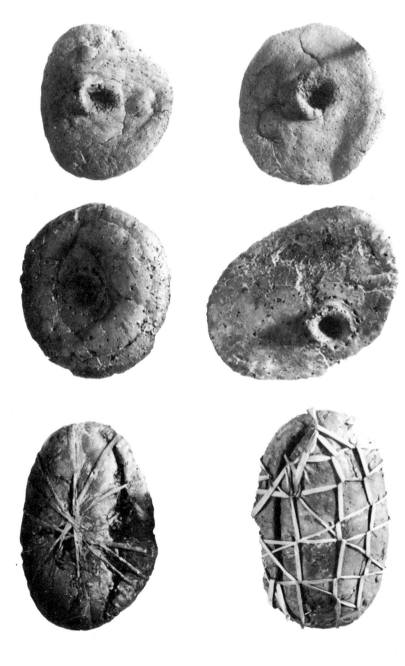

Fig. 12.13. A selection of loaves of the New Kingdom at the Dokki Agricultural Museum, Cairo. From Deir el Medineh) New Kingdom. (Left) Ovoid loaves with lateral slashes still in their wrapping of papyrus. (Right and middle) Loaves with a central crater.

fellaheen women who, in order to prepare a quick meal, carve in the centre of a loaf, before baking it, a hole that they fill with an egg or other garnishing. Other loaves, examined by Grüss (1932) had been sprinkled with flour or overlaid with fresh dough after a preliminary baking, and had then been rebaked to a brown dextrin.

Especially under the New Kingdom, fancy loaves and cakes were rolled into spirals like Swiss rolls, or were given the shape of a goose, cow (Fig. 12.14), or female figure (Fig. 12.17), either as a toy cake or loaf, or with a votive or magic purpose, like the phallus-shaped cake of the London papyrus (*L.*, 13, 3–7) on which a spell against the disease *áaâ* had to be pronounced before giving it to a cat, or the many cakes in the shape of Sethan animals or imprinted with their image utilized in the cult. Thus in the rituals connected with the Osiris-Seth cycles, Pultarch relates

> ". . . and when they make cakes at their sacrifices in the months of Payni and Paopki, they imprint on them the device of an ass tied by a rope." (*I. and O.*, 362, 30)

On another occasion, the image was that of a tightly tied hippopotamus (*I. and O.*, 371, 50); and in certain festivals, when pigs had to be sacrificed, the poor who could not afford live pigs formed pigs of dough which they baked and offered in sacrifice (*Her.*, II, 47).

The symbolic meaning of eating (Chapter 3, p. 85), the holiness of bread, the magic notion of the identity of images with their models, gave these "bread-dolls" an essential significance in festivals, magic or cult. It is just this significance that the Council of Leptines, in forbidding in A.D. 743 the fashioning of human figures from flour dough (Hefele, 1910), reserved for the holiest Christian mystery.

Many other varieties of bread are enumerated in records of Pharaonic Egypt (see page 503), but their characteristics are unknown. In Graeco-Roman times, there was an ever wider variety. Cakes were sweetened, flavoured, and enriched with honey, sesame, anise and fruits. The all-fruit *pankarpian*, that was well known in Alexandria, consisted of crumbled seed-cakes cooked in honey, formed into balls, and wrapped in thin papyrus (*Deipnos.*, 14, 648, B), and Strabo wrote of an Egyptian cake, *kakeis*, that checked diarrhoea (17, 2, 5). Theophrastus mentioned three special kinds made in Egypt, which were made from doum fruits (2, 6, 10), sebesten (4, 2, 10), and lotus (4, 8, 11); the last also was mentioned by Diodorus (1, 34, 6) and Pliny (*H.N.*, XIII, XXXII, 108 and XXII, XXVIII, 56).

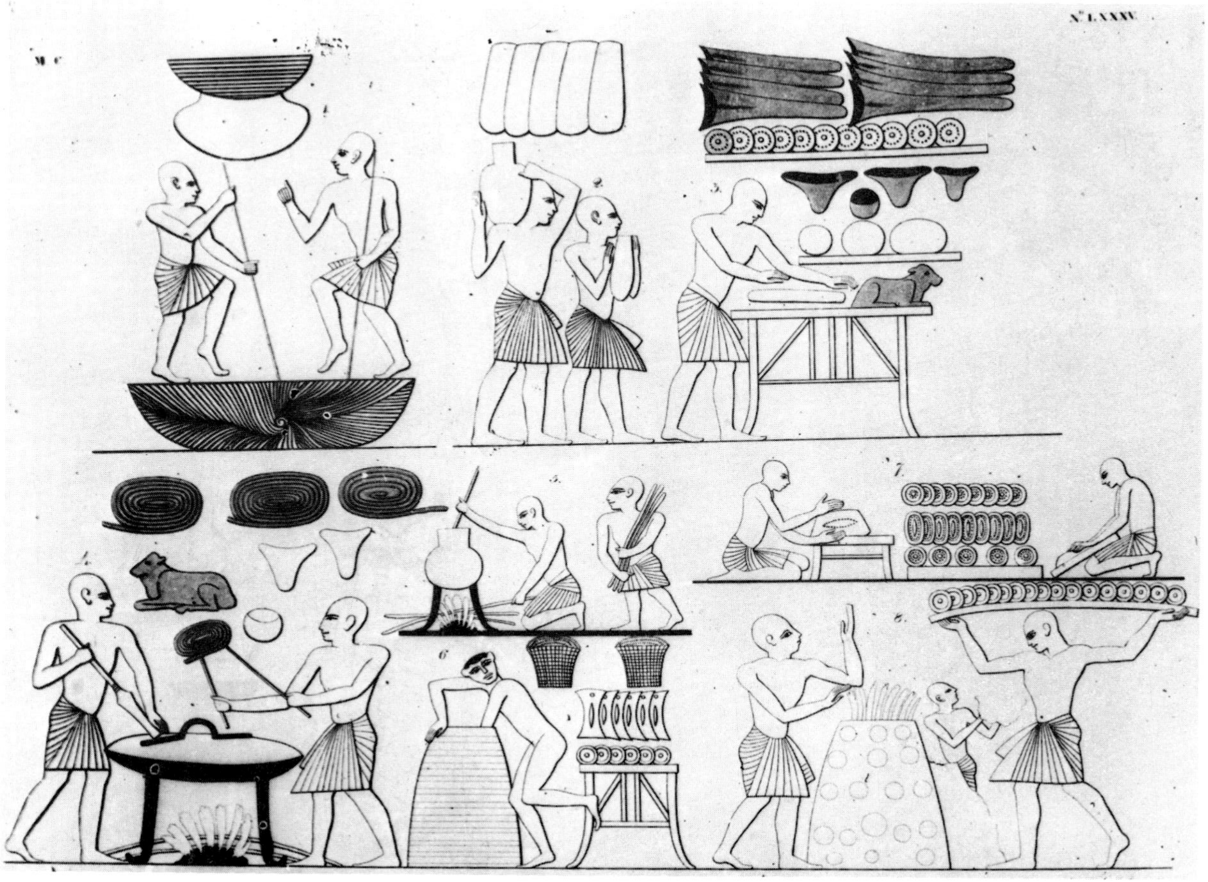

Fig. 12.14. A bakery in Rameses III's tomb. Thebes. After Rosellini, II, plate LXXXV. Note the cakes of various shapes.

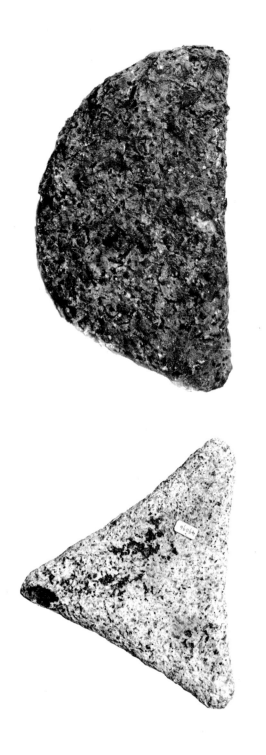

Fig. 12.15. (Left) Triangular loaf from Deir el-Bahari. Eleventh dynasty. Cairo Museum. No. J. 49096.

Fig. 12.16. (Right) Semi-circular loaf or cake from the tomb of Tut-ankh-Amon. Cairo Museum.

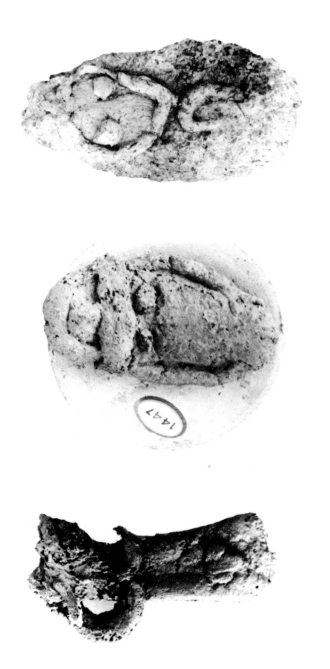

Fig. 12.17. Cakes or loaves in the shape of a feminine figure. From Deir el-Medineh. Eighteenth dynasty, around 1400 B.C. Dokki Agricultural Museum, No. 1447.

According to a statement of Pontanius reported by Athenaeus (*Deipnos.*, 3, 109, B–C), Tryphon of Alexandria enumerated raised bread, unleavened bread and breads made of white wheat flour, of groats, of unbolted meal (said to be laxative), of rye (?), of spelt, and of millet. The groat bread, he said, was made of rice wheat, because it could not be made of barley. It is known, however, that neither rice nor rye were grown in Ancient Egypt.

Elsewhere, Athenaeus enumerated an impressive list of varieties known to Egyptians, of which a wafer-bread probably baked over charcoal like the ash-bread of the Athenians, and consecrated by Alexandrians to Cronus in whose temple it was offered to visitors (*Deipnos.*, 3, 110, B). The *obelias*, he said, was so called either because it cost an obol, or because it was baked on a spit and by a pun on *obolos*, which meant both an obol and a spit (3, 111, note *c*).

Pliny, who cited *kyllestis* and an Alexandrian bread garnished with cummin (*N.H.*, XX, LVIII, 163), gave us a fine insight into the origin of these different appellations and into the influence of a leisurely class upon culinary refinement

> "In some places, it [bread] is called after the dishes eaten with it, such as oyster bread; in others, from its special delicacy, as cake-bread; in others from the short time spent in making it, as hasty bread; and also from the method of baking, as oven bread or thin loaf or baking-pan bread; while not long ago there was even bread imported from Parthia, called water-bread because by means of water it is drawn out into a thin spongy consistency full of holes. The highest merit depends on the goodness of the wheat and the fineness of the bolter. Some use eggs or milk in kneading the dough, while even butter has been used by races enjoying peace, when attention can be devoted to the varieties of pastry-making." (*N.H.*, XVIII, XXVI, 105)

Other Uses of Bread

Apart from its alimentary use which, naturally, predominated, bread was one of the ingredients with which the bodies of sacrificial kine were filled (*Her.*, II, 40). After light cooking, bread was fermented to make beer (see Ch. 13, Beer). Mixed with other ingredients, it was also used in medicine, mainly *per os*. For example, to break "pain matter" (*wḫdw*), it was compounded with fresh beef, frankincense (? terebinth) juniper, and sweet beer (*Eb.*, XXIII, 86); and, against rectal prolapse, it was combined with goose-grease, honey, colocynth, to be taken in one day (*Eb.*, XXXIII, 149).

Toasted bread, with manna, honey and water, improved appetite (*Eb.*, LI, 289, 290). Double-bread (or *bread of two breads?*) with red ochre, costus, rock oil and sweet beer, was credited with anthelminthic virtues (*Eb.*, XXII, 76). *Stt* bread could expel illness from the interior of the body (*Eb.*, LXXVI, 589), while bread of *Zizyphus spina Christi* was used against jaundice (*Eb.*, LXVII, 480), and the mysterious *áaâ* (*Eb.*, XLV, 225).

Less commonly, bread was to be used locally. Thus, *prsn* bread (a variant of *pzn*), mixed with vegetable mucus and various fruits was applied to fractures (*H.*, 218, 220). Barley bread, with oil and salt, formed a dressing for burns, (*Eb.*, LXIX, 509); and sour wheaten bread was applied to the scalp to expel obstinate dandruff (*Eb.*, LXXXVI, 712 b).

Other Cereal Products

Actually, many preparations other than bread and cakes were made from cereals, e.g. *ntt* (?), *nd̲* flour (?), *d̲d̲w* meal (?), and *d̲w*(?) (Edel, 1970). There is no indication, however as to their nature.

Alexandrians prepared a special kind of starch (*N.H.*, XVIII, XVII, 77; *Diosc.*, 11, 125). But, despite Ebbell's questionable translation of *ns.ty n bš̯* (i.e. *nsty* (?) of wheat) as starch, (*Eb.*, LXXXI, 650; LXXXIV, 682), this commodity, according to Pliny, was made first in Chios, whence the best quality came; next came that made in Crete; and only in the third rank came the Egyptian produce. He described its manufacture in the following way

". . . next to the starch made from three-month wheat is the kind made of the lightest sort of wheat. This is soaked with fresh water in wooden tubs, with the grain completely covered, the water being changed five times in the course of a day, and preferably in the night time as well, so as to get it mixed up evenly with the grain. When it is quite soft but before it goes sour it is strained through linen or wicker baskets and poured out on a tiled surface that has been smeared with leaven, and left to thicken in the sun . . ." (*N.H.*, XVIII, XVII, 76–77)

A kind of pap was also made from hulled-wheat grains by a method common to Campania and Egypt (*N.H.*, XVIII, XVI, 76).

The quality of groats was controversial. Athenaeus saw them prepared in the Egyptian manner, served at a Greek wedding (*Deipnos.*, 4, 131, D). This would suggest that they were appreciated. On the other hand, Pliny wrote that

> "they were no doubt also made in Egypt but of a rather contemptible quality"

and he described their method of preparation

> ". . . alica (groats) is made from *zea* which we have already called by the name 'seed'. Its grain is pounded in a wooden mortar so as to avoid the hardness of stone grating it up, the motive power for the pestle, as is well known, being supplied by the labour of convicts in chains . . . after the grain has been stripped of its coats, the bared kernel is again broken up with the same implements. The process produces three grades of alica; very small, seconds, and the largest kind which is called in Greek 'select grade'. Still these products have not yet got their whiteness for which they are distinguished, though even at this stage they are preferable to the Alexandrian alica . . ." (*N.H.*, XVIII, XXIX, 109–113)

Notes: Chapter 12

1. Second king of the twelfth dynasty (*c.* 1970–1936 B.C.). Sesostris is the Greek form of his Egyptian name Senusret.
2. Sometimes portrayed as a mother goddess and considered a goddess of childbirth, Nekhbet bore the head of a vulture.
3. The ancient goddess of the Delta, usually represented as a cobra.
4. A term that may mean malt (see Chapter 13).

Chapter 13   Beer

Myth, Religion and Superstition

The invention of beer (a), even in the earliest Egyptian times, was so deeply lost in the abyss of irretrievable memories, its making and use were so inextricably knit in the fabric of daily life, while its exhilarating powers appeared so mysteriously supernatural that human imagination readily weaved around it the most incredible, albeit significant tales.

Egyptians never forgot that Ra had dulled Hathor-Sekhmet's rage thus saving mankind from destruction, by fooling her with a red-dyed beer that she took for blood (see Volume 1, p. 125). Once a year, the gentle form of this fierce feline goddess was feasted in Bubastis and, although Herodotus said that people revelled with wine (II, 60), the fact that he erroneously said elsewhere that there was no wine in Egypt (II, 77) indicates that he probably meant any intoxicating drink, wine being nearer to his Greek heart than beer.

The general character of these celebrations is fairly well known. A text on Mut's gate at Karnak (Mut and Sekhmet being different functions of one goddess) recalls Sekhmet's legend by transposing it into the ritual

> "In honour of the goddess, beer, red with Nubian ochre, is poured in these days of the Feast of the Valley, so that, having become different from the usual aspect of beer, it could appease the anger in her heart." (translated from Sauneron, 1968)

Many hymns to Hathor depict her as the goddess of inebriety and as the inventor of beer whereby she was turned from a wild lionness into an amiable fun-loving lady. A Roman emperor in the temple of Isis at Philae sang to her

> "Mistress of Both Lands, Mistress of Bread,
> Who made beer with what her heart created
> And her hands prepared
> She is the Lady of Drunkenness, rich in Feasts
> Lady of Music, fond of Dances"

(Junker and Winter, 1965, p. 271)

(a)

ḥḳt

529

Another poem, the Hymn of the Seven Hathors, exalted the happiness she brought

> "Our hearts exult on seeing thy Majesty
> For thou art the Mistress of Wreathes
> The Lady of Dance
> And of Drunkenness without end"   (Junker, 1906)

Drunkenness was thus a source and a symbol of mirth and forbearance, possibly also of religious ecstasy. Besides Sekhmet's, it intervened in the worship of other gods, as in the cult of Tefnut, where wine played a large role (Bonnet, 1952). As to Pharaohs, being gods, they could be neither good nor bad, they were mere forces; though humans from their mortal angle, could look at them otherwise. Like gods (Sekhmet-Hathor) they could have many aspects, all justified. This consideration points to the correct way of looking at such otherwise, absurd or blasphemous names as "How drunk is Mykerinus" (Reisner, 1931, p. 275), "Cheops is drunk" (Smith, W. S., 1952), or "Sahoure is drunk" (Borchardt, 1910, Vol. II, p. 86).

But there were, besides Hathor-Sekhmet, other goddesses of beer, like *Mnq.t* whose name could well have been a pun on, or a deification of, the *mnq.t* jars where beer was stored, and *Tnmy.t* (*Wb.*, V, 312) possibly also a punning deification of a *tnm* beverage or beer (*Wb.*, V, 312) that is mentioned exclusively in religious texts (*Pyr.*, 106).

If a man dreamt of beer, the omen varied with the kind of beer and the dream context. It was of good augury to dream of drinking sweet beer: the dreamer would rejoice; or to drink bakery-beer, he would live; or stored beer, he would be healed (Volten, 1942, p. 91). But it was a bad portent to dream of drinking warm beer, it forebode suffering; or of brewing in one's house, the dreamer would be turned out of his house; or of putting beer into a vessel, it meant the removal of something from the house (Gardiner, 1935, pp. 16–19). On the other hand, to drive away evil dreams, the face of the dreamer had to be rubbed with herbs moistened with beer while uttering a spell (Gardiner, 1935, p. 19).

History

Diodorus (IV, 2) attributed the invention of beer to Dionysus whom the Greeks identified with Osiris (*Her.*, II, 42), and he credited Osiris with spreading it in countries where wine was unknown (I, 20). Egypt was thus, in Greek opinion, the originator of beer, although the Sumero-Akkadians, another agricultural people who prepared it since the dawn of history, may share the claim.

One may even surmise that its invention came as a result of the accidental discovery in household bakeries of the euphoria experienced after consuming cereals prepared to make gruels or bread, when left to ferment. This is supported by the use in Sumero-Akkadian of the word *lahamu* that originally probably meant to make loaves (*cf.* Hebrew *laham*, bread) to indicate brewing, and by the constant association of baking and brewing in Egyptian art.

In fact, brewing seems to have been, at least in its beginnings, a woman's calling. The divinities presiding over it were goddesses, and girls and maids are prominent in the processes of kneading, sieving and actual brewing, as represented in tomb art. In large domains, they were under the supervision of some kind of Chief Brewer, like the high official Kha-bau-Seker who bore the title of "Controller of the Brewing Women" (Murray and Sethe, 1937, p. 11).

Prehistoric jars examined by Petrie (1920, p. 43) were found to contain residues of beer, and this drink is mentioned in texts, as early as the third dynasty (Murray, 1905, p. 39). From the fifth dynasty, Hotep-iry-akhet a priest of Ne-Woser-Re's Sun-temple at Abusir, tried to induce visitors to his tomb to make mortuary offerings of beer, by promising to commend them to the god

> "Whosoever shall make offerings to me therein, I shall do for them; I will commend them to the god very greatly; I will do this for them, for bread, for beer . . ." (*A.R.*, I, 251)

The Pyramid Texts, which are much older, although known only from sixth dynasty versions, mention several varieties of this beverage, "beer", *dšrt*, *ḥnm.s*, and Nubian. From the succeeding periods one has only to scan the impressive list of instances of beer donated as food, as divine offerings, evening offerings, mortuary offerings, oblations, or offerings to obelisks (*A.R.*, V, index: Beer), to be convinced of the importance of this drink in daily life.

Social Standing

Beer, however, was the usual drink of commoners, while wine was the beverage of the rich. Athenaeus indicated this difference in the tale of its invention, citing an "academic" philosopher, Dio, as his authority

> "The Egyptian [nobility] became fond of wine and bibulous; and so a way
> was found among them to help those who could not afford wine, namely,
> to drink that made from barley; they who took it were so elated that they
> sang, danced, and acted in every way like persons filled with wine."
> (*Deipnos.*, 1, 34, B)

This distinction may be the reason why, in Egypt, less is known about
beer than about wine, since the customs and food habits of the poor
were less carefully recorded by the chroniclers than those of the rich.
The Greek and Roman travellers equated beer with poverty, while they,
themselves, understood and appreciated wine. Even Aristotle is
credited with a discriminatory comment

> "Men who have been intoxicated with wine fall down face foremost,
> whereas they who have drunk barley beer lie outstretched on their backs;
> for wine makes one top-heavy, but beer stupefies." (according to Athenaeus;
> *Deipnos.*, 1, 34, B)

With the financial means to cater to their more refined tastes, it
might be surmised that the Egyptian kings and nobles would scorn
beer. But the extensive lists of offerings and donations that have
survived, do not bear this out. In certain funeral texts the deceased was
promised "beer that would not turn sour", indicating the wish of the
nobility to pursue their beer-drinking habits in eternity, and the
concern over spoilage and storage problems (Montet, 1958, p. 87). In
fact, Diodorus acknowledged the pleasant taste of the drink made from
barley that, he said,

> "For smell and sweetness is not much inferior to wine." (1, 34, 10–11)

The reason of the social discrimination between wine and beer was
probably, therefore, the cheapness of beer, that was due, on the one
hand, to the abundance of grain in a country that was not only able to
cater to its own needs, but that could export a surplus, and on the other
hand, to the ease of its production in comparison with the extensive
technology and care required by the vine and the vinification process.

Beer was thus next in preference to water, the popular beverage *par
excellence*. Often combined with bread in paintings and bas-reliefs, it
was also associated with it in common parlance which, metaphorically
(b)   used the phrase "bread and beer" like today in the East "bread and
   salt", for food in general. In writing, the combined hieroglyphs for
bread and for beer (b) formed the generic determinative of food as, for

example, after *s3b*, food, or *prt-ḥrw*, invocation offering (c). An even   (c)
more striking custom was the common use of the greeting formula
"bread and beer" (Montet, 1958, p. 93).

Beer recurs in each of the tales told and retold around Ancient
Egyptian hearths, and copied and recopied by successive generations of
scribes. Wine is mentioned only in the *Adventures of Sinouhe* and then
when the hero was in Asia (Lefebvre, 1949, p. 11).

The universal popularity of beer as a general beverage, even in
preference to water, may in part be explained by the state of sanitation
that made water, usually contaminated, a risky drink until the last
century. The fear of contamination from pond water is illustrated in the
present-day Egyptian expression

"With its mud rather than washed in pond water"

when choosing an uneducated person in preference to one brought up in
a doubtful milieu.

A proper perspective is given to this problem by the care given by old
authors, like Hippocrates, to correlate water, along with winds and
other ecological factors, with health, temperament, and disease. The
theme of unwholesomeness of water recurs again and again in the
history of early settlers in the United States, when official reports
ascribed sickness to lack of beer and consequent reliance on water.
Those of the colonists who could not make their own beer were the
quickest to complain. A letter written in 1613 says of these sturdy
colonists

". . . nor do they drink anything but water—all of which is contrary to the
nature of the English—on which account they wish to return and would
have done so if they had been at liberty." (quoted in Baron, 1962, p. 5)

The result was the publication of advertisements to induce brewers to
emigrate. But home brewing remained a well-established custom in
both English and Dutch settlements well after the first licensed commercial breweries were established in the first third of the seventeenth
century, and no lesser persons than Presidents George Washington and
Thomas Jefferson were among the most prominent gentlemen brewers
(Baron, 1962, p. 96). These traditions served the country well during
the crucial years of friction between the rulers and the colonists, when
the fear that imported supplies be cut off led to the publication of
numerous family recipes; then home brewing thrived again, as it did
later under the Prohibition.

Method of Preparation

The preparation of beer, as described in late Egyptian documents and in tomb art of all periods, did not materially differ from the methods of preparing present-day *booza* (see below), or its African homologues variously called *tij*, *bojalwa beer*, or *merissa*, but all basically identical preparations.

The basis of all beer production is the fermentation of starch in amylaceous cereals. Grain always contains a small quantity of directly fermentable sugar, but this is inadequate in amount to produce an alcoholic drink. As starch, itself, cannot ferment unless first split into fermentable sugars, it is usually first subjected to malting; i.e. letting grain germinate, a process during which starch is converted into maltose, and considerable amounts of diastase are developed. In modern processes, malt is then heated and dried to stop germination, then boiled with water, strained and incubated with yeast.

In antiquity, however, malt was immediately worked into a dough and processed. In some countries, like China and Japan, starch splitting moulds or other microflora, either deliberately added onto the brewing mash or growing in it spontaneously, are responsible for the production of alcohol from rice or bran. This forms the basis of the modern Amylo method of production of alcohol (Owen, 1933). However, the Egyptians, wittingly or not, relied on malting.

Malt bš (ꜣ)(?)

Several substances drawn in Egyptian tomb paintings have been said to represent malt, a substance with which Sumerians are known to have been familiar. Much discussion has centred in particular around a word, *bš(ꜣ)*, mentioned in the Ebers papyrus (*Eb.*, LXXXIV, 682), and found associated with wheat and dates on steles, on granary labels and especially in the Moscow Mathematical Papyrus (Struve, 1930, p. 59).

In Ti's tomb, the wall facing the entrance of the storeroom is covered with pictures showing the various stages of bread making and brewing, with at their centre, scenes of grain storage and milling (Fig. 12.3). In these scenes, only *bš(ꜣ)* and *zwt* grains, but mainly *bš (ꜣ)*, are mentioned

as sources of beer, while *zwt* is identified in connection with a process
that could well be malting, according to Wild (1966).

Struve, after a lengthy analysis of the Moscow Mathematical
Papyrus, concluded that *bš(ꜣ)* was some kind of grain, a conclusion
with which Gardiner (1947) agreed (*Ancient Egyptian Onomastica*, II, 223).
In some tombs, where this word is found in texts accompanying bread
and beer-making, one such caption discusses "grinding" *bš(ꜣ)*, where
the particular word used for grinding is a term utilized only in relation
to making beer (Wild, 1966).

Another inscription, in Neferhotep's tomb at Thebes (eighteenth
dynasty), indicates the

". . . day of moistening the *bš(ꜣ)* and spreading out the bed of Osiris . . ."

a clear reference to the grain-sprouting Osiris bed mentioned in
Chapter 11 (p. 483). On that account, Nims (1958), who stated that
Helbaek had examined malt from Old Kingdom tombs, suggested that
bš(ꜣ) signified any grain kept or prepared for brewing, and that this
could be malt (Nims, 1950). But an important objection to this view
was raised by Wild (1966) who noted that in Ti's tomb, *bš(ꜣ)* is measured
pounded, cribbled, and then used in bread making, while *zwt* wheat is
subjected to germination.

According to the latter author, *bš(ꜣ)* could be a special quality of
barley. In several tombs of the Old Kingdom, it is being reaped by
harvesters who sing

"Beer for he who reaps *bš(ꜣ)*"

whereas *t-wꜣd* (green bread, erroneously read green grain, *wꜣdt*) could
have been the mass of malt that, in Fig. 12.3 (middle panel, right), a
standing workman is drawing out of a reclining jar while another is
working it up with his hands into a loaf.

The Use of Yeast and Leaven

Whether yeast was known in a pure form is debatable. Grüss (1932)
found material from beer jars, and the residue of mashing from various
periods, to consist of grains of Emmer starch, yeasts, moulds and
bacteria. The yeast consisted of a previously unknown species, and was
accordingly named *Saccharomyces winlocki*, after Winlock who provided

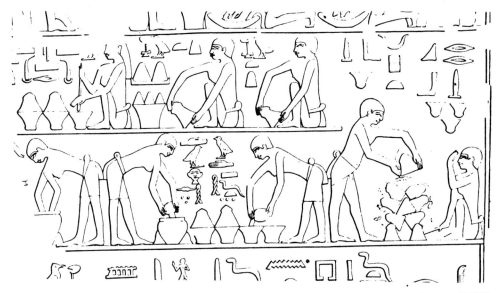

Fig. 13.1. A scene of brewing. See Text. Reproduced from Daumas and Goyon (1939), plate LXVII.

the material. In addition, yeast specimens in eighteenth dynasty finds were sufficiently uniform and pure to suggest that pure yeast could be prepared at that time. In Ptolemaic times, yeast was well-known, and the profession of yeast maker, the *Zymourghos*, is well attested.

In brewing illustrations, Montet (1925, p. 239) was the first to recognize leaven. In his commentary on the scenes in Ti's tomb he noted two workmen pouring something from a small vessel, one into a mould, the other into a differently shaped container (Fig. 13.1 third and fourth from the right). The legend says

"to pour [a word for dough] onto [another word for dough]".

Montet, as well as Vandier (1964, IV, p. 287) concluded that one of the two terms for dough designated leaven (*heza*), and the other ordinary dough. Vandier supported this interpretation by quoting a legend from a mastaba at Giza where a woman kneading tells another worker

"Heat well, for the dough has received *heza*"

and he concluded that, under the Ancient Empire, *heza* must have designated leaven, but that later it came to mean the leavened dough and, finally, just dough.

Grain Use in Brewing

Greek authors nearly all stated that beer in Egypt was made of barley (*Her.*, II, 77; *Deipnos.*, 1, 34; *Diod.*, 1, 3; *Strabo*, 17, 2, 5). An exception is Pliny who merely said that it was made of corn (wheat) (*N.H.*, XIX, XXIX). On that account, the Greeks regarded the drink as unmanly

> "Males, aye, but males well ye find the inhabitants of this land; men whose drink is no barley-brew"

was the King's reply to the herald who announced an Egyptian attack (Aeschylus, *The Supplices*, 953).

Helck, calculating from the daily supplies to the Court as listed in different papyri, and on the assumption that these constituted the basic materials of brewing, found that *bš(ꜣ)*, dates, and wheat were utilized in the proportion 2:2:1 in certain papyri, but that the proportions were different in other texts, one giving a ratio of dates to *bš(ꜣ)* equal to 2 :1 (Helck, 1971).

Grüss's analyses, however, did not confirm the use of barley. As mentioned previously, the brewing residues he examined were uniformly made of Emmer starch. Harris, however, found three specimens from Deir El Medineh to be residues of barley (Lucas, 1962, p. 16), and a pottery vase from Deir El Medineh, filled with barley remnants of beer strainings is kept in the Agricultural Museum at Dokki, Cairo (Fig. 13.2). It is therefore, the more surprising that the scenes in Ti's tomb mention only *zwt* and *bš(ꜣ)*, neither of which are the usual names of wheat or barley.

Production Methods

The actual process, as carried out in the third to fourth centuries A.D. was described in a text ascribed to Zosimos of Panopolis in Upper Egypt. Though this text stems from a late period, and despite the need for a revision of the existing translation (Wild, 1966, p. 99, n. 6), it may provide an idea of earlier techniques (see Montet, 1958, p. 253; Lucas, 1962, p. 14).

In one method, barley was first macerated in water for a day, after which it was spread and well aerated. It was then re-moistened, ground, worked into a dough, and yeast was added. When it was judged that fermentation had proceeded sufficiently, the whole mass was strained through a cloth or a sieve, and the filtrate recovered.

The second method utilized dried bread, soaked in water, and left to ferment in a warm place.

Iconography of Beer

In Ti's tomb, the following manipulations, as interpreted by Wild (1966), may be recognized (Fig. 12.3).

In the lowest register, to the left, grain is being withdrawn from the stores, measured (second man in lower half, as indicated by a legend) and registered (first man in upper half). Two men at the other end of the panel hold pole-like pestles with which they alternately pound grain ($z\dot{h}$) in a mortar. The remaining workmen are composed of groups, each made of a kneeling woman grinding grain on a hollow stone and realistically spilling it onto the floor, facing a squatting companion holding a rounded object that, from the legend, may be identified as a cribble (nk (r) $b\check{s}(\hat{3})$). The grain in all these scenes is $b\check{s}(\hat{3})$.

In the middle register, to the right, grain (called zwt) is moistened by a standing workman plunging his arm in a reclining ovoid jar. Below him, to his right, a kneeling man is kneading into dough a mass of t-$w\hat{3}\underline{d}$ (green bread), possibly malt from the jar above. The third man is working a batter into an oblong loaf called in the legend pzn. The fourth carries to the brewer and to the baker pzn, and loaves of other shapes on a tray. From left to right, moulds are being heated (see Chapter 12: Bread); a worker is pouring a liquid or semi-liquid preparation (? malt) into a jar; and the third is macerating bread, probably with water, into a basket that filters into an earthenware jar. Finally, the uppermost register illustrates addition of a substance called $sgnn$ (possibly an aromat), (see p. 547), supervision by a scribe, brewing, filtering and filling and sealing the jars.

Filtering beer is mentioned in the Ebers papyrus in prescription *Eb.*, LIII, 311 which recommends straining a mixture "as is done for beer"; confirming some of the above interpretation are many models of strainers found in Ancient tombs. An Old Kingdom limestone model of a perforated basket superimposed on a receiving jar is on view at the Dokki Agricultural Museum, Cairo (Fig. 13.3); and two strainers, made of gesso-covered wood, with a central disc of perforated copper, were found in Tut-ankh-Amon's tomb (Fig. 13.4).

To come back to the illustration in Ti's tomb, Wild, comparing this fifth dynasty sequence with similar eighteenth dynasty reliefs, noted no great differences, except in the shape of the loaves and jars, the loaves having become broader and flatter after baking moulds had been replaced by ovens; and the jars being of many different shapes.

As has already been mentioned, two different cereals are used in these operations: $b\check{s}(?)$ to prepare loaves, and *zwt* to obtain malt. The same duality recurs in other tombs, e.g. in those of Sou-em-niwt and Ken-Amon, both of whom lived under Amenophis II (Wild, 1966, p. 15); as it does in the problems of the Moscow Mathematical Papyrus (Gardiner, 1947, *Ancient Egyptian Onomastica*, II, 226).

In Ken-Amon's Tomb, at Thebes, Wild surmised that the whitish flaky material contained in two baskets in one of the illustrations could well represent malt (Fig. 13.5 above, right). One of the baskets is capped by a small pot that could be a measuring vessel. The substance supposed to be malt is withdrawn from an obliquely placed, large-bellied jar that could have been used to germinate grain; and a workman is plunging his hands into it, possibly to mix grain with the loaves that his fellow to the left is breaking into pieces; the mixing is being carried out before or after these have been tramped in a large vat by other workers (Fig. 13.5, person in the middle).

Similar scenes are found in Antefoker's tomb at Thebes, the discussion of which in Chapter 12 stopped at the production of bread. Figure 12.9 shows the continuation of the process into the manufacture of beer. In the flames (upper left), the dough is soon rough-baked. It is taken out, crumbled into water, and left to ferment. The former operation may be shown in the lowest register, where a man stoops over a mass and works it with his hands. The process of fermentation is left to the onlooker's imagination, unless it be represented by a man with his hand in a jar (second from the left) who mutters something about "his lucky day". When it is completed, we see the liquor being pressed out of the mass through a fine sieve into a large jar (second person from the right below). The lees seem to have been tempting, for a child brings his little bowl to the brewer and begs a portion.

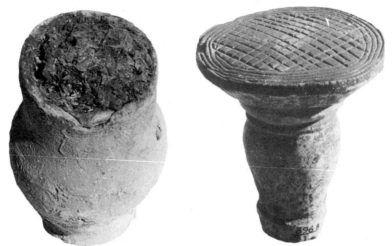

Fig. 13.2. (Left)Pottery vase with remnants of barley strainings. Deir El-Medineh. New Kingdom. Dokki Agricultural Museum, Cairo.
Fig. 13.3. (Right) Limestone model of squeezing mill and vessel for beer production. Old Kingdom. Dokki Museum.

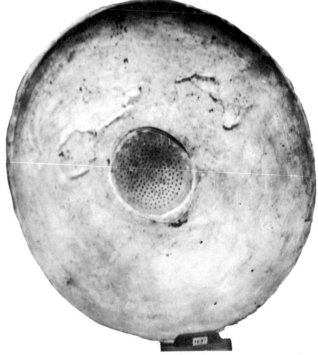

Fig. 13.4. Beer strainer. Gesso-covered wood with, in the centre, a perforated copper disc. Found in the tomb of Tut-ankh-Amon. Cairo Museum.

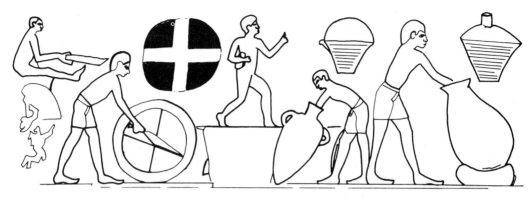

Fig. 13.5. Preparation of bread and beer. Ken Amon's tomb. Middle Kingdom. Thebes. (Davies and Gardiner, 1930.)

"Give me some *seremet*; I am hungry."

(For a different interpretation of the whole scene, see p. 546.)

Many statuettes of the Old Kingdom and models of daily life, likewise illustrate persons performing these operations (Fig. 13.6).

Modern Preparation of Booza

The whole process as illustrated above, and as described by Zosimos, in particular the use of two different cereal preparations, appears very similar to the preparation of booza, a common drink nowadays in Nubia and the Sudan. Booza is also made all over Egypt by Nubians but it is drunk only by the poorer classes. The present-day method of preparation consist first in kneading ground wheat, barley, or other cereal with water and yeast. After a short leavening, this dough is lightly baked into thick loaves. Separately, another fraction of wheat is moistened, exposed to air for some time, crushed, and then added to the previously prepared loaves after they have been crumbled. The fermentation is then promoted by the addition of some old *booza*. No flavouring material and no hops are added. The result is a thick beverage with a strong yeasty odour.

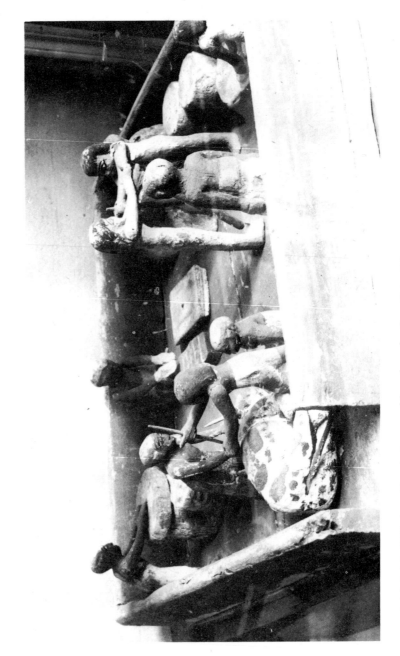

Fig. 13.6. Model of Kitchen. Dough, beer, and bread production, Cairo Museum.

Flavouring Agents

Hops were unknown in Ancient Egypt; in fact, even in England where ale was prepared as early as the third century, they became known only in the fifteenth century when Dutch brewers introduced hopped "beer"; the distinction being that beer was a weaker, but more bitter and less perishable drink than ale.

Graeco-Roman authors seldom mentioned the use of flavouring agents; when they did, the spiced and flavoured beers they described were more like medicated or "processed" beers than genuine "fictitious" beers, to use Pliny's expression in regard to wine (see Chapter 15, p. 613).

Strabo stated simply that

"beer is prepared in a peculiar way among Egyptians." (*Geo.*, 17, 2, 5)

Nor do the medical papyri, which cite at least seventeen varieties of beer, indicate any distinguishing characters that might have reflected either different proportionings of various grains or the addition of different aromats.

The only evidence is a difficult passage of Columella which is usually quoted as indicating that lupine, skirret, and the root of an Assyrian plant (? radish) were added to beer. Other translations, however, merely indicate that these relishes were eaten to arouse thirst

"'Tis time for squirret and the root which, sprung
From seeds Assyrian, is sliced and served
With well-soaked lupines to provoke the thirst
For foaming breakers of Pelusian beer."
(Columella, *On Agriculture and Trees*, X, 114–116)

Egyptian beer was almost certainly, enriched or flavoured with dates. This is attested by several documents: the Moscow Mathematical Papyrus (Struve, 1930) in which dates are the object of interesting calculations, a papyrus in the Louvre (Gardiner, 1947, *Ancient Egyptian Onomastica*, II, pp. 225, 226), a brewing scene in Antefoker's tomb at Thebes where dates are expressly mentioned (Fig. 12.9, bottom of column of hieroglyphs at the extreme right), a bas-relief in the Karlsruhe Museum (Fig. 13.7) and by the common sequence of dates and ceresal in lists of offering ever since the second dynasty (Wild, 1966, p. 99), and of daily supplies to brewers (Megally, 1971, pp. 34 ff.).

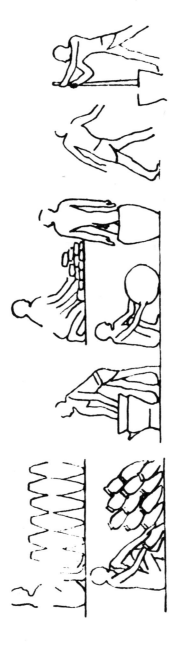

Fig. 13.7. The preparation of date juice to enrich or flavour beer. Redrawn from Wiedemann and Portner (1906), plate VI. See text. The hieroglyphic writings have not been redrawn.

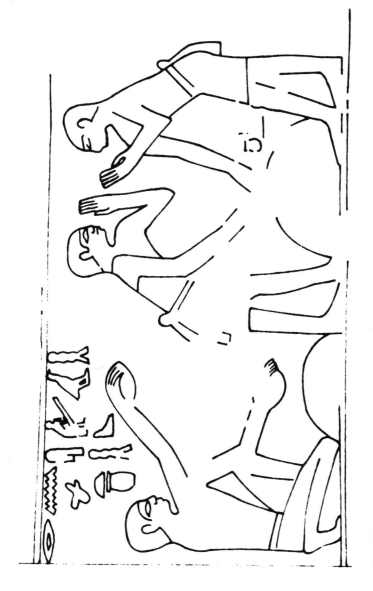

Fig. 13.8. Beating clay to smear the insides of jars of beer. Meir. Redrawn from Blackman (1924), Vol. IV, plate XIII.

In that respect, some brewing scenes described above have received new interpretations. Some see in Antefoker's illustration (Fig. 12.9) the production of date wine (Vandier 1964, IV, pp. 294–295 and 305). Helck (1971) interprets it as a continuation of a process depicted in a bas-relief in the Karlsruhe Museum (Wiedemann and Pörter, 1906, plate VI). In the latter scene, according to Montet (1925, p. 250), dates are first trampled in a large jar, as indicated by a legend that he read '*hm3bnr in* "to trample the dates by . . ." (Fig. 13.7 extreme right) The resulting mass is then cleaned by a woman who picks out the stones (legend: "to clean the dates; the servant"). A man works the mass into small balls which another man puts into a large vessel.

In Helck's opinion (1971) the man who, in Antefoker's tomb (Fig. 12.9) forms a heap, is saying

"The dates from the old granary are now here. I can now make something good out of them."

Vandier (1964, IV, p. 295) translates this legend differently

"These dates, that come out of the granary, are very old. If only I could see them all out, this would be a happy thing to me"

and he comments that this part of the scene is not always connected with brewing, which deprives it of a great part of its value.

According to Helck again, the heap is a date cake (possibly similar to today's '*agwa*?) that is then sieved into a large jar; the *srm.t* that the young boy is begging is a piece of that cake (see p. 541); and the *sgnn* poured at the extreme left into the basketwork container is date juice made from *srm.t*.

The whole interpretation rests on the correct reading of the word read *bnr* by Montet, and on the translation of *srm.t* and *sgnn*.

Undoubtedly *bnr* is correctly read in Antefoker's tomb, but Wild (1966) entertained some doubt as to the reading of this word in the Karlsruhe relief. He suggested two alternatives that seemed to him more plausible, either "the sweet servant" (*bnr* meaning both sweet and dates), or the girl's name, since the names of the other workers are written beside them.

The *srm.t* which the boy is begging, is translated by Faulkner (*F.*, 236) as a food and a beverage. Petrie (Tell el Amarna, 1894, p. 34) recorded the expression "good *srm.t* of the Queen" and stated that its equivalent in Coptic means wine lees. In the papyrus Anastasi (Caminos, 1954, p. 81) the expression "sweet *srm.t* brew of Great of Victories" suggests that it was a sweet beverage or juice. Wallert (1962, p. 30) interpreted the whole scene as showing the production of date wine and translated it *Gegorenes*, something fermented.

As to *sgnn*, this was, since the New Kingdom, the name of an oil or of a scent, a meaning that it kept in Coptic (*Wb.*, IV, 322, 333). But Montet (1925, p. 250) and Helck (1971) are of the opinion that it was prepared from dates.

That dates were utilized in brewing is, indeed, supported by many documents that enumerate the large quantities delivered to brewers, like the accounting papyrus *E.* 3226 of the Louvre (Megally, 1971, pp. 34 ff.), but their use in quantities equalling or exceeding the cereals (see p. 537) indicates that they constituted, not an aromat, but a source of additional sugar to enhance fermentation, as in the modern practice of adding sugar to many beers.

Treatment of Jars Before Bottling

In numerous scenes, a man is depicted with his arms plunged deep into a jar, to introduce a product called in the legends *sin*, clay (Wb., IV, 37–38). This is made clearer in a tomb at Meir (Fig. 13.8) (Blackman, 1924, IV, plate XIII) where a legend says of a seated workman holding something above an undefined heap lying in front of him "beats *sin* for the jars". It has been concluded that the jars, before being filled, had their inner surfaces smeared with clay to ensure their impermeability and possibly to clarify the fermented product.

The resultant brews were certainly different from modern beers, which have been improved by important developments that removed the element of chance and permitted the consistent production of a beer with constant characteristics. Among these were the isolation of a pure strain of yeast by German brewers in the nineteenth century; mechanization; the use of steam for heating; pasteurization; and refrigeration. Many of the beers of the Ancients probably resembled those produced at home today widely throughout Africa south of the Sahara.

Other Uses of Beer

Cooking

Beer seems to have been considered a household and kitchen necessity rather than a superfluous luxury. Theophrastus (4, 8, 12) wrote that *malinathalle* was boiled in beer to make it sweet and edible. But by far the greatest consumption of beer was for the pleasure and good humour it imparted. Hence, "to make a beer hall" or to sit in the beer hall", used in common parlance for "to carouse, to have a jolly time" (*A.R.*, IV, 451, 880).

Medical Uses of Beer

The discussion of the medical uses of beer covers twelve pages of von Deines and Grapow's Wörterbuch der Drogennamen (1959, pp. 372–383). Like wine, but more often, it was used as a constituent of mixtures (*Eb.*, LIII, 312, *Eb.*, XXXII, 150, etc.), as an after-drink (*Eb.*, XVIII, 60; LII, 302), or as an aid to dispensing (*Eb.*, II, 4; XIX, 63). But although its mild sedative or euphoric action was recognized, there are reasons to believe that in all these prescriptions it was utilized as a vehicle or base. These reasons are the large amounts in which it is prescribed, or its prescription without any indication of dosage; its usual mention at the end of the prescription or, less commonly, at the very beginning; and its frequent occurrence in the part of the prescription connected with dispensing or preparation.

In many cases, "sweet" beer is specified. But von Deines and Grapow point to the frequent interchangeability of "beer" and "sweet beer" in alternative or repetitious prescriptions, e.g. *Eb.*, III, 9 (*ḥḳt*, beer) that is repeated verbatim in *Eb.*, IV, 14 (*ḥḳt ndmt*, sweet beer).

Beer was also included in medicines to be chewed, e.g. (*Eb.*, LXXXIX, 745); "to treat the gums with rinsing of the mouth": bran (?) sweet beer (?) chewed and spat out; or "to strengthen the gums and treat the gums"; celery, sweet beer, chewed and spat out (*Eb.*, LXXXIX, 749). It was injected in enemata (*Eb.*, XLIX, 265), or in vaginal douches (*Eb.*, XCVI, 830); it formed part of anal fumigations to treat diseases of the anus (*H.*, 7) and of dressings (*Eb.*, XXX, 130; LXXVII, 605; LXXXV, 690).

In addition, unidentified "parts" of beer, or lees, were used; nearly always internally (e.g. *Eb.*, XCIV, 794); except in two cases "marsh-water, pignon (?), *i'jt* of beer; leaves of cucumber, fresh dates . . ." (*Eb.*, XLIX, 271), and "(?) boiled with *hrwt* of beer (*Eb.*, LXXII, 548).

A further discussion of the official use of beer will be found in the section dealing with the medicinal uses of wine.

Importation of Beer

There was no need to import beer as it was available to the smallest purses, in the most modest households; and cereal was everywhere abundant. Nevertheless, the papyrus Anastasi contains two references to an imported *Kedi* beer. In the first, an officer, complaining of his having nothing to do on a frontier post where he is supposed to erect buildings instead of marching to meet the enemy, writes

> "If ever one openeth a bottle, it is full of beer of Kedi." (Erman, 1966, p. 204)

The second sings the praise of the amenities of the "House of Rameses", the newly founded residence of Rameses II which lay on the site of the later Pelusium

> "The draughts of Great of Victories are sweet . . . beer of Kedi from the port, and wine from the vineyard." (Erman, 1966, 207)

Apparently, this was a well-known beer since a letter quoted by Lutz (1922, p. 83) describes a thirst that empties the Kedi countries.

This is striking, in view of what must have been an enormous local production.

Beer and the Authorities

Several important officials had to deal with the administrative and financial problems raised by this imported product. One thus hears of an "Inspector of the Brewery" and of a "Royal Chief Beer Inspector", both titles implying the existence of many more subordinate employees.

About taxation in Pharaonic Egypt we know little, but under the Ptolemies and the Romans, beer was subjected to producer taxes paid in copper (see also Hunt, *S.P.*, 2, 395, n.A.).

Chapter 14   Wine (Part I)

Mythological Beginnings of Wine (a)*

(a)

irp

"... and the discovery of the vine, they say, was made by him Dionysus near Nysa, and that, having further devised the proper treatment of its fruit, he was the first to drink wine and taught mankind at large the culture of the vine and the use of wine, as well as the way to harvest the grape and to store the wine . . ." (*Diod.*, 1, 15, 8)

A recurrent difficulty in the retrieval of the past is the intertwining of myth, tradition and fact in a manner seldom easy to unravel. Most of our knowledge of the ancient origins of vine growing and of wine production in Egypt represents Greek and Roman interpretative thought rather than true Egyptian mythology or history. Indeed, botanists are not certain where the vine (*Vitis vinifera*) originated, though some believe that this was in southern Russia in the mountainous vicinity of the Black and Caspian Seas (Candolle, 1886, pp. 191–194). The Biblical account of Noah (Genesis, 8, 4) situates the point where the ark came to rest not far from that region, on the mountains of Ararat, traditionally located in eastern Turkey (formerly Armenia). It was presumably there that

"... Noah began to be an husbandman, and he planted a vineyard: and he drank of the wine, and was drunken; and he was uncovered within his tent . . ." (Genesis, 9, 20–21)

It is known, however, that by historic times (*c.* 3200 B.C. in Egypt) the vine was widely distributed throughout the Middle East and the eastern Mediterranean areas; and the hieroglyph of the wine-press (b) and its variants, which are attested as early as the Pyramid Age in the name of *šmu*

(b)

"the god of the Wine, of the oil-press and of cellars" (*Wb.*, IV, 537)

offer additional evidence that wine was already produced at that time.
  Greek and Roman mythology, however, are far from agreeing on

*In Ptolemaic times *sha*.

the district of original vine cultivation. As has been seen, Diodorus placed it near Nysa, the name of various sites in the Ancient World; on the Greek island of Euboea, in Aethiopia (*Her.*, II, 146), or in Asia (Barguet, 1964, p. 1395).

Nevertheless, there are many other conflicting statements. Hecateus of Miletus wrote that the vine was discovered in Aetolia (*Deipnos.*, 2, 35, A); Theopompus of Chios related on one occasion that it was discovered at Olympia along the banks of the Alpheius River (*Deipnos.*, 1, 34, A); and, on another, he could not differ from the claim that the vine had been discovered on his own island (*Deipnos.*, 1, 26, B). Philonides of Athens listed the Red Sea region as a possible origin (*Deipnos.*, 15, 675, A); while Achilles Tatius (2, 2, 2–6) located it in the vicinity of Tyre in Phoenicia. Our interest, however, is specially drawn to an account by Hellanicus of Mytilene, who wrote that the vine was discovered first in the city of Plinthine in Egypt (*Deipnos.*, 1, 34, A–B). Cosson (1935, pp. 108–109) places Plinthine 4·5 kilometers east of Taposiris, on the northern coast of Egypt, i.e., approximately 15 miles west of Alexandria. But, though this site has not been located with absolute certainty, the reference moves one to investigate more thoroughly the mythologic history of the vine and wine in Egypt.

Moreover, the possibility of a southern route of introduction of the vine into the Nile Valley cannot be ignored. Grapes have been encountered in Nubia and Central Africa by several explorers. Burckhardt (1822, p. 133), commenting on the general sparsity of fruit there, noted

"Except for date trees and a few grapes there are no fruit trees in Nubia."

Schweinfurth (1873a, Vol. II, pp. 234, 235) found wild vine loaded with ripe clusters on which he could refresh himself on his way from Marra to Gumango.

It is, therefore, the more to be regretted that excavation in the vicinity of the Nile in Nubia has become impossible now that these localities have been submerged by the waters of the High Aswan dam.

The main leitmotiv of Egyptian mythology centred round Osiris as the good and benevolent god who taught his people agriculture, and the production of grain and grapes. Much later, Greek tradition equated him with Dionysus, and asserted that the rather uninhibited festivities of Dionysus worship, the Dionysia or Bacchanalia, had been introduced into Greece by the Egyptian king Danaus, who, with his fifty daughters, had fled his twin brother, Aegyptos, and settled in the Argive region of the Peloponnesus.

The inconsistent Herodotus wrote that the Egyptians had no vines in their country (II, 77); although, in other passages, he mentioned several instances of wine drinking (II, 60, 121, 133, 168) and considered Osiris to be Dionysus (II, 42, 144).

Plutarch (*I. and O.*, 353, 6) likewise ignored these traditional beliefs when he wrote

". . . before the reign of King Psammetichus, they [the Egyptians] did not drink wine nor use it in libations as something dear to the gods, thinking it to be the blood of those who had once battled against the gods, and from whom, when they had fallen and become commingled with the earth, they believed vines to have sprung."

Without stopping to comment on the identification of wine with blood and on its possible relevance to the tale of "The Destruction of Mankind" where beer was dyed red to mimic blood (pp. 125, 533), or to the ritual transformation of wine into blood in certain modern religions,[1] one is struck by the frequency of this comparison in folkloric traditions

". . . Where did you get this purple water, my friend? Wherever did you find blood so sweet . . ." (Achilles Tatius, 2, 2, 4–5)

Plutarch (*I. and O.*, 353, 6) even believed that this relation was the cause of the intoxicating properties of wine

". . . this is the reason why drunkenness drives men out of their senses and crazes them, inasmuch as they are then filled with the blood of their forbears . . ."

The statements of Herodotus and Plutarch as to Egyptian ignorance of wine are, however, some of those blatant mistakes of Greek authors which remain incomprehensible. Unless Plutarch meant only that wine was not used in religious ceremonies, and unless Herodotus thought that all wine in Egypt was imported, one is led by such statements to doubt wholesale the reliability of these two "historians".

Had Psammetik been one of the early kings of Egypt, Plutarch's report would have been credible. Psammetik, however, ruled approximately twenty-five centuries after the first appearance of the wine-press as a hieroglyph and the introduction of Osirian beliefs into Egyptian religious thought. Plutarch apparently used as his authority the Greek traveller and historian, Eudoxus of Cnidus (not to be confused with Eudoxus of Cyzicus who failed in his attempted circumnavigation of Africa, *c.* 130 B.C.). This Eudoxus is known to have lived in Egypt during the Late Dynastic Period *c*. 366 B.C., and he must have realized that wine in Egypt had a history longer than a mere 300 years.

This was true also of Plutarch 400 years after Eudoxus: for, even if he were not cognizant of Manetho's *History of Egypt*, his Greek and Roman sources must have told him that it had been in production in Egypt long before Psammetik. A legend had developed, however, that connected Psammetik with wine, possibly based on a pun on the name of Psammetik (*Pa-s-n-mtk*) that could have meant "the man of the diluted wine" *mtk* being variously translated "a beverage" or "diluted wine." According to Herodotus (II, 151) an oracle had prophesied that the next king of Egypt would be the one to offer a libation to the god of Memphis in a bronze vessel, although golden goblets were always used for that purpose. It then happened that, on one of the god's festivals, twelve contenders attended to pay their homage, but that the priest miscounted them and prepared only eleven goblets. When the turn of the last in line came, this prince, finding himself denied the honour of offering his libation, spontaneously offered his bronze helmet and thus fulfilled the prophecy of the oracle.

Diodorus (1, 66, 7–10) dismissed this story as a fabrication of Herodotus. He believed Psammetik to have been a merchant who aroused the envy of the eleven other princes by acquiring near the sea large tracks of land that enabled him to carry on extensive trade with Phoenicia and Greece and, thereby, amass great riches.

Speaking of Psammetik as a "man-of mixed drinks", a Greek legend concerning the origin of "mixing" wine,[2] which was recorded by Philonides of Athens in his *On Perfumes and Wreaths*, has fortunately been preserved by Athenaeus (15, 675, A–C)

> ". . . after the vine had been brought by Dionysus from the Red Sea into Greece, most men perversely turned to unmeasured enjoyment of it, and drank it unmixed; some in their insane perversity became delirious, others became like corpses in their stupour. But, once upon a time, when some men were drinking at the sea-shore, a rain-storm fell upon them and broke up the party, but filled up the bowl, which still had a little wine left in it. After the weather cleared they returned to the same place and tasting the mixture of wine and water, they found pleasant and painless enjoyment. For this reason, when the unmixed wine is poured during the dinner, the Greeks call upon the name of the Good Divinity, doing honour to the Divinity who discovered the vine . . ."[3]

In Greece, the discovery of wine was at first credited to Dionysus, son of Zeus by Semele, the daughter of Cadmus, but, after the innocent era of mythologic credulity, there came sceptics who sought more rational explanations of the association of Dionysus with wine and asserted that

> "there was never any birth of him in human form whatsoever, and the word Dionysus means only 'the gift of the wine'." (*Diod.*, 3, 62, 2–3)

But mythological tales need not be "sacred monsters", intangible in the dusky imagination of their inventors. There still live many heirs to these fabulous creations of the human mind. Dionysus had companions,

> ". . . men who were experienced in agriculture, such as Maron in the cultivation of the vine." (*Diod.*, 1, 18, 2)

Maron died in Egypt while travelling with Osiris/Dionysus, and the region near his burial was fertile in vine. How many travellers on the desert highway between Cairo and Alexandria have but glanced at the dusty mounds that surround the modern settlement of Mariut, and given a thought to Maron who is said to survive in the Arabic name that has replaced the earlier *Marea*, and the still earlier Egyptian *Pa-mer*, although Cosson (1935, p. 68) doubts this derivation.

More fascinating is the shimmering lake of the same name[4] whose silver face mirrors the ever changing sky and the two low ridges that protect its sleeping beauty. There, one almost hears the poet whisper

> "Phantoms of sound: of ripple, voice, and bell
> But mirage marks the lake, dry troughs, the well
> Great wind-worn stones and pot-sherds mark man's hand"
>
> (quoted by Cosson, 1935, p. 195)

Excellent wines are still produced from the rich vines of the region, renewing a noble tradition which dates back thousands of years, and many villagers feel confident that old Maron's soul is indeed pleased with the Egyptian beverage they produce today.

History and Production Techniques

As early as the first dynasty, written records distinctly specified wine and associated it with Horus. The first Pharaoh of that dynasty, Den (or Udimu) called his vineyard "The Enclosure of the Beverage of the Body of Horus". Khasekhemui, last king of the second dynasty named his "Praised be the Souls of Horus". Zoser (third dynasty) called it

"Praised Horus who is in the Front of Heaven", and we read in the biography of Methen, a noble of that period (*c.* 2723 B.C.)

"Very plentiful trees and vines were set out, a great quantity of wine was made there in." (*A.R.*, I, 173)

Further excavations may even unearth texts and other evidence from earlier periods, an expectation fully justified by the numerous finds in tombs of the first two dynasties, like the discovery by Emery (1962) of sealed jars of wine . . . (long evaporated) among the remains of a meal in a second dynasty tomb, and the obvious familiarity of first dynasty scribes with the sign of the "wine-press".

Tomb illustrations add to this evidence another dimension. Most illuminating are the Old Kingdom tombs at Saqqara and Giza that show the stammerings of the wine-production industry at its beginning; while the Middle and New Kingdom paintings, through their use of colour, pulsate with an uncanny vitality.

Representations of vineyards usually show vines growing on trellises (Fig. 14.1); but they are occasionally depicted as short stubby bushes, as described by Pliny (XVII, XXXV, 185)

". . . the greater part of the world lets its vintage grapes lie on the ground inasmuch as this custom prevails both in Africa and in Egypt and in Syria."

Lutz (1922, p. 51), from an examination of the many coloured tomb paintings, concluded that there grew grapes with a colour spectrum ranging from white through pink, green, red and blue.[5] But a conclusion based solely on the colours used in paintings does not take account of other factors, like the availability of pigments at different times or localities, or the conventions and set canons that traditionally dictated their use, and ordered for example, painting men a brown-red and women a light yellow.

Lutz, himself, was not expressly firm on this point. He wrote

". . . whenever the grapes are painted black as, for instance, in the tomb of Sennofri at Thebes, blue or dark blue is naturally intended"

and he added, that Egyptians, as all Orientals, have difficulty in distinguishing between these two colours (1922, p. 51). One wonders where he obtained his unfounded information.

Along with this lack of certainty in the evaluation of the colour of grapes, a similar uncertainty exists as to the colour of wines. Lucas (1962, p. 18) wrote that there are no known dynastic literary records which indicate the colour of Egyptian wines, and Ricci (1924, p. 61) stated that wine colour is not discussed in the known Greek and Roman papyri found in Egypt. In point of fact, an early inscription does mention '*irp dšr*, red wine; but, as we shall see later, the word *dšr*, admits of other interpretations.

It may be argued also that New Kingdom paintings vividly show a dark red juice pouring out of the treading vats. Such representations, however, need not be true to life, since the juice even of purple grapes is usually colourless. But as the colour of red wine is derived from the grape skins from which it is extracted by the alcohol produced by fermentation, the yield of the treading vat may be coloured if fermentation has sufficiently proceeded during the early stages, which is quite possible in hot weather.

The first mention of colour as colour is the second to third century A.D. appraisal of Mareotic wines by Athaeneus

". . . the vine is abundant in this region and its grapes are very good to eat. The wine made from them is excellent; it is white and pleasant, fragrant, easily assimilated, thin, does not go to the head, and is diuretic." (*Deipnos.*, 7, 33, D–E)

One would conclude that both white and red wines were made in Egypt, although archaeological information is not conclusive.

Montet (1958, p. 106) wrote that grapes were individually picked, but many authors consider the illustrations quoted by Montet as simplified sketches of a difficult subject, for picking grapes, grape by grape, would be very time-consuming[5]; although this might be practised for some high quality wines like the best French vintages at present.

The harvested grapes were transferred in baskets to the treading vats, of which no specimen has survived, although they are abundantly illustrated. The fact that no vat has been found indicates that no religious meaning was attached to them, in spite of the Osirian connections of wine. It has also raised the possibility that they were temporary constructions of wood, and Lutz (1922, p. 53) has specified that they were made of acacia wood, without indicating how he arrived at this conclusion.

Montet (1958, p. 106) believed, however, that they were made of soft hewn stone, although in that case one might have anticipated finding hewn objects that matched the illustrations, especially when one considers the amount of wine produced throughout Egyptian history by some vineyards, like the one reported by Posener that, about 1200 B.C.,

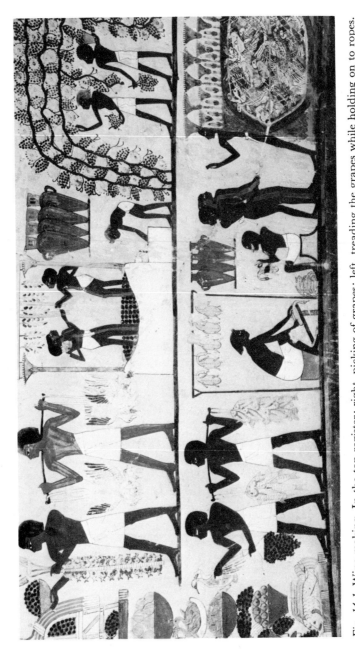

Fig. 14.1. Wine making. In the top register: right, picking of grapes; left, treading the grapes while holding on to ropes. The juice is seen to run out through a spout into a container. Tomb of Nakht. Thebes. New Kingdom.

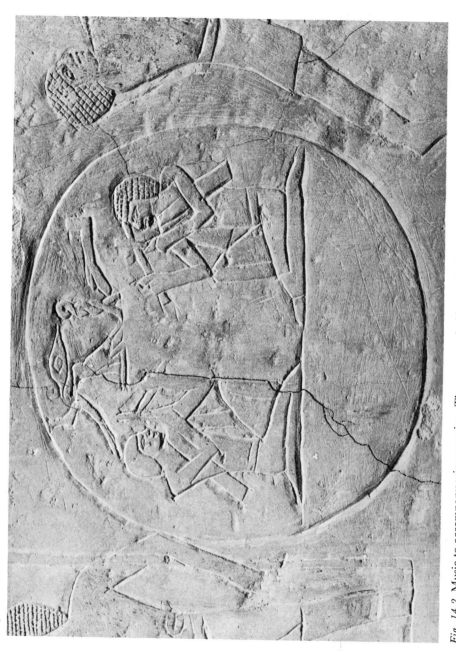

Fig. 14.2. Music to accompany wine-pressing. The two men inside the circle are keeping rhythm with sticks. Fig. 14.5 is a continuation of this relief. Mereruka's Tomb. Saqqara. Old Kingdom. Photographed 1969.

delivered in one year 1200 jars of good wine, and 50 of medium quality (Posener, 1962, p. 300).

The grapes were then squeezed by treading, as is still done in some small wineries in Europe. In some illustrations, the treaders are shown maintaining their balance while treading the slippery must by holding onto ropes hanging from the ceiling or from a cross-beam that forms a frame with two vertical poles attached at each end of the vat (Fig. 14.1). In others, the treaders take support on each other's hips, the first and last of the row leaning on two sticks outside the vat. The treaders then went merrily round and round accompanied by music and the clapping of the onlookers. Regarding the treading method of pressing grapes, it has been commented that, because it does not crush the skins and seeds, it is less likely than the modern mechanical press to release undesirable astringent matter.

In Greek times, the hiring of workmen and musicians was a business of middlemen. A contract dated A.D. 322 is informative on this point

> "I acknowledge that I have contracted and agreed with you the landlord to present myself at the vintage of the vineyards which are there, along with the appointed grape treaders, and without fault assist the grape treaders and the other workers by my flute playing, and not leave the grape treaders until the completion of the vintage." (*S.P.*, I, 22)

This may be the subject of an enigmatic relief in the tomb of Mereruka (Fig. 14.2) showing seated figures holding sticks, possibly performing some rhythmic beat by which the treaders could keep time or chant.

After treading, the lees were transferred to a cloth bag for further squeezing. In one technique, one end of the bag was tied to a fixed support, and the other end was fixed to a pole which was twisted by several men (Fig. 14.3). In another, both ends of the bag were tied to poles, and two groups of workmen wrung the bag by turning the poles in opposite directions (Figs 14.4 and 14.5). In between the two groups, a fellow was busy with hands and feet keeping the poles apart. The artist, no doubt a humorist, often added a note of his own. A huge baboon played the latter's role (Moussa and Altenmüller, 1971, Fig. 14.6). It is typical of rural conservatism that a similar technique utilizing cloth bags was observed in the nineteenth century by members of the Bonaparte scientific staff (Girard, 1813, p. 608).

We do not know whether the products of treading and of squeezing were mixed, or whether they were allowed to ferment separately producing wines of different qualities, the second carrying with it colouring and other matter from the grains, seeds and stalks.

Lutz (1922, p. 56) made the interesting observation that tombs thus far excavated in and south of Thebes show neither of the techniques of secondary extraction discussed above. These are depicted only in tombs to the north of the Theban necropolis. He prudently draws no conclusions. Further excavations may indeed reveal such scenes, although their absence hitherto allows speculation as to the quality of Thebaid wines.

The expressed juice was then strained through cloth into fermentation jars. In some cases, the process was quickened by warming; and when it was over, the product was decanted or siphoned (Fig. 14.7) into containers, small and circular for religious or funerary use, larger for domestic consumption.

Some archaeologists believe that the inside of the jars was coated with an impermeable substance, either "bitumen" or "resin" (Lutz, 1922, pp. 56–57), and have interpreted some illustrations as depicting this process. But the size of the wine jars, the enormous amount of wine produced, coupled with the lack of adequate local supplies of either bitumen or resin, have thrown doubt on the "coating". Montet (1958, p. 88) arrived at this negative conclusion from the description of Egyptian wine as "very sweet," "tends to spoil early" (Strabo, 17, 1, 35), in contrast to the heavily resinated Greek wines that were said to withstand better the acidic change because of the coating. Lucas (1962, p. 20), confirmed this conclusion for, in the large number of wine jars of all epochs that he examined, he found no evidence of coating before the Greek Period. This is not surprising, for their extensive forests provided the Greeks with the pitch necessary for this procedure, whereas Egypt was not blessed with any such reserves. (For coating beer jars see p. 547 and Fig. 13.8.)

Finally, when fermentation was over, the wine vessels were sealed with opercula of straw and clay (Fig. 14.8), in which were impressed the official stamps, with the year of the king's rule, the district, the name of the wine and, sometimes, the name of the gardener (Kees, 1961, p. 82).

In many of the jars, safety holes were drilled either in the stopper caps or in the necks, to prevent bursting by accumulation of gases. These were plugged with straw or wax (Lucas, 1962, p. 19), or with a plug of clay stamped with the owner's seal (Fig. 14.9).

At some stage in the final processing, wine was tasted and its quality

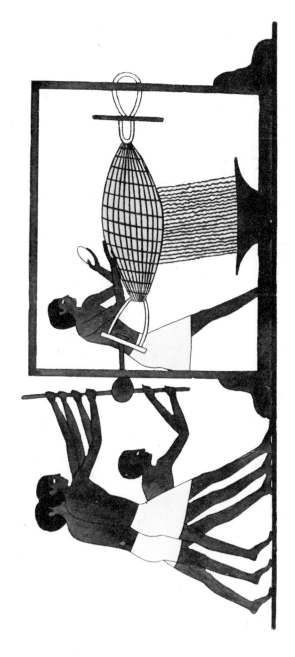

Fig. 14.3. Expressing the juice of grapes in a bag tied at one end, and twisted at the other. Beni Hassan. Reproduced from Caillaud (1831), plate 5A. Darby collection.

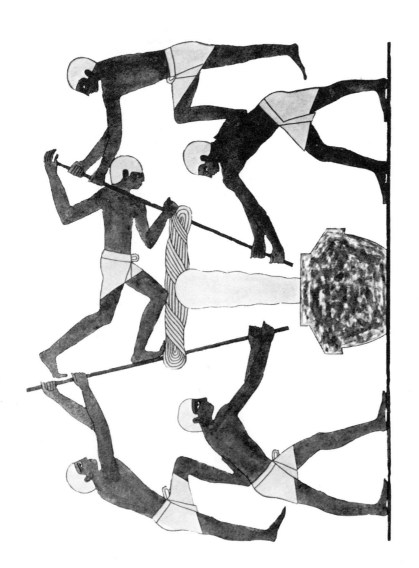

Fig. 14.4. Pressing grapes in a bag twisted at both ends by means of poles. After Caillaud (1831), Darby collection

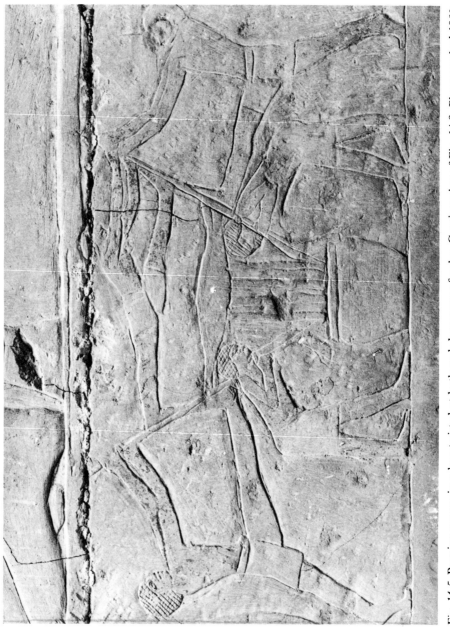

Fig. 14.5. Pressing grapes in a bag twisted at both ends by means of poles. Continuation of Fig. 14.2. Photographed 1969. Mereruka's tomb. Saqqara. Old Kingdom.

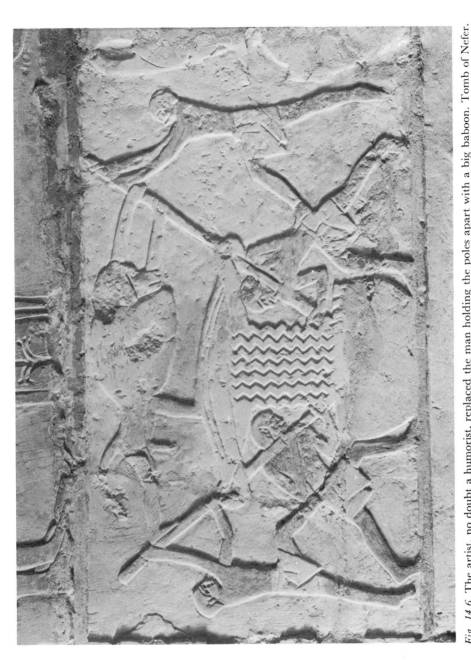

Fig. 14.6. The artist, no doubt a humorist, replaced the man holding the poles apart with a big baboon. Tomb of Nefer. Saqqara. Old Kingdom. Photographed 1969. Courtesy of Dr R. Stadelman, Director of the German Institute of Archaeology. Cairo.

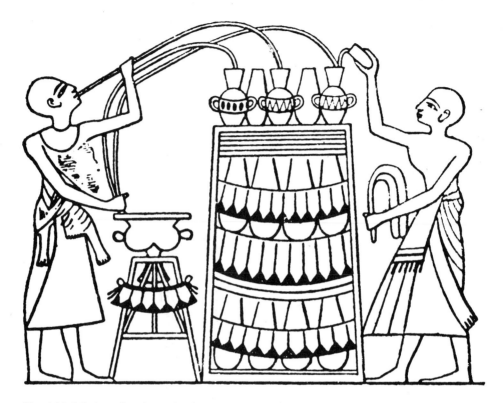

Fig. 14.7. Mixing wines by syphoning them into a cup. The elaborate decoration of the stand suggests that the mixing was carried out in a banquet hall. Reproduced from Erman and Ranke (1952), Fig. 74.

assessed. In Antef's tomb at Thebes (Fig. 14.10), a naked girl wearing only a string of pearls round her loins is standing in front of an aged supervisor and says

"Take this and drink to the health of the herald Antef."

The pictures of the cup that she presumably presented, the flask from which she filled it, and the cup that the supervisor probably raised to his lips have perished, but the old man's answer is still legible

"How sweet is this wine. To the *ka* of the herald Antef as a gift of *Rnwt.t*[6]

(Save-Söderbergh, 1957, plate XV and p. 18).

The grade was then indicated on the lids, classing the vintage in its proper category, good, twice good, three times good,[7] sweet and so forth.

An interesting painting from the tomb of Amenemhat, the Theban architect who served Amenophis III (1405–1367 B.C.), shows a servant "fanning" a rack of wine jars, perhaps cooling them by evaporation. If this interpretation be correct, it supports the view that the jars were not internally coated.

Blending of wines is suggested by a drawing showing a servant siphoning wine into a cup from three different jars (Fig. 14.7). As the mixed product is not run into a storage jar, it is to be presumed that in this case blending was carried out according to taste just before drinking, and that no brands of blended wines were on sale.

A contract dated to the Roman Period, A.D. 208, sheds a side light on these final stages of wine production

> ". . . and further we agree to assist you in the vineyard and we will perform the testing of the jars intended for the wine, and will put these, when they have been filled with wine in the open-air shed, and plaster them, and move the wine, and strain it from one jar into another . . ." (*S.P.*, I, No. 18)

The same papyrus likewise tells that the workers were paid well in silver and in wheat; and that they were allowed four jars of wine daily from the vat for their own pleasure.

Most wines were consumed locally, although we shall meet with evidence that wines of quality were transported. Little is known concerning transport of this fragile merchandise, but tomb reliefs depict the movement of huge wine jars on sleds, with workmen pouring liquid in front of the skids to reduce friction, as well as their storage in cellars. One of these illustrations (Fig. 2.5) recorded an amusing dialogue which we quoted in Chapter 2.

In the temple of Khnum at Esna, an inscription dated to Ptolemaic times indicates where the wine was stored

> "This is the place of wine and wine jugs when one gets drunk. Happiness is in it, joy of heart comes out of it. The products of Buto of Arabia, of the oasis of Farafra [*Ḥt-sha-Ḥor*] as well as the country of *Knm* [? Dakhla] and all the products of *Dsḏs* [Bahariya] brought as taxes to this pleasant chapel." (Sauneron, 1959–1969, Vol. II, No. 124, p. 2)

Thus was the annual promise of Osiris/Dionysus continuously fulfilled.

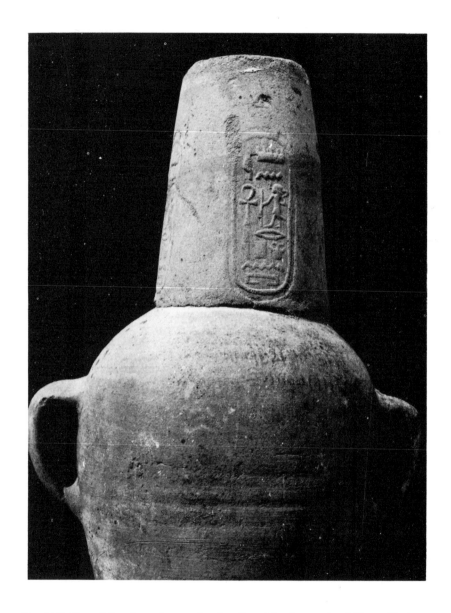

Fig. 14.8. One of the three dozen wine jars found in the tomb of Tut-ankh-Amon. The lid bears the stamp of the Pharaoh. Cairo Museum.

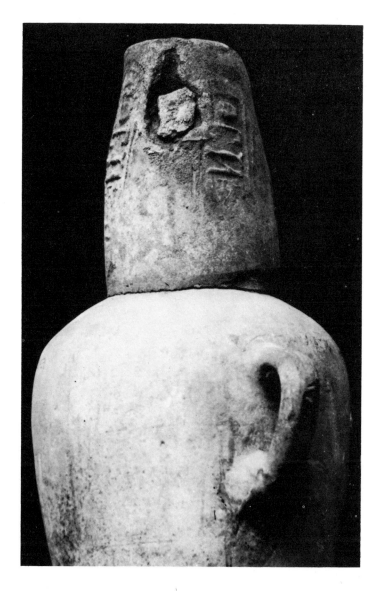

Fig. 14.9. One of the wine jars found in the tomb of Tut-ankh-Amon. Note the seal of the pharaoh imprinted on the lid, and the safety opening, made in the lid to allow gases out, later closed with a plug of clay. Cairo Museum.

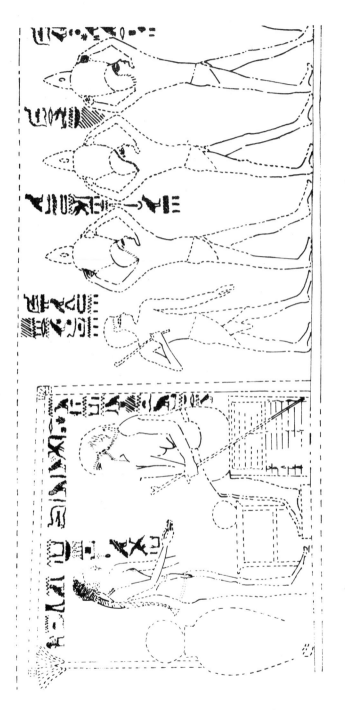

Fig. 14.10. A naked girl presents to an elderly man what is presumed to have been a cup of wine, saying: "take this and drink to the health of the herald Antef". The elderly man answers: "how sweet is this wine". Tomb of Antef. Thebes. Redrawn from Save-Söderbergh (1957), plate XV.

Religious Use of Wine

Festivities

"There are two liquids that are specially agreeable to the human body, wine inside, and oil outside." (*N.H.*, XIV, XXIX, 150)

The ritual use of intoxicating drinks and the theological significance of the euphoria and disordered behaviour induced by them were discussed in the section on beer (Chapter 13, pp. 529–537). People drank also much wine during these festivities; at Busiris,[8] Sais, Buto, Heliopolis, Papremis (near Saïs), and especially at Bubastis[9] where Herodotus, by his vivid description (II, 60), seems to have been an eye-witness

"Men and women come sailing all together, vast numbers in each boat, many of the women with castanets, which they strike, while some of the men pipe during the whole time of the voyage; the remainder of the voyagers, male and female, sing the while, and make clappings with their hands. When they arrive opposite any of the towns upon the banks of the stream, they approach the shore, and, while some of the women continue to play and sing, others call aloud to the females of the place and load them with abuse, while a certain number dance, and some standing up uncover themselves [see Fig. 14.11]. After proceeding in this way all along the river-course, they reach Bubastis, where they celebrate the feast with abundant sacrifices. More grape-wine is consumed at this festival than in all the rest of the year besides. The number of those who attend, counting only the men and women and omitting the children, amounts, according to the native reports, to seven hundred thousand."[10]

If the remarks of Herodotus are true, there must have been an abundance of cheap wine. The most impressive description to survive from antiquity relative to wine and festivities in Egypt was recorded, however, by Athenaeus, the Graeco-Egyptian from Naucratis, who wrote during the Roman Period. He described the magnificent spectacle celebrated in honour of the god Dionysus at the stadium of Alexandria. The date of this celebration cannot be fixed with certainty; but it occurred during the reign of King Ptolemy Philadelphus and cannot, therefore, be considered purely Egyptian. The following extracts from this very lengthy passage in which Athenaeus melted his memories with

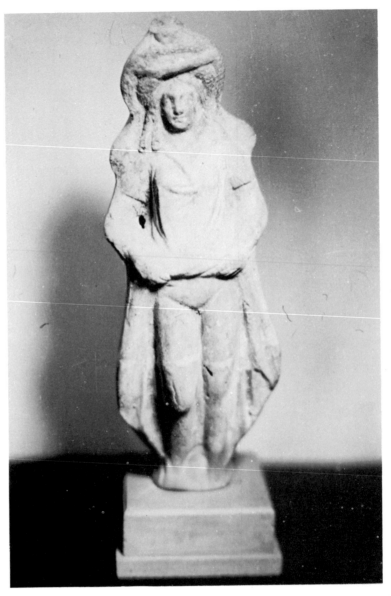

Fig. 14.11. Terracotta statue of a woman raising her "chiton". Such statues, placed in tombs, are sometimes called "concubines of the dead". They may, however, illustrate the ritual custom, attested by Diodorus (I., 85) of women stripping themselves in front of the new Apis during the forty days that follow its discovery, or the gesture of women baring themselves, standing on barges, during the Bubastis festivals (*Her.*, II, 60). Personal collection of the authors.

those of the lost text of Callixeinus of Rhodes, illustrate the exorbitant riches, pageantry and luxury displayed on this occasion (*Deipnos.*, 5, 196, A–5, 203, B).

". . . after these came a four-wheeled cart, twenty-one feet long and twelve feet wide, drawn by one hundred and eighty men; in this stood a statue of Dionysus; fifteen feet tall, pouring a libation from a gold goblet—in front of him lay a gold mixing bowl holding one hundred and fifty gallons [of wine]—next came the Macedonian Bacchants with hair streaming down and drowned with wreaths, some of snakes, others of vine leaves and ivy—next there followed another four-wheeler, thirty feet long, twenty-four feet wide, drawn by three hundred men; in this was set up a wine-press thirty-six feet long, twenty-two and one half feet wide, full of grapes. And sixty Satyrs trod them while they sang a vintage song to the accompaniment of pipes—next came a four-wheeled cart thirty-seven and one half feet long, twenty-one feet wide and drawn by six hundred men; in it was a wine skin holding thirty thousand gallons, stitched together from leopard pelts; this also trickled over the whole line of march as the wine was slowly let out[11]—following the skin came one hundred and twenty crowned Satyrs and Sileni, some carrying wine pitchers, others shallow cups, still others large deep cups everything of gold—immediately next to them passed a silver mixing bowl holding six thousand gallons in a cart drawn by six hundred men—and two silver wine-presses—a table of solid silver eighteen feet long—one hundred and sixty wine coolers; all these vessels were of silver—after all this there marched one thousand six hundred boys; two hundred fifty carried gold pitchers, while another band of three hundred twenty bore gold or silver wine coolers—twenty four elephant chariots, seven of gazelles, eight teams of ostriches—then came camels some of which carried three hundred of myrrh, two hundred of saffron, cassia, cinnamon, and all other spices—[then came] peacocks, guinea fowl, leopards, panthers, giraffes, and an Ethiopian rhinoceros—in the procession also were many thrones constructed of ivory and gold—on one lay a crown made of ten thousand gold coins—a very large number of gilded figures were there, wild beasts of extraordinary size, and eagles thirty feet high—further there were four hundred cartloads of silver vessels, twenty of gold vessels, and eight hundred of spices—then came the infantry forces (57,600) and cavalry (23,200) . . ."

Callixeinus concluded his description by a statement of total expenses involved

". . . the total expense in currency, amounted to 2,239 talents and 50 minas,[12] and all of this sum was paid in to the managing officials *before* the exhibition was over . . ." (*Deipnos.*, 5, 203, A–B)

Even if Callixeinus was prone to exaggerate, and there are arguments both for and against this point, this festival offered by Ptolemy Philadelphus to the citizens of fair Alexandria must have been one of the most exotic and spectacular ever witnessed by man.

Sacrifice

Pouring wine on libations has always been part of religious ritual in the East. Although the description given by Herodotus (II, 39) of the use of wine during sacrificial offerings of animals is late, it was true, as attested by sacrificial scenes, of all periods

> ". . . the victim, marked with their signet, [is led] to the altar where they are about to offer it, and setting the wood alight, pour a libation of wine upon the altar in front of the victim and at the same time invoke the god . . ."

There is practically no temple devoid of illustrations showing kings offering wine in the special round jars affected to the purpose (Fig. 14.12), nor are texts lacking in such records. King Sesostris II (*c.* 1906–1888 B.C.), included wine in his offerings to the gods

> ". . . I followed my statues to the temple; I devoted for them their offerings; the bread, beer, water, wine, incense, and joints of beef credited to the mortuary priest . . ." (*A.R.*, I, 630)

Rameses III's religious or sacrificial offerings of wine were truly sumptuous; 22,566 jars of wine to various temples at Thebes, 103,550 jars to the temples of Heliopolis, and 25,978 jars of wine to the temples of Memphis (*A.R.*, IV, 172). He considered this gift significant since, in a comparative time, the previous kings of Egypt had offered only 2,385 jars of wine to the temples of Heliopolis, and a mere 390 jars to those at Memphis (*A.R.*, IV, 168).

In respect to the non-ritual consumption of wine by Egyptian priests, Herodotus (II, 37) noted that priests were given a daily allotment of wine with their food. They appear, however, to have subjected themselves to certain restrictions in this respect, for Plutarch (*I. and O.*, 353, 6) stated that some of them avoided wine

> ". . . as for wine, those who serve the god in Heliopolis bring none at all into the shrine, since they feel that it is not seemly to drink in the day-time while their Lord and King[13] is looking upon them . . ."

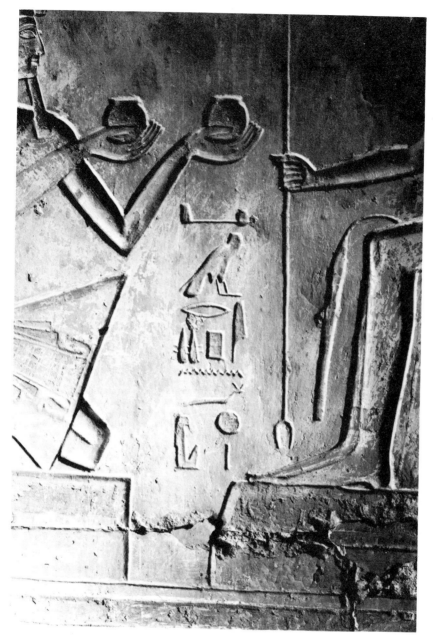

Fig. 14.12. Rameses II offering wine to Re-Harakhty. The vertical legend below the offering hand says: an offering of wine (*irp*). Ramesseum. Centre of Documentation, Cairo.

Such abstinence among priests appears, however, to have been a regulation of only the Heliopolitan order. Elsewhere, or at times other than services, this restriction was not followed, for Plutarch (*I. and O.*, 353, 6) further noted

"... the others use wine, but in great moderation. They have many periods of holy living when wine is prohibited and in these they spend their time exclusively in studying, learning, and teaching religious matters..."

Over one hundred years after Plutarch, Porphyry of Tyre, on the authority of Chaeremon of Cyrene, confirmed the moderation or abstemience of priests

"... for with respect to wine, some of them did not at all drink it, but others drank very little of it, on account of its being injurious to the nerves, oppressive to the head, an impediment to invention, and an incentive to venereal desires..." (Porphyry, 4, 6)

Funerary Use of Wine

To assure a plentiful supply of wine on which the deceased could draw, at least enough to last an eternity, tomb walls were adorned with the scenes of viticulture and vinification which we have already described, and with lists of gifts that, upon recitation of certain spells, were destined to be "activated".

The Pyramid texts of King Unas (*c.* 2423 B.C.) listed five varieties of wine offered in remembrance of his name

"wine-of-the-north", "Abesh-wine", "wine-from-Buto", "Hamu-wine", and "wine-from-Pelusium" (Piankoff, 1968; *Utt.*, 153–157)

Emery (1962) found at Saqqara, amid second dynasty tombs, large stores of wine jars that served funerary needs, but the wine had long since evaporated.[14]

Later, several Greek and Roman authors wrote that wine was employed in embalming, although they identify the variety as "palm-wine" rather than grape wine. Greek funerary custom required the body of the deceased to be washed with wine before interment, and this tradition was, of course, practised by the Greek community in Egypt, and it persists among the Greek minority now living in Egypt.

Medicinal Use of Wine

". . . in medicine it is most beneficial; it can be mixed with liquid drugs and it brings aid to the wounded . . ." (Athenaeus, 2, 36, A)

". . . the advantage of wine is that it excites the secretion of urine, thus removing the bilious humour with it, and that it moistens the joints . . ." Avicenna, No. 735).

The medicinal, or rather the magic-medical, use of wine followed closely upon its discovery; for early healers must have been impressed by the bubbling and quickening of fermenting liquids and could have scarcely overlooked the mysterious change in behaviour and personality of those who partook of the new product—hence, possibly, the association of wine with gods.

In the medical papyri,[15] wine is frequently listed, though less commonly than beer, possibly on account of its higher cost, or its more powerful effects. But it was relatively given more frequently internally.

Externally, lees were the usual medium, as in *Eb.*, LXXXII, 657 that prescribed

"Dregs of wine, grease of ox, onion, soot, terebinth, myrrh"

with which the body had to be rubbed and then exposed to the sun. The use of lees was also possibly a function of cost, but it limited this medicine to the vining season. In that respect, the Berlin papyrus differed in that it always mentions for external application wine, never dregs (see von Deines and Grapow, 1959, Vol. VI, p. 50). This invites the speculation that the patron who commanded this papyrus was wealthier than the sponsor of the Ebers papyrus.

In the medicated enemas which the Egyptian forerunners of the Greek *iatroklystis* and Molière's clyster givers called "The Physician's Art" (*Eb.*, XXXIII, 156; *Ber.*, 163; *H.*, 164), wine was simply a vehicle, although the alcohol it contained, which was readily absorbed through this route, certainly contributed a soothing effect

"Remedy to cool the anus, 'The Physician's Art', styrax, wine, brain of a fat ox,[16] *sdr* drink, honey, are strained and injected into the anus." (*Eb.*, XXXIII, 156)

Lesser systemic effects were to be expected from the following

"Onion, wine, mixed, and injected into the vagina" (*Eb.*, XCVI, 828)

although a rubefacient action was certainly achieved. It was prescribed for oral use in many ways:

a) as an after-drink to facilitate swallowing a dry medicine

"Another, to regulate the urine and cause purgation, goosefat, sory, are boiled to finger-warmth and swallowed with wine." (*Eb.*, X, 27)

b) As a dispensing aid

". . . to kill tapeworm . . . colocynth, heart of *ms* (? a bird), honey, wine, thyme (?)[17] sweet beer, are shaped into a cake, and eaten." (*Eb.*, XXII, 81)

c) Sometimes, a specific soothing action was sought, as suggested by the nature of the other ingredients, and by the inclusion of other liquids in sufficient volume to make it unnecessary as a vehicle

". . . hyoscyamus, dates, beer, fruit of sycamore, wine, ass's milk, boiled, strained, taken for four days." (*Eb.*, XXXIV, 98)

This mixture was prescribed for the mysterious illness, *whdw*, for which no better translation than "materia peccans" has yet been found.

d) As a vehicle

"Testicles of an ass,[18] ground fine, put in wine, and drunk." (*Eb.*, XC, 756)

Two indications stand out as particularly common for wine and beer. For anorexia, out of ten prescriptions in the Ebers papyrus (*Eb.*, Ll, 284–293), three contain wine alone, one beer and wine, and four only beer. Against a disease marked by cough, out of ten Ebers prescriptions (*Eb.*, LV, 326–335), five contain wine only, one wine and beer, and two beer alone.

Some medicated wines were specifically used to ease childbirth, like *Eb.*, XCIV, 799 and 804 which were supposed to "loosen the child in the belly of the woman". Such preparations recall the abortifacient wines mentioned by the Greeks. One was cited by Athenaeus

". . . in the region of Cerynia in Achaea, he [Theophrastus of Eresus] further says that there is a kind of vine, the wine from which causes pregnant women to miscarry, and if they but eat of the grapes, he declares, they miscarry." (*Deipnos.*, 1, 31, F)

Another, called by Pliny *ecboladic* (ejector) wine, was credited by him with similar properties (*N.H.*, XIV, XVIII–XXII).

Lutz (1922, p. 4), commenting on Pliny's statement, wrote that this must have been a particularly strong wine, and as such, avoided by women in Egypt.

Other prescriptions into which wine entered were noted by Greek and Roman travellers. Pliny (XX, LVIII, 164) recorded that scorpion stings could be relieved by drinking wine into which linseed (?) and powdered ami (*Carum copticum* or *Ammi visnaga*) had been stirred.

But of all Egyptian wines the Thebaid ones were the most appreciated for hygienic reasons

". . . [they are] thin and assimilable, so easily digested, that [they] may be given even to fever patients without injury." (*Deipnos.*, 1, 33, F)

Fashionable physicians, however, prescribed foreign wines to their wealthy clients. Apollodorus recommended to Ptolemy Pontine and Preparthian wines as being more curative than Egyptian ones (Pliny, *N.H.*, XIV; IX; 76). Athenaeus (*Deipnos.*, 1, 31, E–F) wrote of some medical wines from Greece in a manner that indicates that several foreign varieties were appreciated for their "special" qualities. One, from Thasos, made men sleep; another caused insomnia; and a vintage from Arcadia, the country of blissful innocence, was credited with two properties, to impregnate women, and to drive men insane, without, however, establishing any causal relationship between the two (*N.H.*, XIV; XXII, 116).

Temperance and Excess Among Egyptians

"My heart is not yet happy with your love
So be lascivious unto drunkenness"

(Faulkner *et al.*, 1972, p. 299)

In antiquity, as today, wine was principally a source of pleasure. There was in Egypt a wide variety from which to choose. The Mareotic, Sebennytic, and Taeniotic were particularly noted during Late Dynastic and Ptolemaic/Roman Periods, and their fineness provoked connoisseurs' demands, thus raising their price above what could be afforded by the average citizen of Egypt whose taste and purse could only afford ordinary or "poor" vintages (Strabo, 17, 1, 14), or beer.

A parallel situation prevailed in Rome around 89 B.C. when the price of Greek wine soared so high that a maximum price had to be fixed by edict. It was highly esteemed, but only one cup was given to each guest at banquets. Pliny further added, on behalf of Marcus Varro, that

"... when Lucius Lucullus was a boy he never saw a full-dress banquet in his father's house at which Greek wine was given more than once."
(*N.H.*, XIV, XVI, 96)

It is evident that fine wines have remained throughout history the characteristic drink of the affluent, whereas beer and cheaper wines have been the lot of common man. This stratification of drinking habits continues in modern society, though the differences between "beer-drinkers" and "wine-amateurs" may transcend social and economic boundaries oftener than in antiquity.

Athenaeus (1, 34, B) wrote that beer was in fact invented to help those who could not afford wine. This statement, of course, is legend; but it does support the thesis that in Egypt those of little means could scarcely afford wine, particularly the finer varieties. It would appear, therefore, that when Diodorus Siculus (1, 36, 6) wrote

"... also the land planted with the vine, being irrigated as are the other fields, yields an abundant supply of wine to the natives ..."

he meant certain natives, but not the average peasant. One ethnic minority, however, did enjoy the vine

"... and wherefore have ye made us to come up out of Egypt, to bring us in unto this evil place? It is no place of seed, nor of figs, or of vines ..."
(Numbers, 20, 5)

The psychological aspect of food and drink cravings is beyond the scope of this text; but such occasional references to wine consumption by minorities, and by average citizens, as occur in the Bible, in Diodorus, or in the festival description of Herodotus (II, 60), do not affect the general thesis that these groups were generally denied the better wines because of simple economic constraints.

But whereas it was realized that the company of Dionysus brings pleasure to those who practise moderation, the disasters it brings to others were painfully appreciated. Eubulus (*c.* 375 B.C.) concisely put it thus

"... three bowls only do I mix for the temperate; one to health, which they empty first, the second to love and pleasure, the third to sleep. When this bowl is drunk up, wise guests go home. The fourth bowl is ours no longer, but belongs to violence; the fifth to uproar, the sixth to drunken revel, the seventh to black eyes, the eighth is the policeman's, the ninth belongs to biliousness, and the tenth to madness and hurling the furniture.

Too much wine, poured into one little vessel, easily knocks the legs from under the drinkers . . ." (*Deipnos.*, 2, 36, B–C)

An even more concise description of the stages of drunkenness is that of the much later Arabic parable, the translation of which was twice published in the *Journal of the American Medical Association*, first in 1894, subsequently in 1969 (*JAMA*, 209, p. 845)

"When Adam first planted the vine, Satan came and killed a peacock over it, and the vine drank its blood. When the vine grew and put forth its leaves Satan came again and killed an ape over it, and the vine drank the blood of the ape also. When grapes first formed on the vine he killed a lion over it, and the vine drank up the blood of the lion. When the fruit was fully ripe Satan came again once more and killed a pig over it, and the vine drank up that blood also.

"Hence, he who drinks of the fruit of the vine imbibes these four qualities. When he first tastes the wine, and it begins to crawl in his limbs, the color blooms in his face, and he becomes gay as a peacock. When the first signs of drunkenness come upon him he plays, claps hands, and dances like an ape. When the wine grows stronger within him he grows violent like the lion, and challenges every one else. At last he wallows like a pig in the mire, desiring only to sleep, and his strength is gone."

Diodorus (1, 70, 11) observed that Egyptian custom dictated

". . . for the kings to partake of delicate food, eating no other meat than veal and duck, and drinking only a prescribed amount of wine, which was not enough to make them unreasonably surfeited or drunken . . ."

Plutarch (*I. and O.*, 353, 6) agreed and wrote

". . . their kings also were wont to drink a limited quantity prescribed by the sacred writings . . ."

one of the first records of a "religious dictate" in drinking.

In contrast to this moderation, and apart from the possibly ritual drinking of some pharaohs (Chapter 13, pp. 529 and 530), some kings may have been more than occasionally intemperate. One of them was Mycerinus whose name is included in that curious proper name "How drunk is Mycerinus" (see Chapter 13, p. 530)

". . . Mycerinus[19] the Egyptian pharaoh learned from his soothsayers that he was to live only a short time; so he caused many lamps to be lighted whenever night came on, and drank and made merry without stopping day or night; he even roamed into the swamps and woods and wherever, besides, he learned there were gatherings of young people, and there got drunk . . ."[20] (*Deipnos.*, 10, 438, B)

Although this accusation may be a later fabrication, Mycerinus was the first king of Egypt to be accused of exceeding the limits of propriety.

According to further tales he was not the last. Of all the kings of Egypt discussed by Herodotus, the one he least admired was Amasis (*c.* 588–568 B.C.) who lived about a hundred years before him

"... from early dawn to the time when the forum is wont to fill, he sedulously transacted all the business that was brought before him; during the remainder of the day he drank and joked with his guests, passing the time in witty and sometimes, scarce seemly conversation ..." (*Her.*, II, 173)

When Amasis was rebuked by his friends, he was reported to have answered

"... men that have bows bend them at need only; were bows kept forever bent they would break and so would be of no avail when they were needed. Such too is the nature of men ..." (*Her.*, II; 173)

Elsewhere (II, 174), he further elaborated on the moral personality of Amasis

"... it is said that Amasis, even while he was a private man, had the same tastes for drinking and jesting, and was averse to engaging in any serious employment. He lived in constant feasts and revelries, and whenever his means failed him, he roamed about and robbed people ..."

The known partiality of Herodotus against this king may have had political or nationalistic motives which were considerations that often influenced the "father of History."

Kingship and intoxication in fact were by no means confined to "native" kings; two notable examples were Philip of Macedonia and Alexander. According to Theopompus of Chios

"... Philip, Alexander's father was another drink-lover. Philip was a madcap and inclined to rush headlong into danger, partly by nature and partly because of drink; for he was a deep drinker, and was often drunk when he sallied into battle ..." (*Deipnos.*, 10, 435, A–B)

Alexander, the king who "hellenized" Egypt, was no better than his father for, as told by Carystius of Pergamum

"... he even went revelling in a chariot drawn by asses ..." (*Deipnos.*, 10, 434, F)

Behaviour among members of the Egyptian nobility varied, though Egyptians did not, like the Persians,

"... carry on their most important deliberations when drinking wine ..."

nor did they, like them,

". . . regard decisions then made as more lasting than those made when they are sober." (Strabo, 15, 3, 20)

Athenaeus remarked

". . . Among Egyptians, also, every kind of symposium was conducted with moderation in ancient times—for they sat as they dined, making use of the simplest and most healthful food, and drinking only so much wine as would be sufficient to promote good cheer . . ." (*Deipnos.*, 5, 191, E–F)

Such generalizations are, however, too sweeping; for no group or nation has ever served as a paragon of abstemious virtue.

Lutz (1922, p. 97), however, is wrong in stating that the moral necessity of temperance dawned upon Egyptians only under the New Kingdom. In the *Instruction of Ka-Gem-Ni*, believed to have been composed under the third dynasty, though most extant copies date to the Middle Kingdom as products of constant re-copy and study by generations of Egyptian scribes, a passage prescribes the proper behaviour of guests

". . . if thou sittest with a greedy person, eat thou only when his meal is over, and if thou sittest with a drunkard, take thou only when his desire is satisfied . . ." (Erman, 1966, p. 66)

Later sages, similarly attacked unseemly behaviour due to intoxication

". . . do not warm thyself in the house where intoxicating liquors are drunk . . ."

The Scribe Ani, who gave this advice, was an astute observer

"Take not upon thyself. Boast not that ye can drink to drink a jug of beer. Thou speakest, and an unintelligible utterance issueth from thy mouth. If thou fallest down and thy limbs break there is no one to hold out a hand to thee. Thy companions in drink stand up and say 'Away with that sot'. If there cometh one to seek thee in order to question thee, thou art found lying on the ground and thou art like a child." (Erman 1927, pp. 236, 237)

Several tomb paintings of the New Kingdom offer, however, a graphic rebuttal to the sweeping character of the claim of Appollonius that "all symposia were conducted with moderation". In a banquet, amid scenes of the usual polite behaviour, an almond-eyed beauty, her stomach overwhelmed with the festivities, turns away from the table in need of assistance; but the serving maid unfortunately arrives too late to aid her mistress, giving the unknown proletarian artist whose brush captured this embarrassing moment, an opportunity to illustrate that the nobility were no better than he (Fig. 14.13).

In the tomb of Paheri, (reign of King Thutmose II, *c.* 1520–1484 B.C.), an elegant lady presents her empty cup to the butler and says

"... give me eighteen measures of wine, behold I should love [to drink] to drunkenness, my inside is as dry as straw ..."

A helping servant offers encouragement

"... drink; do not refuse [?]; behold, I am not going to leave you ... drink, do not spoil the entertainment; and let the cup come to me ..." (Tylor and Griffith 1895, plate 7)

Lepsius (1842, 16, 16) recorded another interesting inscription that pulls a familiar string, but over 3,000 years ago

"... do not cease to drink, to eat, to intoxicate thyself, to make love [and] to celebrate the good days"!

The final outcome may be the subject-matter of a scene in the tomb of Khety at Beni Hassan, (eleventh dynasty, *c.* 2143–2000 B.C.) (Fig. 14.14), adjacent to and in association with illustrations of wine and beer production. Newberry and Fraser (1893, pp. 60, 61) interpreted this as a game. But it would appear equally possible, if not indeed probable, that the bearers were supporting one of their number who had passed out from drinking. Indeed, Lutz (1922, p. 98) described the scene as illustrating servants carrying home their inebriate noble master. But as all members of the group are identical in size and dress, they should according to Egyptian canons rather be regarded as his peers.

The entertainers of these merry gatherings were of course the most prone to habitual excess. A harpist who required drink and sustenance prior to playing said

"... I cannot bring the harp in order to chant without having drink [and] eaten from the jar ..."

The musician leaves the hosts aghast at his capacity for food

"... and he uses wine for two, meat for three, food for five together ..."

The result was that the harpist was too loggy and too inebriate to play properly, and could only "strum a few-measures"; the company was so disillusioned that they longed for the "first-harpist"—the same man

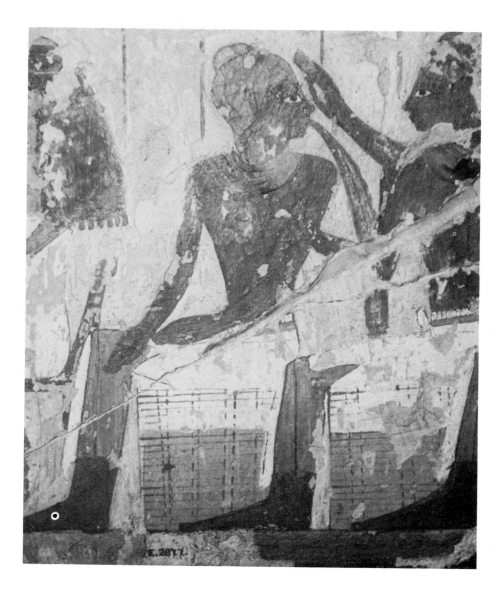

Fig. 14.13. Sick lady at banquet. Brussels Museum, No. E. 2877. Courtesy of Mr Mekhitarian.

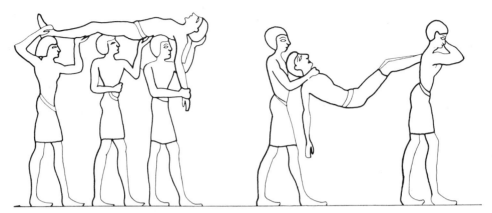

Fig. 14.14. Guests carried away at banquets. Beni Hassan. Redrawn from Wilkinson (1878) Vol. I., Fig. 169.

before he became intoxicated! Other harpists, too, were the butt of literary jokes

". . . the harp-player Stratonicus, whenever he started for bed, would tell his slaves to bring him a drink. 'Not so much because I am thirsty' he said, 'as because I don't want to be thirsty' . . ." (*Deipnos.*, 8, 349, F)

To guard against the undesirable consequences of excessive drinking, cabbage, according to the Greeks, was included in the fare:

"that the Egyptians are wine-bibbers is indicated by the custom, found only among them, of putting boiled cabbage first on their bill of fare at banquests, and it is so served to this day . . ." (*Deipnos.*, 1, 34, C)

There is no support for the existence of this habit earlier than the life-time of Athenaeus, but later historical association of cabbage with drinking is well documented. Avicenna, whose drinking habits are well-known, wrote

". . . it is an advantage to include in the menu cabbage boiled with meat; olives boiled in water, and the like. For this conduces to drinking more wine . . ." (No. 811)

The evidence concerning the date of introduction of cabbage into Egypt is, however, conflicting (see Chapter 17, p. 669). Breasted, in a text of the time of Rameses III translated a word ŝwt, cabbage (*A.R.*, IV, 240), but this is still *sub iudice*. It is thus uncertain whether the observation of Athenaeus held only for the Greek and Roman Periods, or whether this custom existed in pharaonic times.

In some instances, in the Late Dynastic Period, the banquet concluded with a macabre scene that symbolized the frailty of man, and his desire of immediate self-gratification

"... when the banquet is ended, a servant carries round to the several guests a coffin, in which there is a wooden image of a corpse—as he shows it to each guest in turn, the servant says, 'gaze here, and drink, and be merry; for when you die, such will you be." (*Her.*, II, 78)

This attitude of more than one society is found but slightly modified in the First Letter of Paul to the Corinthians

"If the dead are not raised, Let us eat and drink, for to-morrow we die." (Corinthians, I, 15, 32)

But the Egyptians, even in their wildest moments, were reminded of the virtue of moderation:

"Make holiday
But tire yourself not with it"
(*The Harper's Song*, Faulkner *et al.*, 1972, p. 307)

Drinking Habits in the Greek Period

How Greek and Roman customs influenced Egyptian upper class drinking behaviour can be but speculated upon, for the autochthonous Egyptians and the majority of Greek and Roman officials, nobility, and intellectuals, paid little heed to each other. But basic attitudes were not dissimilar. Plato (*Laws*, VI, 775, B–C) defined a code of desirable and undesirable behaviour

"... to drink to the point of intoxication is not proper to any other occasion except the festivals in honour of the god who gave the wine, and it is not safe; neither is it appropriate at the time when one is seriously engaged in the business of marriage, wherein, more than at any other time, bride and groom ought to be in their sound senses,[21] since they are under-going no little change in their lives; and at the same time, because their off-spring ought in all cases to be born of sound-minded parents . . ."

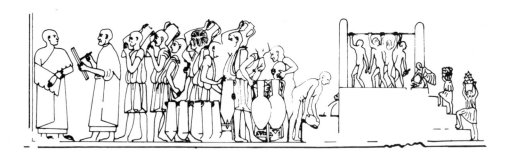

Fig. 14.15. Continuation of Fig. 14.13. Manufacture and registration of wine. Late Pharaonic-Ptolemaic Period, Tomb of Petosiris (Lefebvre, 1923, Vol. III, plate XII).

Elsewhere Plato wrote

". . . boys under eighteen shall not taste wine at all; for one should not conduct fire to fire;[22] wine in moderation may be tasted until one is thirty years old, but the young man should abstain entirely from drunkenness and excessive drinking; but when a man is entering upon his fortieth year he, after a feast at the public mess, may summon the other gods and particularly call upon Dionysus to join the old men's holy rite, and their mirth as well, which the god has given to men to lighten their burden— wine, that is, the cure for the crabbedness of old age, whereby we may renew our youth and enjoy forgetfulness of despair . . ." (Laws, II, 666, A–B)

Greek Views on Drinking

Earlier Greek views that could have affected attitudes towards wine in Ptolemaic Egypt, had been expressed in the sixth century B.C. in the aristocratic "Elegies" of Theognis of Megara

". . . assuredly 'tis a disgrace to be drunken among the sober, but disgraceful is it also to abide sober among the drunken . . ." (Elegy, 627),

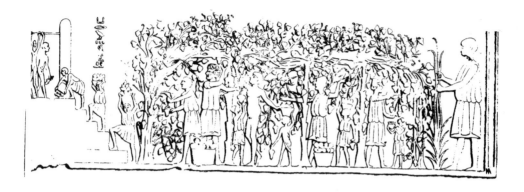

Fig. 14.16. Picking of grapes and wine-making. Late Pharaonic-Ptolemaic Period. Tomb of Petosiris (Lefebvre, 1923, Vol. III, plate XII).

". . . wine maketh light the mind of wise and foolish alike, when they drink beyond their measure . . ." (Elegy, 497).

How remarkably similar are these attitudes to the earlier writings of Ka-Gem-Ni, Ani, and other Egyptian sages who likewise had tried to build up a "drinking-morality"!

Roman Habits

Roman attitudes towards wine were in the main similar to both the previous Greek and Egyptian concepts, but with one striking difference. Throughout Dynastic and Ptolemaic history, there is no indication of any social taboo against wine drinking by Egyptian women. The Romans introduced a new "etiquette" at banquets

". . . among the Romans, neither a slave nor a free-born woman could drink wine,[23] neither could the young men of the free class up to thirty years of age . . ." (*Deipnos.*, 10, 429, B)

This tradition is supported by the writings of Polybius of Megalopolis

". . . among the Romans, women are forbidden to drink wine; but they drink what is called *passum*. This is made of raisins, and when drunk, it tastes like the sweet wine of Aegosthena or like the Cretan; hence they use it to counteract the urgency of thirst . . ." (*Deipnos.*, 10, 440, E–F)

Pliny (*N.H.*, XIV; XIV, 89) concurred

". . . At Rome women were not allowed to drink. Among various instances we find that the wife of Egnatius Maetennus was clubbed to death by her husband for dinking wine from the vat, and that Romulus acquitted him . . . a matron was starved to death by her relatives for having broken open the casket containing the keys of the wine-cellar; and Cato says that the reason why women are kissed by their male relations is to know whether they smell of 'tipple' . . ."

In spite of Athenaeus who told of the fondness of women for wine (*Deipnos.*, 10, 440, E), women certainly had difficulties in that world for the same author added

". . . it is impossible for a woman to drink wine undetected; for, in the first place, the woman has no control over the store of wine; besides this, she must kiss her own and her husband's relations down to cousins' children, and do this every day as soon as she sees them. Finally, since the chances of meeting make it uncertain whom she will encounter, she is on her guard; for the situation is such that if she but take a small taste, nothing more need be said by way of accusation . . ." (*Deipnos.*, 10, 440, F)

If this were the tradition among Roman women, what must have Julius Caesar and Mark Anthony thought of Queen Cleopatra VII whose favourite beverage was said to be wine[24] (Horace, *The Odes of Horace*, No. 37).

All these accounts, however, are warped by the fact that the moderate users of wine were overshadowed by their more boisterous counterparts who added "colour" to history. Wine was indeed liked under the Ptolemies. Reliefs from temples of that period at Edfu and Esna indicate a permissive attitude

". . . the produce of Pelusium, of *Hat-Seḥa-Ḥor*,[25] together with that of the oases *Kenem* and the produce of the oases *Ḏsḏs*.[26] Whenever the delivery occurs, then appears hearty joy and drunkenness in it." (Sauneron, 1959–69, Vol. II, No. 124, p. 2)

This recalls more than one Biblical saying

"Give strong drink to him who is perishing and wine to those in bitter distress
Let them drink and forget their poverty and remember their misery no more" (Proverbs, 31, 6)

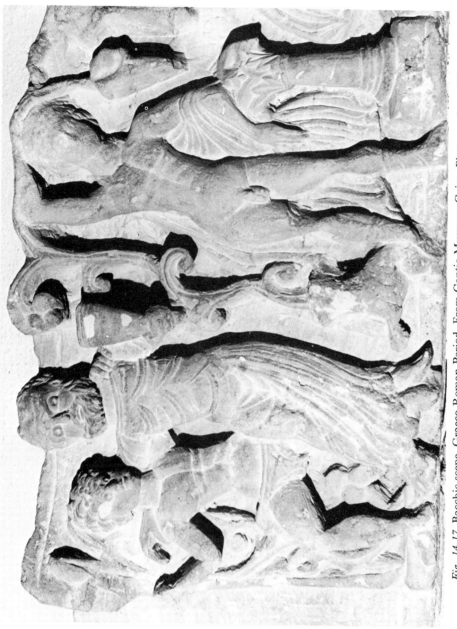

Fig. 14.17. Bacchic scene. Graeco-Roman Period. From Coptic Museum, Cairo. Photographed 1969.

"Bread is made for laughter and wine gladdens life." (Ecclesiastes, 10, 19)

Nor did artists in these late epochs lag in illustrating the various phases of the vining of this hallowed beverage. In the beautiful reliefs of everyday life that may be seen in the tomb of Petosiris at Tuna-el-Gabel (Figs 14.15 and 14.16) they have retained the centuries-old motifs, gracefully tempering the ancient rigidity of the canons with the flowing togas of their characters.

Incidents of lack of restraint, such as that described by Athenaeus (19, 420, E–F) were probably as numerous as anywhere else

"... People who gather for dinner-parties today, especially if they come from fair Alexandria, shout, bawl, and objurgate the winepourer, the waiter, and the chef; the slaves are in tears, being buffeted by knuckles right and left. To say nothing of the guests, who thus dine in complete embarrassment; if the occasion happens to be a religious festival, even the god will cover his face and depart, abandoning not only the house but also the entire city ..."

Such immoderates, well illustrated in Bacchic scenes of the Graeco-Roman period (Fig. 14.17), would have done well to recall the dictum of Alexis of Thurium

"... if the headache only came to us before we drink to intoxication, no one would indulge himself in wine immoderately ..." (*Deipnos.*, 10, 429, E)

Notes: Chapter 14

1. A voluminous literature from decisions of Councils and writings of the Fathers of the Church defines the smallest details of the liturgical use of wine. Many of these were detailed in the 63rd Epistle of St Cyprian who was elected Bishop of Carthage in A.D. 248. In this letter, Cyprian wrote lengthily to a bishop condemning an abuse that was introduced during the persecutions. This was the use of milk instead of wine in Holy Communion. As Mass was celebrated in the morning, the condemned bishop had tried thereby to avoid betraying the participants by their smell. Among other prescriptions, Cyprian added that water should be added to mark the union of Christ with men (Rohrbacher, 1878, Vol. II, p. 544).

Nowadays, Eastern Churches prefer red wine, because it is closer to the blood into which it is said to be transmuted by consecration, whereas Western Churches prefer the less messy and cleaner white wines that better symbolize the holiness and splendour of the sacrifice *Fons omnis sanctitatis et iutoris.*

Wine is used too in other parts of the liturgy, for example, in washing the Chalice, in priestly ablutions, and in the consecration of bells, altars and churches. Its historical connection with and importance to the unreformed churches has been such that the flourishing of wine and vining in Catholic countries, as opposed to beer in reformed churches, has been attributed to these liturgical and monachal activities.

2. In the sense of diluted, i.e. mixed with water or with decoctions of herbs or spices.

   "Unmixed wine" was commented upon by Ancient writers "Now the Sythians and Thracians drink nothing but unmixed wine, their wives as well as all the men; they pour it over their clothes and think that they practise a noble and happy custom . . ." (*Deipnos.*, 10, 432, A). During the reign of Zaleucus, King of Locria, a severe penalty was decreed against that custom ". . . among the western Locrians, if anyone drank unmixed wine without a physician's prescription to effect a cure, the penalty was death . . ." (*Deipnos.*, 10, 429, A).

3. It is interesting to compare this belief with the opinions of Aristotle and Avicenna. Aristotle asked "Why do those who drink wine diluted have a worse headache than those who drink it neat? It is because diluted wine owing to its fineness penetrates farther into more and narrower regions, but unmixed wine to a less extent" (*Problems*, III, 3). Avicenna wrote "Diluted wine intoxicates quickly because the watery constitute takes it quickly into the blood."

4. Maqrizi wrote in the fourteenth century A.D. that lake Mariut was so white that night could not be seen to fall upon it, that travellers fearing for their sight had to hold black rags, and that monks for that reason had to wear black clothes (Ch. XXIV, p. 18). Originally, it was a fresh water lake on whose shores all kinds of fruit grew (Maqrizi, Ch. XXIV, p. 20). It was separated from a salt water lagoon and the Mediterranean by the strip of limestone on which Alexandria was founded. On the 12th April, 1801, Sir John Hely-Hutchinson, the British General who was besieging the town, let in seawater to cut off the water supply and stop the besieged's retreat, creating the weedy salt-swamp utilized nowadays as a saline. Many an old legend surrounds this area of silence and mirage. One attributes it to the punishment of Hatassy, a rich but mean lady who lived in that region and refused, one stormy night, to give shelter to a holy man. The storm was raging; her neighbour, a poor but kind woman by the name of Neferu welcomed the harassed traveller who next morning blessed

her promising that Amon would give her success in anything she attempted. Neferu went to her usual chores, but when she drew out of a
chest an old piece of cloth, she was surprised to find she unrolled an
endless run of linen of the best quality. Whereupon, Hatassu, hearing of
the prodigee, hastened to offer her hospitality to the old man who,
likewise, blessed her. But when she proceeded to wash her hands to count
her money, counting on an endless treasure, the water she drew from her
well flew endlessly and nothing could stop it. It drowned her garden, and
ended by forming the lake.

5. In some figures, vines appear to bear gourds. But such a rendition does
   not necessarily mean that "gourd wine" was being processed. The reliefs
   were simply incomplete, the artist leaving details to a later session that
   was not held.

6. *Rnwt.t* (or *Rnn.t*) goddess of the harvest (see Chapter 11, p. 453 and Fig.
   11.2) presided also over the vine and vineries.

7. A grammatical way of expressing superlatives.

8. The Ancient Egyptian city of *Pr-Wsr-Ddw*, the "House of Osiris".

9. The Ancient Egyptian city of *Pa-Bast*, a name preserved in the Arabic
   name, *Tell Basta*, near Zagazig in the Delta. Bastet, represented as a
   woman with the head of a cat, was worshipped there in several temples
   of which the oldest dated to the fourth dynasty.

10. An incredible number. The conquering army of Alexander the Great
    has been estimated at a mere 30,000 soldiers. It is more reasonable to
    believe that "large crowds" attended, rather than the figure given. This
    statement should also be considered in the light of the statement of the
    same Herodotus (II, 77) that no wines were found in Egypt.

11. Amerine (personal communication, 1968) offered several enlightening
    criticisms of this passage: 30,000 gallons is nearly equal to 125 *tons*. Six
    hundred men might have pulled this amount, but the "four-wheeled
    cart" would have been indeed heavily laden. Moreover, how could
    leopard skins be stitched watertight?

12. Basing himself on the 1927–1928 value of the Sterling Pound, and on its
    relative 1927 purchase power, Gulick (1928, Vol. 2, p. 419) estimated
    that this sum was equivalent to 720,000 Sterling Pounds (or) $3,600,000.

13. The sun-god, Ra.

14. No wine has actually been found in tombs. This is quite natural con-
    sidering the weather and the centuries.

15. For the medical papyri, see Vol. 1, Ch. 3.

16. Or "visceral fat of ox" (Von Deines *et al.*, 1958, Vol. IV, 2, p. 113).

17. Thyme is a known vermifuge.

18. This could be a plant's name. Compare Arabic "testicle of fox" *Khosyet
    el-thaalab*, and Latin *orchis*, for sahleb.

19. Fourth king of the fourth dynasty, builder of the third Pyramid of Giza.

This name is the Greek form of his Egyptian name, Men-Kau-Re.
20. This appears also in Herodotus (II, 133).
21. Athenaeus (*Deipnos.*, 10, 445, E–F) credited Alcaeus of Mytilene with the following anecdote "once a fellow-drinker saw the wife of Anacharsis at the drinking-bout and said to him, 'you have married an ugly woman, Anacharsis'. He answered, 'Yes, indeed, I think so too; come slave, fill up a stronger cup, that I may make her good-looking' . . .".
22. Compare Avicenna's advice (No. 810) ". . . to give wine to youths is like adding fire to a fire already prepared with matchwood. Young adults should take it in moderation. But elderly persons may take as much as they can tolerate . . .".
23. Among the people of Massilia, there was a law that compelled women to drink water (*Deipnos.*, 10, 429, A).
24. "The Queen with her unwholesome crew
       of nasty men, mad to aspire
    And drunk with fortune, till came through
    Scarcely one ship out of fire.

    Then calmed her ardour; and her heart
    Weakened by Mareotic wine
    Caesar with terror made to start
    Driving her on over the brine"
        (Horace, *The Odes of Horace* No. 37)
25. Identified by Sauneron as the oasis of Farafra (*Le Temple d'Esna*, Vol. II, No. 124, p. 2).
26. Two Egyptian oases: probably Bahariya and Dakhla.

Chapter 15   *Wine (Part II)*

> *"How much more ingenious, however, man has been
> in respect of drink will be made clear by the fact
> that he has devised 185 kinds of beverages or, if
> varieties be reckoned, almost double that number."*
>   (*H.N.*, XIV, XXIX, 150)

Tentative Classification of Ancient Egyptian Wines

Wines in Egypt, as elsewhere, were named after the village, town, district or general geographic region where they were produced, but authors have not been consistent in rendering suffixes; for example, "Wine-of-Alexandria", Alexandreotic, Alexandrian and Alexandria, all appear in the literature. We have eliminated the more obvious synonyms and have chosen the form most likely to be encountered by the reader scanning Egyptological texts for the first time, while retaining the more interesting name variants which, as we believe, might facilitate identification. It must be noted, however, that most of our information comes from Greek authors writing at the beginning of our era, and that their reports, at times, may not apply to the Dynastic Period proper.

Vintages of Lower Egypt

Wines of the Delta were known by several generic names, like "wine-of-the-northern-country", sometimes shortened to "northern wine". Some of these general appellations, however, may have designated specific varieties of Delta wines. A "wine-of-the-North" is listed in the Pyramid Texts (Utt. 153) beside "wine-from-Buto", (Utt. 155) another Delta variety (Piankoff, 1968), suggesting that the first term was not all-inclusive. The following are some of the appellations found in the literature, arranged in alphabetic order.

Antyllan or Anthyllan Wine

This wine was highly praised by Athenaeus (1, 33, F)

> "surpassing all others is the wine of Antylla, a city not far from Alexandria, the revenues from which were assigned by the early kings of Egypt and by the Persians to their wives for to buy girdles."

Rawlinson (1885, Vol. 2, p. 89), perhaps basing himself on these remarks, stated that it was a favourite wine of the Egyptians.

Buto Wine

Produced at the northern Delta city of this name, Buto wine was specifically mentioned in the Pyramid Texts. According to Brugsch (1878, p. 91), it was more widely known by the name *Amt*. The close resemblance of this name to those of the villages of *Hmt* and *Imt* in the Delta, where wine also was produced, poses further questions of identification. At present, it is safer to note these problems, and to wait for their solution. For example, one would hesitate to assert that it was the identical *Imt* discussed by Montet (1958), Kees (1961), Lutz (1922) and others.

Hamet

Kees (1961, p. 82) believed Hamet to be a major centre of viticulture under the New Kingdom, quite distinct from *Imt*. Neither of these two regions has yet been identified, and the above-noted resemblance with *Amt* must be taken into account.

Hursekha

This wine district said by Brugsch (1878, p. 91) to lie in the vicinity of Lake Mareotis, should probably be read *Ḥt-sḫa-Ḥor* (Het-sekha-Hor), recently identified as the oasis of Farafra.

Imt

Imt wine is mentioned in several texts (e.g. *Pyr*, 120a). Montet (1958, p. 105) wrote that this wine, variously spelled *Imit, Imet,* or *Ymet,* was one of the most popular during the New Kingdom. Petrie (1888) located a town called *Amt* at the modern village of Nebesheh close to Tanis. It is possible that *Imt* and *Hamet* were identical, although Kees (1961, p. 82) considered them distinct.

Iwnw

Brugsch (1878, p. 92) discussed briefly wine produced in *Annu*, his spelling of the more generally accepted *Iwnw*, which was the Heliopolis of the Greeks.

Mareotic Wine

This wine, also called Alexandrian, was one of the most appreciated (Athenaeus, 1,33,D–E), and Strabo praised it as highly as did Athenaeus

> ". . . and the vintages in this region are so good that the Mareotic wine is racked off with a view to ageing it." (17, 1, 14)

and Horace suggests that Cleopatra indulged in it (see Chapter 14, note 24). Rawlinson (1885, Vol. 2, p. 89) implied that Mareotic was distinct from Alexandrian wine and he, accordingly, listed them separately. This is difficult to accept unless he meant that Alexandria wines were a variety of the Mareotic, or that some vineyards to the north of Lake Mareotis, west of Alexandria, had their natural market in that town. These we shall discuss later under the label "Egypto-Libyan wines".

It is also tempting to equate the fine Mareotic wines with the so commonly mentioned wines-of-the-northern country. Erman (1894, p. 196) wrote that the first ones were products of the New Kingdom, while the second were made in other Delta districts, in addition to the Mareotic.

Another vintage, the *nh꜄mw* of the Pyramid Texts was believed by Lutz (1922, pp. 12–13) to have been a product of that same region.

Mendesian Wine

Lutz (1922, p. 4) speaks of a Mendesian wine, quoting Athenaeus (*Deipnos.*, I, 30) and Pliny (*N.H.*, XIV, 9), but there appears to have been some confusion with the Mendaean wine of Athenaeus, a Greek type, and with other Egyptian wines cited by Pliny.

Pelusium

Although produced far from the Delta, and east of the Suez isthmus, Pelusiac wines may conveniently be discussed here. It is generally agreed that Pelusium was built in Graeco-Roman times at the site of the Egyptian border post *Sin*, variously spelled *Sajan, Senu, Sjn, Suni, Sunu* even *Syene*, but not to be confused with southern Syene, where Aswan today stands. *Sin* wines were produced during the Old Kingdom and were of the highest quality. Nevertheless, they are called "Pelusian" wines by some of the most careful authors, possibly for the sake of clarity; but this may confuse the unwary. Piankoff (1968, Utt. 157) translated one of the wines of Unas's Pyramid Texts as "Pelusium-wine", and Kees (1961, p. 82) listed Pelusian wines among the best of the nineteenth dynasty, although the site was not named Pelusium until over a thousand years later.

It is interesting that the high respect gained by Sin/Pelusium wines persisted through dynastic to modern eras. Was their appreciation enhanced by the pivotal position of Pelusium, a starting and re-entering post for anxious and extenuated soldiers?

Sebennytos

This town, the *Tjeb-Neter* of the Ancient Egyptians, was particularly renowned for having fine soil for grapes. Pliny (*N.H.*, XIV, IX, 74) spoke of the fame of its wine

> "this last is grown in Egypt, being made from three famous kinds of grapes that grow there: the Thasian, the soot-grape, and the pine-tree [or pitchy] grape."

He elsewhere said of the Thasian that it was the best of all Egyptian grapes in sweetness and medicinal properties (see later).

Taeniotic

This wine is not to be confused with wine from Tanis. The term *taenia*, a strip or ribbon, as a qualification, implies that this wine was produced in the sandy cultivated strip on either side of the "black land" Delta, where the soil is ideally suited to the vine. According to Athenaeus, the Taeniotic was even better than the Mareotic

> "wines made there are somewhat pale, disclosing an oily quality in them which is dissolved by the gradual mixture of water, like the honey of Attica—this Taeniotic wine, besides being pleasant, has also an aromatic quality, and is mildly astringent." (1, 33, E)

This variety is usually included by recent authors among the wines that were most popular in the later periods (Rawlinson, 1885, Vol. 2, p. 89; Erman, 1894, p. 196).

Wine of the Fisheries(?) *Irp Ḥ m*

Geographic confusion mars the history of this product. It is mentioned, in several texts, as being among the best known wines of Lower Egypt.

Erman and Grapow (*Wb.*, III, 32) translate *ḥȝm* as a wine-growing district, possibly an oasis. Faulkner (1962, p. 163) translated *Ḥȝmw* by both "fisherman" and "a kind of wine", according to the determinative used. Montet listed it as one of the best nineteenth dynasty vintages. Breasted (*A.R.*, IV, 734) in his translation of a tribute to Osorkon I (*c.* 929–893 B.C.), which included *Hemy* wine, believed this to have been produced in the western Delta, in the vicinity of Lake Mareotis.

It is evident that the term was applied to a specific wine of great repute and with a long history. The name implies that it was produced near one of the many fishermen's paradises strewn along the shores of the northern lakes, of Lake Moeris, and of the Nile and its canals. Provisionally, considering the high quality wines produced near Lake Mareotis, the likeliest site is somewhere there, but the evidence is slim.

Wine of the Marshes

The two marshy regions in Egypt are the northernmost and the eastern-most parts of the Delta. Brugsch (1878, p. 91) believed this name, however, to be a generic for northern wines. One must admit to a close similarity between the words *Mḥw*, Lower Egypt; *Mḥt*, the Delta marshes, and *Mḥty*, northern.

Wine of the Region of Amun

Šȝ-imn, translated as "Vine-region of Amon", was a vine-growing area, probably the property of New Kingdom kings, situated in the region called "The City of the Apis Bull", the westernmost city of the third Libyan nome. It is mentioned with different kinds of wine in an inscription at Esna. There is no further information on it.

Vintages of Upper Egypt

As with northern wines, there were generic names for Upper Egyptian vintages—for example, *'irp rs*, "wine-of-the-South", an appellation sometimes applied to a specific vintage, possibly "the" southern one.

The wines designated by these terms, however, were distinct from wines produced in the oases, which bore their own names.

Rawlinson (1885, Vol. 1, p. 87) stated that *Thebaid* wines were known for their lightness and wholesomeness though, in fact, he was specifically discussing Coptos wines (see below). As noted previously, Lutz (1922, p. 56) remarked that Thebaid tombs do not illustrate the technique of "secondary" extraction through a cloth bag as depicted in tombs north of Thebes. As already pointed out, this difference in technique might have reflected itself in a difference in colour and quality.

Coptos Wine

This wine, praised by Athenaeus (1, 33, F), was

"thin and assimilable, so easily digested that it may be given even to fever patients without injury."

Rawlinson repeated nearly verbatim these words (1885, Vol. 2, p. 89). Calling them "Coptic" as he did is confusing; for they were, obviously, not produced by Copts, since the Coptic religion had not yet appeared.

Šft.t

S'*ef-ti*, according to de Rougé (1867), a mountain in the seventh nome, may have been a wine-growing area

"The vine branches of *Šft.t* flourish in their hands." (Dümichen 1865–1885, Kal. Inschr., 103)

The seventh nome (Diospolis parva) was known for its vines, and Lutz (1922, p. 13) placed *šft.t* there. Brugsch (1878, p. 92) thought *Sef* or *Seft* to be produced in Kharga or Dakhla, but there is no support for his contention.

Syene

Lutz (1922, p. 14) contends that wine was not produced at Syene (or

Elephantine) before the Ptolemaic Period, because an inscription attributed to Nesuhor, commander of the garrison under the twenty-sixth dynasty, informs us that he

". . . gave very fine wine of the Southern Oasis, spelt, and honey into [their] storehouses." (*A.R.*, IV, 992)

This report, incidentally, shows that existence of trade routes between the oases and the valley only forty to fifty years before the loss of the army of Cambyses between Kharga and Siwa. But it does not exclude the existence of local wines.

Vintages of the Western Oases

The western Egyptian oases are scattered in a north-south chain from Siwa, approximately 180 miles south of the Mediterranean, to Kharga and Dakhla, at about the same latitude as Esna. In antiquity, Siwa was called the "oasis of Amon", Bahriyah was the "northern oasis", and the ensemble Kharga-Dakhla was included in the term "southern oasis". Oasian soil is, in general, ideal for viticulture; it produced excellent wine and, in spite of the tremendous difficulties of wine transport, these were widely distributed to all points of the valley.

The Fayoum: Arsinoitic Wines

The Fayoum is separated from the valley by a mere 60 miles. It is connected to it by several roads, and to the Nile by a canal. Wide stretches of cultivated land on each side of the waterway give it, on a map, the appearance of a bulge of the valley, This is why it is not usually classed as an oasis. The Fayoumis, at times, think of themselves as a separate ethnic group, but continuous contact with the people of the valley, and with Greeks in the Graeco-Roman period, has all but erased their distinctiveness.

The wines of the Fayoum were called *Arsinoitic*, for the major settlement named after the wife of Ptolemy II Philadelphus, Queen Arsinoe II, who was deified after her death.

Strabo, in his *Geography* (11,1,35) recorded the abundance and fine quality of these wines, adding (17,1,38) that they were mixed with honey and fed to the sacred crocodiles. He does not comment, however, on the possible effects of this beverage on the saurians!

Wine of the Northern Oasis

It seems permissible now to identify the "northern oasis", or Bahariya, with *Dsḏs*. Wine of *Dsḏs* was mentioned together with those from the other western oases in the previously quoted inscription of Esna (Sauneron, 1959–1969, Vol. II, no. 124, p. 2)

> "This is the place of wine . . . the products of Buto of Arabia, of *Ḥt-sḥa-Ḥor* [Farafra], as well as the country of Knm [? Dakhla], and all the products of *Dsḏs* [Bahariya], brought as taxes to this pleasant chapel."

Wine of the Southern Oasis

The two oases of Kharga and Dakhla were called by Egyptians *Knm* and, sometimes, by the Greeks the "Island of the Blessed". Strabo (17, 1, 42) accurately placed Kharga at seven days' journey from Abydos, and commented on its wealth of water and wine. But the earliest mention of its wines dates to the offerings of Osorkon I (*c.* 928–893 B.C.) (*A.R.,* IV, 734); and we know from the above-quoted inscription of Nesuhor (*A.R.,* IV, 992) that it was sent to Syene.

Siwa

It may be presumed that wine was utilized at Siwa, at least under the New Kingdom, in the celebration of the Amon rituals; but there are no documents attesting Siwan wine production. Nowadays, vines grow there in profusion; but, possibly on account of the limited archaeological research hitherto conducted, the date of introduction cannot be determined.

Other Oasian Wines

Of the several wines of the vast areas covered by those oases, the most colourful in its appellation is the "Green-Eye-of-Horus" (the white eye being milk). The eye of Horus that, in the legendary fights with Seth, had been torn to pieces, and had then been restored by the power of Thot, was the symbol of health, healing and perfection. The Green Eye of Horus must have, therefore, enjoyed the highest regard.

Two wines, *Tbui* and *Nhamt*, have been the subject of much divergence of opinion, Lutz (1922, p. 14), placing them in these oases, and Brugsch (1878, p. 92), placing *Tbui* near Lake Mareotis. Pendlebury (1951, part III, Vol. 1, p. 166) also considered as a Dakhlan variety the *s3-wh3t* wine, of which he found seals at Akhetaten (modern Tell el Amarna), the capital of Amenophis IV. This is plausible since the word *wh3t* means oasis.

Egypto-Libyan Vintages

Throughout history, the Egypto-Libyan border has been difficult to define. Even now the term "Libyan desert" designates all the Egyptian desert west of the Nile, even though parts of it lie hundreds of miles away from the political boundary.

Antiphraean Wine

According to Strabo (17, 1, 14), the wines in this region were poor, especially that from *Antiphraea*

> "The whole of this country is without good wine, since the wine jars receive more sea water than wine; and this they call 'Libyan' wine, which, as also beer, is used by most of the tribe of the Alexandrians."

With this derogatory comment, Strabo placed this wine within the price range of beer as a beverage of the common people, the "tribe" being, according to another passage (17, 1, 12), the third class of Alexandrians, a mixed group of Greek origin coming after the indigenes and the mercenaries.

In spite of this condemnation, this geographic appellation included the Mareotic wines which, generally, were reputed to be excellent. Neither should the statement of Hellanicus be overlooked, as to the discovery of wine in Plinthine, about fifteen miles west of Alexandria along the coast. Thus, unless their quality had immensely improved in the two centuries between Strabo (66 B.C.–A.D. 25) and Athenaeus (A.D. 170–230), these wines were probably misjudged by Strabo.

Plinthic

Cosson (1935, pp. 108–109) referred to several ancient maps that pinpoint the debated site of Plinthine, where Athenaeus placed the origin of wine, 4·5 km east of Taposiris, which is directly north of Borg el-Arab. With the exception of Taposiris and nearby Abu Mena, there are few coastal sites of any magnitude. But as one travels in spring in that desolate region one is struck by the contrast between the dusty tan of the poor cultivated land and the rich pageantry of flowers, ablaze with reds, yellows and greens, covering the humus of ancient mounds, under one of which Plinthine may still be buried.

Egyptian Vintages of Uncertain Identity

Apart from the above, a variety of wines is mentioned in texts with little or no information as to their origin. Some designations refer to colour; others had medicinal implications; other wines, though bearing individual names, remain undefined.

Colour Designations

Three wines were called white, black and red, although these epithets may possibly refer to attributes other than mere colour. For the black arable land of the Delta and valley was repeatedly contrasted with the red desert; and the "red crown" and "white crown" stood, respectively, for Lower and Upper Egypt. Such symbolism was not merely academic; it permeated everyday language.

White Wine. This was listed by Erman (1894, p. 196) among the six major varieties of the Old Kingdom; but it was given a geographic meaning, i.e., it signified wine of Upper Egypt. Nevertheless, Athenaeus wrote that Mareotic wines (Lower Egypt) were white in colour (1, 33, D–E). This was the earliest such report. He added that

> "the vine is as abundant in the Nile Valley as its waters are copious, and the peculiar differences of the wines are many, varying with colour and taste."

Black Wine. The ancient name of Egypt being *Km.t* (the Black Land), black wine could be understood as a generic name for all Egyptian wines, to differentiate them from imported foreign varieties. There is evidence, however, that it served a funerary use in the Old Kingdom (Budge, 1960, pp. 211–212), an implication that it applied to a specific product.

Red Wine. The word *dšr* (red) had in Egypt many connotations. It meant red when modifying a flamingo; desert, if written with a hill; and the crown of Upper Egypt, with a northern crown. It does not seem to have been used in its literal sense for wine.

One "red wine" was a specific kind highly appreciated during the New Kingdom (Erman, 1894 p. 196), but the bulk of information indicates that it was only a regional description of Lower Egyptian wines, as opposed to "white" Thebaid wines. On the other hand, red being the colour of Seth and of the desert, red wines could have been oasian wines, had these not been called by specific names. They could further be names of products of towns and villages that persisted in Seth's worship, like Ombos, Kom Ombo, or Tanis. This raises the question of which wine was meant in a prayer, used during the New Kingdom

> "I drink my fill of Seth wine every evening." (Budge, 1960, p. 543)

"Abesh" Wine. This wine, mentioned in the Pyramid Texts (Piankoff, 1968, Utt. 154), was translated by Lutz (1922, p. 7) as white wine, for no obvious reason. Montet (1958, p. 105) wrote that it was one of the traditional delicacies of the nineteenth dynasty, and that special precautions were taken during its transport by padding the jars with basketwork. Brugsch (1878, p. 56) found *Abesh-ti* wine recorded in an

inscription on the Kharga temple of the Persian Darius II. Although it is not known precisely where it was produced, abesh wine was clearly a distinguished beverage with a prestigious history.

Medicated Wines

Brya. Pliny (*N.H.*, XXIV; XLII, 69–71) described the local use of a decoction of brya leaves in wine, with rose oil and wax, as soothing and as a cure for epinyctitis, a condition translated by Jones (Pliny, Vol. 7, p. 550) as either a sore on the eyelid, or an eruption due to fleas or bugs. Brya has been translated as *Tamarix africana* and/or *T. orientalis* by Jones (*loc. cit.* p. 494), which would equate it with Egyptian '*isr* (*Gpfl.*, 155) of which the fruits, twigs and leaves were in officinal use (*Eb.*, XXIV, 96; *H.*, 102; *L.*, 24).

"*Delivery*" *Wine.* Unidentified ingredients mixed with wine are said in the Ebers papyrus (XCIV, 804) to empty the uterus. This is not suggestive of any intrinsic abortifacent properties and is, therefore, insufficient to equate this composition with the ecboladic Egyptian wines described by Pliny (XIV, XIX, 110 and XIV, XXII, 118).

Š3iw. This is listed by Lutz (1922, p. 7) as a medicinal wine. This word, however, is nowadays translated otherwise.

To the class of medicated wines must probably be added some or most of the so-called "fictitious or artificial" wines, to be described later.

Undefined Wines with Specific Names

Several names of wines are enumerated in the ancient texts, without any information as to their quality or origin. Such are *w3*, *k3y*, *irp-w* (Weill, 1908, p. 251), *sdw-ib*, the quenching or satisfying beverage (Weill, 1908, p. 420). A poetic "Morning Star of the Sky" is cursorily mentioned by Brugsch in a wine list from Abydos (1878, p. 92). Other fermented drinks were possibly, but not necessarily, wines.

Imported Wines

Among the products imported through trade or tribute, wine was not the least.

"Twice a year wine is brought into Egypt from every part of Greece as well as from Phoenicia, in earthen jars." (*Her.*, III, 6)

As the political boundaries in the Near East have been characterized by their parennial fluctuations, all the production of that area may well be considered here.

Syrian wines especially those of Damascus and the Orontes valley were as reputed in antiquity as they were later, when the Arab bards sang their praise even before conquering Syria

"Awake, sweet damsel, and bring me my morning draught; nor hoard
    the rich wines of Enderein[1] . . .
Your cup, Om Amr, passed me by, though t'was going towards me
But the least of us, Om Amr, is not the friend you skipped
For I have drunk a cup in Baalbek and others in Damascus and Qaiserein"

(Translated from Zawzani, 1970)

Much later, in Bagdad, the delightful Abu-Nowas, the débauché Court poet of wine and merriment of Harum Ar-Rashid (A.D. eighth to ninth centuries), facetiously claimed the authority of the famed physician Gabriel ibn Bakhtayshuh, whom he calls also Abu Eissa, in prescribing as the proper intake four pints of wine, corresponding to the four temperaments and humours

"I asked Abu Eissa, for Gabriel is a man of judgment
Wine pleases me. He said 'Abuse is killing'.
I said 'Direct me'.
He answered, and his say is decisive,
I found human natures to be four,
Four to four, to each nature a pint."

Syrian wines were also lauded by the Biblical prophets

"Damascus was thy merchant in the multitude of the wares of thy making
. . . in the wine of the Helbon . . ." (Ezekiel, 27, 18)

"They that dwell under his shadow shall return; they shall revive as the corn, and grow as the vine: the scent thereof shall be as the vine of Lebanon."
(Hosea, 14, 7)

Wines from Tyre were mentioned by Heliodorus (1587, Vol. V, p. 27) and Pliny (*H.N.*, XIV, IX, 74), as well as wines of Gaza, of Tripoli and Berytus (actual Beyrut). Arvad, overthrown by Thutmose III, was said to be filled with the products of all Zahi (Asia); its wines were found

"remaining in its presses as water flows." (*A.R.*, II, 461)

And an Asiatic people called *Fenekh* or *Fenkhou* (see *A.R.*, II, 30, 120, 439; IV, 719, etc.), possibly the *Fenekh* of Brugsch (1878, pp. 81, 91) and Müller (1893, p. 208), were said, in an inscription, to travel southward to Egypt with their wine.

Strabo (16, 2, 9) described Laodicea as a territory abounding with wine, of which the greater part was exported to Alexandria. And very much earlier, Sinouhe, the hero of a twelfth dynasty classical tale, recounted how he was received in Upper Retenu, variously identified as Lydda or as the whole of Syria and Palestine (Lefebvre, 1949, p. 8, n. 25), where, he said, wine was more plentiful than water, and where he was given every day victuals and wine.

Later we know that Syrian wines were brought from Zahi (*A.R.*, II, 461, 462) and from Retenu (*A.R.*, II, 473), as tribute for Thutmose III.

Brugsch (1878, p. 91) mentioned *Sangar* wine, called in Ptolemaic times *Sankal*, from the Biblical town of Sinear in eastern Mesopotamia. The Mesopotamian tradition was maintained under Moslem rule, when Abu Nawas chanted his love of wine

"Come, pour it out, ye gentle boys
  A vintage ten years old
That seems as though 'twere in the cup
  A lake of liquid gold

And when the water mingles there
  To fancy's eye are set
Pearls over shining pearls close strung
  As in a carcanet"   (Alevi, 1924, p. 169)

Wine was imported also from the Greek islands, particularly from Chios, Lesbos, Rhodes and Thasos. Greek style wine jars stamped with the royal stamp of pharaoh Ahmes were found at Defenneh in the north-east of the Delta by Petrie (1888, p. 64) who commented that either Greek potters were employed to make the jars for the royal vineyards, or the wine was transported in skins and then poured into Greek jars and sealed in the palace at Defenneh, or that it was Greek wine imported in these jars and sealed in Egypt.

An Egyptian papyrus dated to 259–257 B.C. recorded the import of wine from Chios and Lesbos (*S.P.*, 1, 170). Johnson and West give several references to imports of the fifth or sixth centuries A.D. from Rhodes (1949, p. 147). Pliny's information on Thasian wine is somewhat confusing.

"Egypt gives the name of 'wine of Thasos' to an extremely sweet native vintage which causes diarrhea." (XIV, XXI, 117)

It is difficult to judge whether this native wine was prepared from grapes imported from Thasos, or from locally grown Thasian grapes. Other comments of Pliny (XIV, IX, 74) suggest the latter alternative (see p. 601).

Strabo, on his part, incidentally mentions Lesbian imports in his version of the legend of the third pyramid, allegedly called "The Pyramid of the Courtesan", for having been built, so the story went, by the lovers of the famed Doricha.[2] This notorious hetaera, was, he said, beloved by Charaxus, the brother of Sapho the poetess,[3] who was engaged in transporting Lesbian wine to Naucratis for sale (17, 1, 33).

Dioscorides called Chios wine well-nourishing, potable, less intoxicating, useful in eye medicines, while Lesbian was more easily digested, being lighter than Chios wine, and good for the belly (V, 10).

Export of Wines

Local production being hardly adequate, little was left for foreign trade. The only evidence for export is found in *The Periplus of the Erythrean Sea* (Schoff, 1912, p. 28), an anonymous compilation by an Alexandrian merchant, of all the ports of call on the way to India, and of the merchandise traded in each. This compendium states that Egypt exported wine to a city of the frankincense country.

Taxation of Wines

Much is known on the modalities of wine taxation during the Graeco-Roman period (see Ricci, 1924). In addition to local customs duties, taxes were levied at the producer's level. The tax rates were apparently based on the evaluation of the quality of the grapes and wine by authorized assessors.

Of the Dynastic Period, Lutz (1922, pp. 20, 21) adduces two documents that, in his opinion, prove this practice. The first is a stele where a

Bilgai, an "Overseer of the Fortress of the Sea" boasts of his people having delivered an amount of wine far in excess of its assessment. The second is a letter from an Asiatic prince asking that his men be exempted from paying customs duties. Despite the facts that the first document does not specifically mention taxation, and that the second does not speak of wine, there is a practical certainty that some kind of wine tax was exacted, witness the wines brought as taxes to the Temple of Esna (see p. 605).

Miscellaneous Fermented Beverages

This heading includes two separate categories: the genuine products of fermentation of various fruits, and the products of maceration of herbs and fruits in wine, corresponding to the "perfumed wines of Athenaeus" (*Deipnos.*, I, 31, F). Pliny calls the whole class "fictitious" (XIV, XVIII, 98), which has been translated "artificial", although they are no more artificial than grape wine. They do not appear to have been of major consequence in the nutrition of the Ancients, but they are included here for the sake of completeness. There is no suggestion that they were brandies or liquors, for the art of distillation was unknown, and the production of alcohol in concentrations higher than those produced by natural fermentation was, therefore, impossible.

Of these beverages Pliny (XIV, XVIII, 98), commenting on the prices fetched by some wines, said

"I am not surprised therefore that many centuries ago almost innumerable kinds of artificial wine have been invented, which we will now specify, all of them being used to medicinal purposes."

He then proceeded to enumerate over 60 kinds, many of these with therapeutic indications.

Dioscorides (V, 28–83) mentioned over fifty of these "wines", but one should more justifiably place them in a category other than wines (the class of galenic tinctures of classical pharmacopoeias), since pure alcohol being as yet unknown, wine was used merely to extract the active or odoriferous substances in the plants. This property is clearly stated by Pliny

"vines having a remarkable property of drawing into themselves the flavour of some other plant." (XIV, XIX, 110)

He also added his usual dash of fiction

"Similarly in Thasos, also, hellebore is planted among the vines, or else wild cucumber or scammony; the wine so obtained is called by a Greek name denoting miscarriage, because it produces abortion." (XIV, XIX, III)

Of the genuine fruit wines, some may have been popular in Egypt: date, palm, fig and pomegranate wines.

Date Wine

The papyrus Ebers (*Eb.*, X, 28) prescribes, to cause purgation, ground senna and fruit of *mnwḥ* (?) to be put on honey and swallowed with sweet wine of dates (Grapow and Westendorf, 1958, Vol. IV, 1, p. 121). Other paragraphs of the same work mention fermented grape juice, as translated by Ebbell, a genuine date wine (e.g. *Eb.*, LXXIII, 561; *Eb.*, LXXVI, 592; *Eb.*, LXXVII, 607). In addition, date juice was very probably added to some kinds of beer to sweeten it and to assist fermentation (see Chapter 13, Beer). Date wine was also known to Babylonians who grew the richest date-palm groves in the world. It must not be confused with palm wine. Rawlinson (1881, Vol. 1, p. 26) was not justified in stating that Egyptians made date brandy, a one-time popular but now forbidden drink in Upper Egypt and in the oasis.

Of the wine, Pliny said that it was used by the Parthians and Indians and by the whole of the East, a peck of the rather soft dates called in Greek "common dates" being soaked in water and then pressed (XIV, XIX, 102). Dioscorides also mentioned it (V, 40).

Palm Wine

Until recently, it was common practice in the oases and in palm-growing areas, to tap the growing top of a date palm tree in order to gather its sweet sap (the *labke*) and offer it to honoured guests. This practice, which signed the fate of the tree, was meant to show how much more valued was the guest than years and years of date harvests. In hot weather, *labke* ferments with incredible rapidity and produces all the fun and disagreements of intoxication. It was drunk, on an unorthodox interpretation of a Koranic *surate* (The Cattle) which maintains that all products of the date-palm are without fault. The practice was slowly increasing the desolation of these areas, and aggravating the depressive effects of hot weather on human productivity. Its production and use now have been completely forbidden by the Egyptian Government.

Herodotus (II, 86) described the use of palm wine in embalming, a subject on which Diodorus (1, 91, 5) expanded

> ". . . when they [the embalmers] have gathered to treat the body . . . one of them thrusts his hand through the opening in the corpse into the trunk and extracts everything but the kidneys and heart, and another one cleanses each of the viscera, washing them in palm wine and spices . . ."

Pliny (*N.H.*, XXIV, CII, 163) recorded a strange property of palm wine as an antidote to *ophiusa*, a plant which grows at Elephantine and causes visual hallucinations of threatening serpents, the fear of which causes suicide.

However, palm wine is nowhere mentioned as being drunk for pleasure, although today it is widely appreciated in black Africa, and is sold in local markets in Nigeria and elsewhere. Its ravages are vividly painted in a description of the delirium tremens of a native addict, in a modern Nigerian novel by Tutola, entitled *The Palm Wine Drinkard.*

Fig Wine

Fig wine is mentioned in both the Pyramid Texts (*Pyr.*, 146a, T117a, N454a, Pepi II), and the Papyrus Anastase (3, 3, 5). Pliny presumably referred to it in his chapter on wines, directly after his discussion of date wine

> "Also fig syrup is made from figs by a similar process, other names for it being pharnuprium and trochis, or if it is not wanted to be sweet, instead of water is added the same quantity of grape-skin juice."

He hinted immediately afterwards at its preparation in Egypt

> "Also excellent vinegar is made from the Cyprus fig, and an even better quality as well from that of Alexandria." (XIV, XIX, 102)

Glg Wine

Glg wine is mentioned once on a potsherd found at Medinet Habu (Lichtheim, 1957, p. 60).

Pomegranate Wine: Shedeh

Pomegranate wine was one of the "fictitious" wines of Pliny (XIV, XIX, 103), and one of the fruit wines of Dioscorides (V, 34). It has been immortalized by the Song of Solomon (8, 2)

> "O that thou wert as my brother of my mother sucked the breasts . . .
> I would lead thee and bring thee into my mother's house
>   Who would instruct me
> I would cause thee to drink of spiced wine of the juices of my pomegranate."

Loret (*Fl.*, 131), because a text concerning an orchard said that it produced two kinds of fruit, grapes and pomegranates, and three beverages, wine, must, and *shedeh-it*, concluded that *shedeh* could be nothing other than pomegranate syrup or wine. Breasted called it an intoxicating drink of uncertain character (*A.R.*, IV, 213, n. c), perhaps pomegranate wine (*A.R.*, IV, 168, n. e); but Keimer (*Gpfl*, 105) thought the evidence inadequate.

Shedeh recurs in Egyptian literature. It was warned against by wise men

> "Would that thou knowest that wine is an abomination, that thou wouldst take an oath in respect to *shedeh* that thou wouldst set not thine heart on the bottle . . ." (Erman, 1966, p. 191).

However, it was among the products of Kharga and Dakhla offered by Osorkon I at Bubastis (*A.R.*, IV, 734), and among the numerous offerings of Rameses III

> "I gave *shedeh* and wine as daily offerings, I made for thee great gardens . . . bearing *shedeh* and wine in the great house of Atum." (*A.R.*, IV, 262)

Lutz remarked that it must have been an expensive beverage since it generally preceded grape-wine in wine lists.

Funeral Wines

Finally several fermented drinks are cited by Budge (1960, p. 216) without further details, as funeral wines: *Hebnet, Heten, Khenemes*.

Vinegar

It is a frustrating fact that, although Egyptians could not have ignored vinegar (the result of overfermentation of alcoholic beverages) they did not leave a single mention of this relish in any text we know, be it historical, religious, secular or medical; and yet, their wines were said to turn easily sour, and their beer could not have stayed long without turning into vinegar. Pliny (*N.H.*, XIV, XXVI) said that whole volumes had been written on how to prevent wines from turning sour, and he added that excellent vinegar was made from the Cyprus fig, and an even better quality from that of Alexandria (*N.H.*, XIV, XIX, 102–103).

Athenaeus credited the philosopher Chrysippus with saying that the best vinegar is the Egyptian and the Cnidian (2, 67, C). Apicius mentioned it as a cooking ingredient (3, 4, 3; 10, 1, 6–8) and he was not the only one to do so. Pliny mixed vinegar medicinally with two Egyptian plants: the clematis (*N.H.*, XXIV, XL, 141) as antidote against asp bites, and the Nile Valley duck weed (*N.H.*, XXIV, CV, 169), to heal wounds. Dioscorides (V, 21–25), who travelled in Egypt with Nero's armies and quoted a large number of Egyptian drugs in his work, prescribed vinegar alone or with honey, brine, thyme or squill, for an extraordinary array of diseases, ranging from anorexia to bleeding wounds, noma, phagedena, worms in the ears, mushroom poisoning, etc. It is hard to believe that all this knowledge came to Egypt only after its hellenization.

Notes: Chapter 15

1. Enderein. Name of a Syrian village.
2. In another version, she was called Rhodopis, i.e., the rosy-cheeked(*Her.*, II, 134), which was merely an epithet. Doriche was brought by a Samoan to Egypt to ply her trade, but she was redeemed for a vast sum of money by Charaxus. Thereafter, she remained in Egypt and, as she was very beautiful, amassed great wealth (*Her.*, II, 135). Herodotus doubted, however, that she could have amassed enough wealth to build a pyramid. Besides, she lived about fifteen hundred years after the pyramid was built. There was an obvious confusion with another rosy-cheeked lady, possibly Nitocris the queen with "flaxen hair and rosy cheeks", Eusebius having stated that the third pyramid had been built by Queen Nitocris of the eighth dynasty, a queen who may have had a share in the building of the monument (Rawlinson, 1885, *History of Herodotus*, Vol. II, p. 208, n. 2).
3. Probably the same poetess after whom Saphic or Lesbian love was named.

Chapter 16

Aquatic Marsh Plants

Literary sources tell us that the seeds, roots or stems of various aquatic marsh plants entered into the diet of Ancient Egyptians of the poorer classes. In view of the similarities, however, that these plants present, and of the sketchy or often contradictory descriptions furnished by ancient authors, it is extremely difficult to distinguish with certainty between them. This difficulty is compounded by differences between ancient and modern terminologies, and by the disappearance of many of these plants from general cultivation in Egypt.

Discussion of marsh plants, particularly colocasia, "Egyptian bean", and lotus, will be seen to involve considerable terminological overlap.

To take lotus as an example, we know of no plant or animal that has been the subject of more confusion, except possibly corn. Such a confusion usually indicates a long history and separate acquaintance by people who belonged to different cultures, with no fixed points of reference for comparison.

Classical mythology embraced the lotus only recently, relative to the antiquity of Egyptian history. When the Europe of nebulous Homer was just emerging from the darkness of history, the lotus had already been through a distinguished career in the Nile Valley. This was the time when Odysseus met the lotus-eaters (The Lotophagi) on his fabulous voyage to Libya.

Later, when Greek and Roman travellers emerged from their "cultural centres of the world" into the outer world, they reported that Egyptians ate lotus. Thus began the confusion, for the lotus the Egyptians were said to eat was not the magic tree upon which the Libyans fed.

In the following pages a distinction will be attempted between the different terms utilized; but it is useful to consider the following approximation suggested by examination of Greek and Roman texts:

Colocasia as used today is *Colocasia antiquorum*. In antiquity it was confused with both lotus and Egyptian bean.

The so-called Egyptian bean was probably *Nelumbium speciosum*, (*T.*, II, 374).

Sedge, as used today, constitutes a group that includes a large number of varieties of *Cyperus*, *C. esculentus*, *C. auricomus* and others.

Papyrus was always referable as *Cyperus papyrus*.

Lotus was distinctly recognized as being of three kinds: an aquatic, a herbiferous and an arboreal form. The existence of many forms of lotus was recognized at least since Homer's time since he mentioned a lotus herb, in addition to his lotus tree. The following may be distinguished:

the aquatic lotus in the sense used today and as applied only to Egypt, covers *Nymphaea lotus* and *Nymphaea coerulea*. In antiquity, in addition to the above, it covered also the Egyptian bean and colocasia;

the lotus tree, as we shall see, has been variously identified with several North African trees. There is, to our knowledge, no way of reducing this confusion in spite of the voluminous literature on the subject;

the herb lotus is an unclear entity. It could have represented one or both of *Trifolium fragiferum* or *Lotus corniculatus*.

Lotus

Aquatic Lotus

One of the plants most characteristically associated with Egypt is the (aquatic) lotus. Even the casual tourist is struck by the regularity with which this plant recurs in Egyptian art and architecture[1] and modern artists, architects and publishers utilize its delicate flower, both the white and blue varieties, as an easy and sure way of creating an Egyptian atmosphere.

Possibly because it closed its petals at night and reopened them with the rising sun, the lotus flower came to symbolize the sun and the eternal resurgence of life. At Heliopolis, where the sun was worshipped, the priests explained the origin of the world as the emergence of the god Atum—a personification of the sun—from a lotus growing out of the primordial waters, and they taught that at sunset the god entered the flower, which folded down its petals on him, and that he was reborn as the flower unfolded, morning after morning.

Thus in Egyptian mythology the lotus played as prominent a role as it did in India and the Far East. As an amulet, it signified the divine gift of eternal life. It capped the head of Nefertum (the Accomplished Beauty) who was qualified in the *Book of the Dead* (Budge, 1949, p. 595) as

". . . the lotus at the nostril of Re when he comes forth from the horizon each day."

(see Fig. 16.1). Also the deceased was often illustrated like Tut-ankh-Amon (Fig. 16.2), emerging from a lotus (Figs 16.3 and 16.4), saying

"I am the pure lotus which springeth up from the divine splendour that belongeth to the nostrils of Re." (Budge, 1949, "The Chapter of making the transformation into a lotus," p. 263)

This was an allusion to an Ancient Egyptian belief that the journey to the Other World occupied the deceased all night of the day of his death, and that he did not emerge into the realms of the blessed until the following morning at sunrise (Budge, 1949, p. LXXXVIII), a ritual embodied in another chapter of the *Book of the Dead*, the "Chapter of Coming Forth into the Day".

Thus related to the gods, the delicate beauty of the fragrant lotus decorated practically all Ancient Egyptian illustrations; it is seen in ponds and marshes (Fig. 6.7), in offerings (Volume 1, Frontispiece and Fig. 12.11), or in the hands of elegant ladies who daintily carried it to their nostrils (Fig. 16.5).

Another legend told how the lotus rose out of the "Sea of Two Knives" and, on opening, unveiled a scarab which metamorphosed into a child from whose tears sprang mankind.[2] The lotus also participated in the Horus-Seth saga, for when Seth tore out Horus's eyes, lotus flowers immediately grew out of the empty sockets and were miraculously changed into eyes (Ames, 1965, p. 73).

As a geographic symbol, the lotus represented the South, while the papyrus was the symbol of the North. Hapi, the Nile god (Fig. 2.6), was always characterized with one or both of these flowers which were often knotted as a sign of the union of the two halves of the land under one sceptre (Fig. 16.6). These omnipresent plants inspired architects

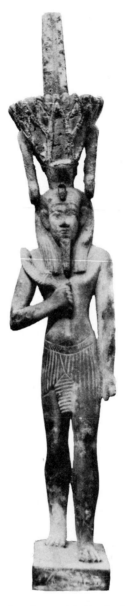

Fig. 16.1. The god Atum, bearing on his head a lotus flower. Cairo Museum.

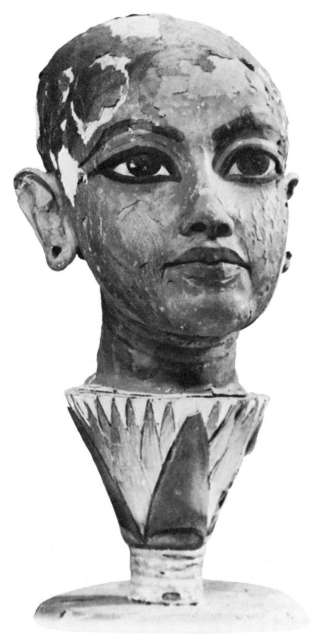

Fig. 16.2. Tut-ankh-Amon emerging out of a lotus flower. Cairo Museum.

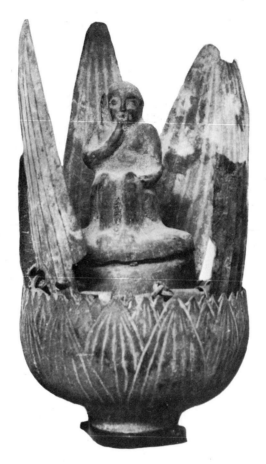

Fig. 16.3. Rebirth out of a lotus flower. Cairo Museum.

who decorated the palace of the esthete Akhenaten with their gracious lines (Fig. 16.7), and built the columns of sacred and profane buildings in their shape (Figs 16.8, 16.9), though they gave them such a conventional treatment that it is difficult at times to distinguish between the two, giving specialists matter for discussion. But in this way, buildings were seen as gardens from which these giant flowers surged, and some authors boldly contrast these representations of a vegetal world rooted in the floor of the sanctuary, with the Greek temples, whose columns were treated as actively supporting limbs of a zoomorphic structure (Helck and Otto, 1956, p. 312).

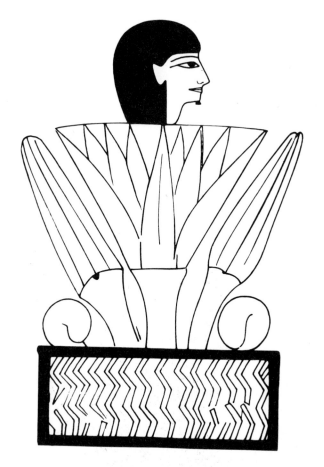

Fig. 16.4. The deceased being transformed into a lotus. Redrawn from the Papyrus of Paqrer (Budge, 1949, p. 264).

Täckholm and Drar, however, consider the flower of the South to be, not the lotus, but *Kaempferia aethiopica*, on account of some of its pictorial characteristics: its short stem, its curved blue or violet outer petals, with an inner, erect, orange, red or yellow body, and its growth on land (*T.*, IV, 150).

Another possibility they considered was that the emblem of the South was an artistic composition supposed to represent the famed "silphium"

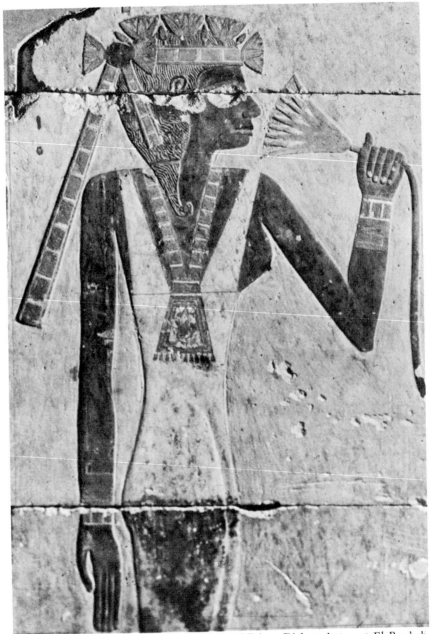

Fig. 16.5. Painted bas-relief from the tomb of Prince Djehuty-hetep at El Bersheh, detail showing a daughter of the prince holding lotus flower, *c.* 1850 B.C. Cairo Museum.

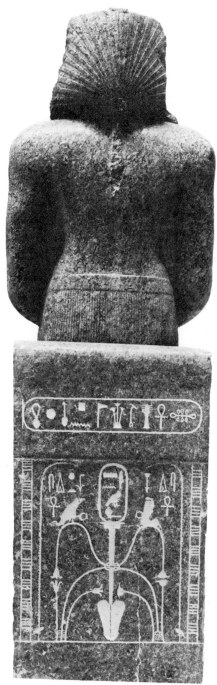

Fig. 16.6. Back of seated statue of Amenemhat I. Cairo Museum. From Tell el-Gin, near Faqus. Papyrus, emblem of the North, and lotus, emblem of the South, are united over the sign *smȝ*, made of the trachea and two lungs, that signifies "union".

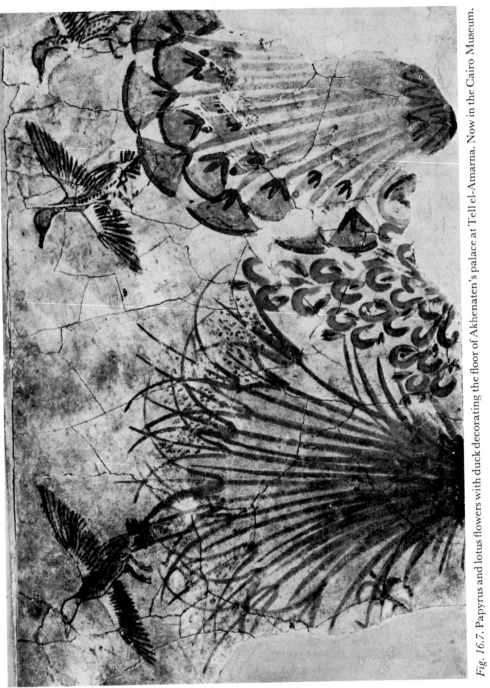

Fig. 16.7. Papyrus and lotus flowers with duck decorating the floor of Akhenaten's palace at Tell el-Amarna. Now in the Cairo Museum.

which was utilized in the Royal jubilees (the *Heb-sed*) to restore to Pharaoh his youthful vigour. In their words,

> "the outer petal-like parts may represent the opposite bracts of leaf-sheaths on a stem, and the middle orange or red part a drop of resin."

If so, the plant in question would be the famed and much discussed *silphion* of the Greeks, the *laserpitium* of the Latins, and the *hantit* or *haltit* of the Copts (*T.* IV, 149).

Confusion with Water-lily, Egyptian Bean and Corsium

Persons who are unfamiliar with aquatic plants easily fall into the error of confusing the lotus with a water-lily; confusion on this point dates back at least to Herodotus who wrote

> "... they gather the blossoms of a certain water-lily which grows in great abundance all over the flat country at the time when the Nile rises and floods the regions along its banks; the Egyptians call it the lotus. They gather, I say, the blossoms of this plant and dry them in the sun, after which they extract from the centre of each blossom a substance like the head of a poppy, which they crush and make into bread. The root of the lotus is likewise eatable, and has a pleasant sweet taste; it is round, and about the size of an apple . . ." (II, 92)

Theophrastus, however, (4, 10, 3) clearly distinguished the lotus from both the Egyptian bean and the water-lily (*sithi*). Of the water-lily he wrote

> ". . . both the flower and the leaves are good for sheep, the young shoots for pigs, and the fruit for men . . ."

He later described the lotus as a plant distinct from the Egyptian bean

> ". . . the plant called the lotus grows chiefly in the plains when the land is inundated. The character of the stalk of this plant is like that of the Egyptian Bean [Kyamon], and so are the hat-like leaves except that they are smaller and slenderer. And the fruit grows on the stalk in the same way as that of the bean. The flower is white, resembling in the narrowness of its petals those of the lily, but there are many petals, growing close one upon another. When the sun sets, these close and cover up the head, but with sunrise, they

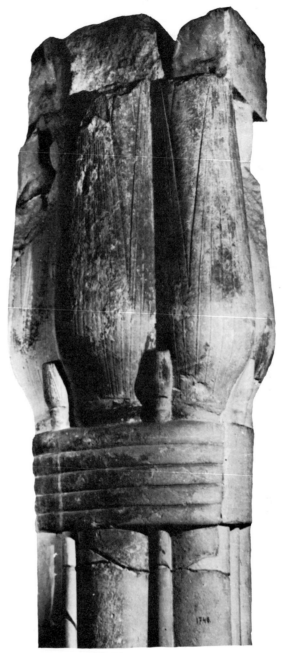

Fig. 16.8. Capitals of a column from the tomb of Ptah- Shepses at Abusir, in the shape of closed lotus buds, sixth dynasty.

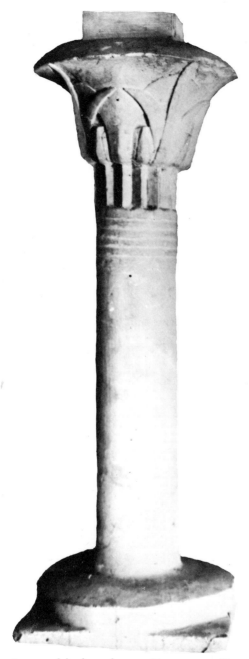

Fig. 16.9. Limestone model of a column with a campaniform capital, made of a number of lotus flowers. Dendera. Height: 42.3 cm. Cairo Museum. Cat. No. 5105.

open and appear above the water. This the plant does until the head is matured and the flowers have fallen off. The size of the head is that of the largest poppy, and it has grooves all round it in the same way as the poppy, but the fruit is set closer in these. This is like millet . . . these heads the Egyptians heap together and leave to decay, and when the pod has decayed, they wash the head in the river and take out the fruit, and having dried and pounded it, they make loaves of it which they use for food. The root of the lotus is call *korsion*, and it is round and about the size of a quince; it is enclosed in a black bark, like the shell of a chestnut. The inside is white but when it is boiled or roasted, it becomes the color of the yolk of an egg and is sweet to taste. The root is also eaten raw, though it is best when boiled in water or roasted . . ." (4, 8, 9–11)

Diodorus (1, 10, 1) differentiated between the roots of "reeds" (*kalamon*), the lotus [*loton*], the Egyptian bean, and the *corsaeum*. The latter is certainly a spelling variant of the *korsion* that Theophrastus (4, 8, 9–11) mentioned as the "root of lotus". Elsewhere Diodorus (1, 34, 6–7) also clearly distinguished the lotus from the Egyptian bean and wrote that Egyptians made from the lotus, bread which could "satisfy their physical needs".

Strabo, like Diodorus Siculus and Theophrastus before him, was aware of the confusion in identification, and clearly differentiated the Egyptian bean from *corsium* (another spelling variation) (17, 2, 4). He did not use the word lotus in his discussion, and spoke of the aquatic lotus only in reference to Aethiopia

". . . some [there] use grass as food, also tender twigs, lotus and reed-roots." (17, 2, 2)

The three- or four-fold division of lotus by Pliny will be discussed later (p. 643). This author, however, distinguished the aquatic lotus from the Egyptian bean (XIII, XXXII, 108) quoting practically verbatim Theophrastus, without giving him any credit, and sounding like one describing a new and exciting species! One passage, however, has raised an interesting question (XXII, XXXVIII, 56)

". . . we have also the lotometra, a plant derived from the lotus. From its rotted seed, which is like millet, are made by the shepherds in Egypt loaves that they knead mostly with water or milk. It is said that no bread is more healthful or lighter than this, so long as it is warm, but when cold it becomes heavy and difficult of digestion. It is an established fact that those who live on it are never attacked by dysentery, tenesmus, or any other disease of the bowels. Accordingly, it is considered to be one of the remedies for such ailments . . .''

What bread and what plant were these?

Varieties Distinguished by Colour

Thus far, the only colour mentioned in regard to lotus has been white (p. 629). Athenaeus, quoting Callixeinus, was among the first to talk of red (or rose) and blue lotus

". . . speaking of Alexandria, I know that in that fair city there is a wreath called *Antinoeios* made from the lotus bearing that name there. This grows in marshes in the summer season; there are two colours, one resembling the rose; it is from this that the wreath properly called *Antinoeios* is twined; the other is called lotus, and its colour is blue. . .'' (15, 677, D)

Athenaeus obviously thrust both red and blue lotus under one heading. There are, however, differences between the three varieties, not only in their colour, but in their meaning and in the uses to which they were put.

The white lotus, *Nywphaea lotus*, was known in Egypt at least as early as the Pyramid Era. It decorated monuments and everyday scenes, and was woven into garlands, some of which were found in thirteenth dynasty tombs, and covering mummies, like that of Rameses II (*Fl.*, 113). Its Egyptian name (a) has persisted in Hebraic *shoshan*, Coptic *shoshen*, Arabic *sousan*, and the Spanish *azucena*, all of which are the names of the lily, and gave the girl's name, Suzan. This was the edible lotus.

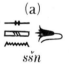

(a)

ssn

Its root, the size of a quince, is covered by a black hard skin (Pliny, *N.H.*, XIII, XXXII, 110; Dioscorides, IV, 414). Its white inner part was eaten raw, but it was much preferred boiled or roasted (*N.H.*, XIII, XXXII, 110).

Many European travellers from the sixteenth to the early nineteenth centuries testified that it was still eaten in Egypt in their time (Wönig, 1886, pp. 29–30).

The pink lotus, *Nelumbium speciosum*, named by Herodotus pink Nile lily, is believed to be the Egyptian bean (Keimer 1932). It is discussed in the following section.

The blue lotus, *Nywphaea caerulea*, was mentioned only by Athenaeus, who called it *kuaneos* (blue). This variety has been found in tombs

(b)

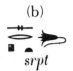

srpt

and was borne by noblemen around their necks as a decoration (Schwein-furth 1886). Its Egyptian name (b) (*Fl.*, 117), in Hebrew *sirpad* (Isaiah, LV, 13), was translated in the Septuagint, *konyza*, and in the Vulgate, *urtica* (*Fl.*, 117).

According to Ruffer (1919, p. 69) this plant almost completely disappeared in later times, and its botanical characteristics were so vaguely remembered by artists that confusion on monuments between it and *Nelumbium speciosum* (see below) became possible. It is, however, very common nowadays in the Delta, even more common than the white lotus (Täckholm, personal communication, February, 1974).

Rawlinson (1881, Vol. 1, 30), wrote, however, that the white and blue species are scarcely more than varieties, as their seeds and roots are closely similar. The Egyptians of his time, he said, distinguished between the blue and the white, preferring the blue, which they called *beshnin araby* (Arabian lotus), to the white, which they called *beshnin el khanzir* (pig's lotus). This implies a distinction similar to that made in some parts of the United States between white and yellow maize.

(c)

nḥb

Egyptian Bean (Nelumbium speciosum?)

Ancient Egyptian: see (c) (d) and (e)
Greek: *Kyamon aegyption*
Other: The pink lotus; the pink Nile lily

(d)

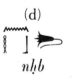

nḥb

The confusion within the immense literature on this plant makes it most unrewarding to try and sort the references to Egyptian bean, lotus and colocasia. Much of the confusion undoubtedly stemmed from the conscious or unconscious plagiarism of travellers and writers that has served to perpetuate errors in identification.

The fruit of *Nelumbium speciosum* (*kiborion*, see below) resembles in section a wasp nest, of which the holes, usually thirty, each nest a bean the size of an olive stone, containing a meaty white kernel (Fig. 16.10 and 16.11)

(e)

nšb

The first mention of what must have been the Egyptian bean appears in Herodotus (II, 92), although the father of History did not call it by this name

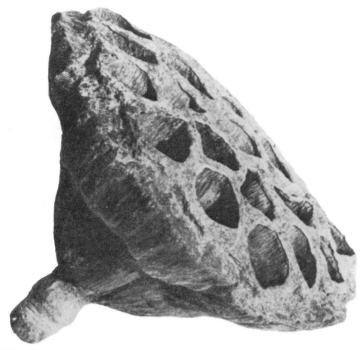

Fig. 16.10. Transversely cut fruit of *Nelumbium speciosum*. Graeco-Roman period. Dokki Agricultural Museum. C.G. 3350. Photographed 1969.

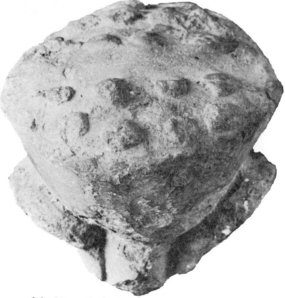

Fig. 16.11. Clay model of lotus fruit. Dokki Agricultural Museum. Cairo. Unknown period. Photographed 1969.

". . . there is also another species of lily in Egypt which grows, like the lotus, in the river, and resembles the rose. The fruit springs up side by side with the blossom on a separate stalk and has almost exactly the look of the comb made by wasps. It contains a number of seeds about the size of an olive stone which are good to eat; and these are eaten both green and dry . . ."

The following are worthy of note: Herodotus gave the colour of the flower as rose; he did not compare the seeds with beans, as did later writers; and he did not assign it a Greek name, an indication that he had not previously seen it in his native land.

As to the term Egyptian bean *kyamon aegyption*, it first appeared about a hundred years later and came then into general use in texts on Egypt. Theophrastus (4, 8, 7–8) gave the first complete description of the plant and its many uses

". . . but the Egyptian bean [*Kyamos*] grows in the marshes and lakes; the length of its stalk at longest is four cubits, it is as thick as a man's finger, and resembles a plain reed without joints. Inside it has tubes which run distinct from one another right through like a honey-comb; on this is set the head which is like a round wasps' nest, and in each of the cells is a bean [*kyamos*] which slightly projects from it; at most there are thirty of these. The flower is twice as large as a poppy's, and the colour is like a rose, of a deep shade; the head is above the water. If one of the beans is crushed, you find the bitter substance coiled up, of which the *pilos* is made. So much for the fruit. The root is thicker than the thickest reed, and is made up of distinct tubes, like the stalk. They eat it both raw, boiled, and roasted, and the people of the marshes make this their food. It mostly grows of its own accord; however, they also sow it in the mud, and if the plant once takes hold it is permanent. For the root is strong and not unlike that of reeds, except that it is prickly on the surface. Wherefore the crocodile avoids it, lest he may strike his eye on it, since he has not sharp sight . . ."

This appears to be the "type" discussion drawn on by other writers who had not seen the plant, but who, nevertheless, wrote with great authority on the plants and foods in Egypt.

Three centuries after Theophrastus, Diodorus (1, 10, 1) detailed an account he had heard from the priests of Egypt, of how man and food came into existence in the Nile Valley. This account clearly differentiated between the Egyptian bean and the lotus

". . . when in the beginning the universe came into being, men first came into existence in Egypt, both because of the favourable climate of the land and because of the nature of the Nile. For this stream, since it produces much life and provides a spontaneous supply of food, easily supports whatever living things have been engendered; for both the root of the reed and the lotus [*loton*], as well as the Egyptian bean [*aegytion kyamon*] and *corsaeum* [Korsaion], as it is called, and many other similar plants, supply the race of men with nourishment all ready for use . . ."

This four-fold breakdown into reed, lotus, Egyptian bean and corsaeum is interesting, for it underlines the non-identity of the lotus of Diodorus with the Egyptian bean. Elsewhere (1, 34, 6–7), Diodorus described the pod that held these beans

". . . and the ciborium [Kiborion], which is found in great abundance, bears what is called the Egyptian bean . . ."

Strabo was a contemporary of Diodorus; they visited Egypt within fifty years of each other, but there is no evidence that they ever met. Strabo, like Diodorus, distinguished between the "Egyptian" and the "Greek" beans

". . . the Aegyptian bean [*aegyptios kyamos*] from which comes the ciborium . . . the bean [*kyamos*] produces leaves and flowers in many parts, and also a fruit like our bean,[3] differing only in size and taste." (17, 1, 15)

Approximately 100 years after Strabo, Pliny, in the middle of a discussion on leguminous plants, in particular on *Vicia faba*, inserted an "excursus" on this riddle plant

". . . it [the bean] also grows in Egypt where it has a thorny stalk which makes the crocodiles keep away from it for fear of injuring their eyes. The stalk is two yards long at most and the thickness of a finger; if it had knots in it, it would be like a soft reed; it has a head like a poppy, is rose-coloured, and bears not more than thirty beans on each stalk; the leaves are large; the actual fruit is bitter even in smell, but the root is a very popular article of diet with the natives, and is eaten raw and cooked in every sort of way: it resembles the roots of reeds. [The Egyptian bean] also grows in Syria and Cilicia . . ." (N.H., XVIII, XXX, 121–122)

In this passage, obviously gleaned from Theophrastus (4, 8, 7–8), Pliny was distinctly describing the Egyptian bean, its colour, stalk, head, leaves and fruit, which clearly distinguish it from *Vicia faba*.

Athenaeus similarly discussed Egyptian bean in several passages, in the longest of which (*Deipnos.*, 3, 72, B–D) he freely quoted Theophrastus, giving him the credit that Pliny failed to give. On the authority of Nicander, he also wrote (*Deipnos.*, 3, 72, A)

"Tubers also to boil and serve at the festival banquet . . ."

clarifying this passage by the following remark

"... by tubers, Nicander means what the Alexandrians call colocasia."

As the same author says

"... peeling and shredding the colocasium from its bean ... and in Sicyon, there is a shrine of Athena Colocasia." (3, 72, B)

This invites a discussion of what plant the Greek authors really meant by colocasia.

Colocasia and the Egyptian Bean

The word "colocasia" appeared first in Dioscorides and Pliny, who seem to have originated the present confusion. In Egypt, said Pliny

"the most famous of wild plants used for food is colocasia called by some cyamos [bean]." (*N.H.*, XXI, LI, 87)

He thus specifically called by the name colocasia a plant that others called a bean. Yet, he did not use in this passage Latin *faba* for bean but the Greek *cyamos*, although earlier (*N.H.*, XVIII, XXX, 122) he had stated that *faba* was grown in Egypt, and attributed to it all the characteristics of the Egyptian bean.

As stated previously, Athenaeus (*Deipnos.*, 3, 72, A–B) identified colocasium with the Egyptian bean

"... the tuber known as *colocasium* belonging to the *Egyptian bean* ..."

and he further differentiated the latter from the lotus (*Diepnos.*, 3, 73, A–B).

Regarding the geographic "uniqueness' of the Egyptian bean, Athenaeus quoted Phylarchus who asserted

"... never before, in any region, had Egyptian beans been sown or, if they were, did they grow except in Egypt." (*Deipnos.*, 3, 73, B)

Athenæus later qualified this statement by saying that some had been grown in Epeirus and at Aedepsus.

This, then, is the evidence on which identification must be made. Three distinct parts of this enigmatic plant were taken as food: the root, the stalk and the seeds. In Roman times, the root was called colocasia, an appellation that was responsible for mistaken identification with *Colocasia antiquorum* (see Chapter 17). The stem remained nameless, but most authors indicated that it was eaten or chewed, as is done with sugar cane today. The pod containing the beans was named ciborium; but the root was the prized portion of the plant, not the bean which was constantly qualified as bitter and was sometimes cursorily dismissed.

The exception to this is the quotation of Athenaeus (3, 72, A) given on p. 638, which, however, is far from being inambiguous. An interesting point is that in none of the passages quoted in this section is the root called corsium, the name under which the root of the lotus was known later. Indeed, both Diodorus and Strabo clearly differentiated corsium from the Egyptian bean.

As to the way in which the confusion arose, Candolle (1886, p. 318) explained it by assuming that the word *kyamos* (bean) originally meant *Vicia faba*; but when the Greeks came to Egypt, they coined the term "Greek bean" to dissipate any confusion between it (*Vicia faba*) and the "bean" they found in Egypt [*Nelumbo nucifera*] and related species.

The misunderstanding about colocasia aroused by Greek authors puzzled all subsequent writers. Thus, Abdaltalif al-Baghdady (1965, p. 51) applied to colocasia what Dioscorides said of the Egyptian bean, that he concluded from his observations to be Egyptian ginger

"According to Dioscorides, this plant has a rose coloured flower. When the fruit begins to form, it is an embryo in the shape of a pouch which one would call a bubble of water, and which contains a broad bean smaller than the Greek bean: on the top of it are seeds. When they should sow the plant, they take this bean and place it in a lump of earth and throw it in water, where it germinates. Dioscorides mentioned that it could be eaten fresh and dry. They can make from it a fine flour, to be drunk in a *tisane*. He says, too, they can make from it a soup which helps to fortify the bowels and intestines to keep them from diarrhoea and dysentery. The green seeds in the centre of the bean have a bitter taste and, being reduced to powder and mixed with oil and dropped in the ear, relieves earache."

Al-Baghdady proceeded to refute the opinion of Israili, a famous Cordoban author of the Islamic period

"Israili said: 'We have never seen the flower of the colocasia'. He added: 'I saw this plant being kept in the houses, and when the time of vegetation comes, there appear several shoots from the bean, which is adhering, and it germinates without producing either flowers or fruit. The colour of the bean itself is pink, but when it produces its seed and commences to shoot, the reproductive part which comes out from the plant is of a beautiful white colour, covered with a slight tint of pink.' He said: 'We could not find this bean dry to the point where one could make flour from it: we found throughout the year it is always fresh like the bulb of narcissus and that of saffron or other similar'. He also said, 'We have not seen in the centre of it the green colour mentioned by Dioscorides: to us it has appeared, at all times of the year, constantly, like a green banana.' . . . I say then by conjecture taken from observation and hearing, that the colocasia is the Egyptian ginger . . ." (1965, p. 53)

The same perplexity was felt by the knowledgeable French traveller Belon who wrote, in the sixteenth century A.D.

"And because this 'Colocasse' is also called lotus and Egyptian bean, after we found that it served nothing to search diligently for its seeds and even that the people of Cairo mocked us for our search wishing to imply that it had none, we had the opportunity of asking why the ancient authors called it the Egyptian bean, well knowing that it produces no beans. We maintain that it grows around the brooks of Crete, for we found it there growing wild, whereas the Egyptians cultivate it with industry. Finally, we discovered the source of the error. This is that Herodotus spoke of two kinds of herbs growing in the Nile. One bears the round root that is 'Colocasse', the other bears in its head something like olive stones. The authors who followed him, copying one another said of them whatever they liked. For although Theophrastus said that its root is spiny, it is otherwise. Dioscorides made nearly the same statements as Theophrastus, and Pliny having translated from them, made identical assertions. This is the reason why we are of the opinion that by Faba Egyptia we mean the true edible beans born in Egypt. Even Galen seems to us to have understood [thereby] common beans when, in the book on foods, he talks of the beans of Egypt. And to clarify what Pliny said, namely, that the Egyptians make various kinds of vessels with its leaves one must understand that these leaves are broad, and that the Egyptians twist them into cones in order to draw and drink Nile water for, after having drunk, they throw them away." (author's translation from: Sauneron, 1970, p. 99b)

The Pink Lotus in Ancient Egyptian Art

An intriguing facet of the pink lotus is that, unlike many animals and plants that profusely illustrated the tombs, the pink lotus was omitted in the Dynastic Period, although Michelangelo chose it as a symbol of Egypt in his monument to the Nile in the Vatican. Schweinfurth (1883) pointed to this absence of the flower from monuments preceding the

Ptolemaic Period. Keimer (1932) commenting on the fact, stated that it came to Egypt from India under the Persian rule; but Wönig (1886, pp. 44–50) who described its leaves as a decoration of the Graeco-Roman temple of Esnah, did not agree with this view.

Nowadays, the plant no longer grows wild in Egypt, and the ecological and climatic reasons for its disappearance have been the subject of lengthy discussions (Wönig, 1886, pp. 45, 46).

According to Loret (*Fl.*, 111), it is on account of its sacred associations that this flower did not appear in profane illustrations. He further asserted that the kind of beans that were, according to Greek authors forbidden to priests, were the fruits of this sacred plant, not those of *Vicia faba*, since the latter were not only found in tombs, but were often prescribed medically (pp. 682–685), and were offered in huge quantities, e.g. by Rameses III to the Theban priests (see *A.R.*, IV, 350). This would also be a creditable reason why the fruit of the pink lotus (Egyptian bean) has never been found in tombs.

The Lotus Tree

". . . for nine long days we were pounded by the howling gale through the teeming sea-water, but on the tenth we reached the land of the Lotus-eaters, who feast on fruit. We went ashore and found water and made a meal beside the swift ships. Then I chose two men and another to act as their herald, and sent them to find what kind of men took their nourishment there. They went, but we got no word from them, for the Lotus-eaters had received them kindly and served them the honeyed fruit of the lotus to eat, a meal, which deprived them of any desire to return or send word. They were content to stay with the Lotus-eaters, consuming the luscious fruit and forgetful of home, but I brought them back to the ships by force, three weeping men, tied them up and dragged them beneath the benches low in the hull. Quickly I ordered the rest of my trusty friends to board the swift ships, lest someone else should happen to eat of the lotus and forget about home." Homer (*Odyssey*, 9, 84–96)

One of the first writers to discuss the lotus tree after Homer was Herodotus (IV, 177), when talking of a people of Libya, whom he was the only writer to mention, and whose geographic habitat remains an open question

. . . a promontory jutting out into the sea from the country of the Gin-
danes is inhabited by the Lotus-eaters who live entirely on the fruit of
the lotus tree. The lotus fruit is about the size of the lentisk berry, and in
sweetness resembles the date. The Lotus-eaters even succeeded in obtaining
from it a sort of wine . . .''

Was that wine the magic medium that made the men of Odysseus wish
to forsake their homes?

Theophrastus (4, 3, 1–2) wrote extensively on this tree and tried to
define the habitat of the ''lotophagi''

". . . in Libya the lotus is most abundant and fairest; as to the lotus, the
whole tree is peculiar, of good stature, as tall as a pear-tree, or nearly so;
the leave is divided and like that of the Kermes-oak, and the wood is
black. There are several sorts, which differ in their fruits; the fruit is as
large as a bean, and in ripening like grapes it changes its colour; it grows,
like myrtle-berries, close together on the shoots; to eat, that which grows
among the people called Lotus-eaters is sweet, pleasant, and harmless, and
even good for the stomach; but that which has no stone is pleasanter, and
they also make wine from it. The tree is abundant and produces much
fruit; thus the army of Ophellas[4] when it was marching on Carthage, was
fed, they say, on this alone for several days, when the provisions ran short.
It is abundant also in the island called the island of the Lotus eaters; this
lies off the mainland at no great distance; it grows, however, in no lesser
quantity, but even more abundantly on the mainland; for, as has been
said, this tree is common in Libya. . .; for in the islands called Euesperides[5]
they use these trees as fuel. However this lotus differs from that found in
the land of the Lotus-eaters . . .''

Theophrastus thus recognized that several kinds of trees bore the
name lotus, and, in another passage (4, 3, 4) he further described a
different variety, but, most of all, he realized that plants, other than
trees, were also called lotus

". . . some plants are found in several forms which have almost the same
name, for instance, the lotus; for of this there are many forms differing
in leaves, stems, flowers, and fruit, including the plant called melilotus.''
(7, 15, 3)

Pliny (*N.H.*, XIII, XXXII, 104–106) gave a lengthy description of
the lotus tree that grows in Africa, stressing its varieties, which differ
chiefly in their fruits, its value as food, its procuring oblivion, its sto-
machic properties, and its source of a wine that does not keep well.

He did not attach a specific label to the tree, however, and, according to Jones (1956, Vol. 7, p. 518), his text represented a confusion between two different species, *Zizyphus lotus*, the Jew's thorn, and *Celtis australis*, the nettle tree.

Elsewhere, in a discussion on "artificial" wines, Pliny (XIV, XIX, 101) differentiated between wines brewed from the lotus tree, the lotus shrub, and herbaceous lotus. In addition, he mentioned the marsh lotus in another context (XIII, XXXII, 107) thus apparently recognizing four groups to which the term lotus was applied.

This makes it difficult to understand another passage (*N.H.*, XXIV, II, 6) where he speaks of an Egyptian plant called lotus, sometimes known as the tree-of-Syrtes (*Syrticam arborem*). The berries of this tree, he added

"which by our countrymen is called the Greek bean [*Faba graeca*] check looseness of the bowels . . ."

Jones (1956, p. 6, note b) noted, however, the possibility that *Syriacam* was meant instead of *Syrtican* and that the passage referred to *faba Syriaca*.

Modern writers have had little success in attributing to these plants generic and specific names. Rawlinson (*Her.*, II, 96, note 9) commented that in the following passage concerning the Libyan lotus

". . . the *acantha*, a tree which in its growth is very like the Cyrenaic lotus . . ."

Herodotus meant the modern *Mimosa nilotica* (Pliny's *spina egypti*, *N.H.*, XIII, XX, 68). As to the Cyrenaic lotus which it was said to resemble, he identified it as probably being *Acacia gummifera* (Arabic *tulh*). This, he thought, was different from the lotus of the lotophagi (*Her.*, II, 96, note 9) which, he suggested, was either *Rhamnus zizyphus* or *Cordia myxa*, but more likely the former (*Her.*, IV, 177, note 7).

Such "authoritative" identifications are numerous in modern literature and it would be uninformative and too cumbersome to list them all. It is evident, however, that the lotus tree is not a single genus or species, but a term applied to a variety of indigenous woody trees found in the desert, i.e. coastal regions of Egypt, and westward into Libya and Tunisia; trees which provided food for desert travellers throughout much of ancient and modern history, whose nature has been confused through misidentification of mythological and historical references, and that continue to be fascinating, but obscure.

The Lotus Herb (Trifolium fragiferum? or Lotus corniculatus?)

In four separate passages, Pliny distinguished a herbal form of the lotus

> ". . . but the same name also belongs to a herbaceous plant . . ." (*N.H.,* XIII, XXXII, 107)
> ". . . it has already been stated where the varieties [of wine] brewed from the lotus-tree, lotus-shrub, and herbaceous lotus are made . . ." (*N.H.,* XIV, XIX, 101)
> ". . . Crepis and lotus have a foliated stem . . ." (*N.H.,* XXI, LIX, 99)

and lastly

> ". . . those who think that the lotus is only a tree can be refuted even by the authority of Homer who among the plants that grow up to serve the pleasure of the Gods, mentions the lotus first. Its leaves with honey cause to disappear scars on the eyes, films on the eyes, and argema . . ." (*N.H.,* XXII, XXVII, 55)

No other writer that has come to our attention discusses the "herbaceous-lotus", and the identification, use, and translation of this form of "lotus" is not evident.

Papyrus (Cyperus papyrus)

(f)

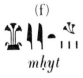

mḥyt

Egyptian: *mḥyt*: see (f)
Greek: *byblos*

"If the lotus is the poetic present of the Nile, the papyrus is the practical gift of the Holy Stream." (Wönig, 1886, p. 74)

The papyrus of Egypt, now found only in gardens and in the Upper Nile marshes, was so typical of the country landscape that it symbolized

Lower Egypt. Its picture and the ideogram (g), a stylized form of the papyrus plant, entered into the composition of several hieroglyphic words connected with the Delta marshes, such as (h), the Delta town of Chemmis, (i), Lower Egypt, and (j), the Crown of Lower Egypt (*G*. 481).

(g)

mḥ

Its use as an article of food was first reported by Herodotus (II, 92)

> ". . . the byblos which grows year after year in the marshes they pull up, and cutting the plant into two, reserve the upper portion for other purposes but take the lower which is about a cubit long, and either eat it or sell it. Such as wish to enjoy the byblos in full perfection bake it first in a closed vessel heated to a glow . . ."

(h)

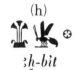

ꜣḫ-bit

Its main use, however, was to prepare writing material. The word "paper" comes from the Greek name of this material *papyrus*, which is supposed to stem from the Egyptian word *papuro*, meaning the Royal, paper being a State monopoly. A variety of papyrus recently discovered growing wild in Wadi Natrun has been utilized by H. Ragab, the founder of the Papyrus Institute to manufacture papyrus sheets according to old formulae.

(i)

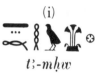

tꜣ-mḥw

On the other hand, the Greek name, Byblos, of the old trading harbour of Jebeil on the Lebanese coast (Biblical *Gebal*; Ancient Egyptian *Kubna*), goes back at least to Mycaenian times; and it gave its name in Greek to the papyrus plant, *byblos*, from the fact that it was the harbour exporting to the Aegean. The name of that city later gave rise to a prestigious progeny of words connected with books; bibliography, bibliophile, and of course, the Bible.

(j)

mḥ-s

This material, tightly packed together, was made into the light boats that one sees depicted on the walls of graves riding the shallow marshes (Figs 6.12 and 6.13). Stronger sea-sailing boats could, however, be made, as the recent transatlantic expedition of the barge of Ra proved: although these boats could not stand too lengthy marine voyages.

Theophrastus writing of this plant said

> "the most familiar to foreigners are the papyrus rolls made of it; but above all, the plant is also of very great use in the way of food. For all the natives chew the papyrus[6] both raw, boiled, and roasted; they swallow the juice and spit out the quid . . ." (4, 8, 4)

Diodorus (1, 80, 5) remarked on the diet of Egyptian children

> ". . . they give them such stalks as the byblos plant as can be roasted in the coals, and the roots and stems of marsh plants, either raw or boiled or baked . . ."

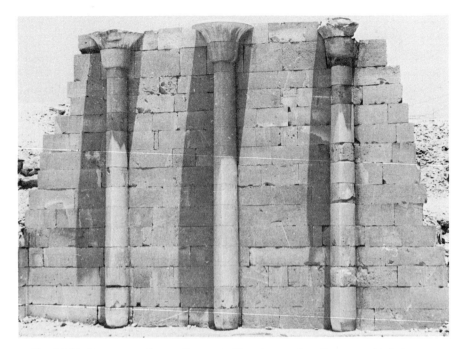

Fig. 16.12. Open papyriform pilasters in Zoser's complex. Saqqara, third dynasty.

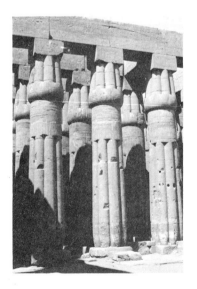

Fig. 16.13. Closed papyriform columns. Temple of Luxor. Centre of Documentation. Cairo.

Pliny (*N.H.*, XIII, XXII, 72) expanded on the varied utilization of this plant without too much reliance on Theophrastus

". . . papyrus then grows in the swamps of Egypt or else in the sluggish waters of the Nile where they have overflown and lie stagnant in pools not more than three feet in depth . . . the roots are employed by the natives for timber and not only to serve as firewood but also for making various utensils and vessels; indeed the papyrus itself is plaited to make boats, and the inner bark is woven into sail-cloth and matting, and also cloth, as well as blankets and ropes. It is also used as chewing-gum both in the raw state and when boiled, though only the juice is swallowed . . ."

Later, Pliny mentioned the plant in connection with paper, giving at the same time, an insight into the possible origin of the medical use of laminaria

"a plant growing in Egypt, the papyrus, which, when it has been dried is especially useful for expanding and drying fistulae and, by swelling, for opening them to admit medicaments. The paper made from it is, when burnt, one of the caustic remedies.[7] Its ash, taken in wine, induces sleep. The plant, itself, applied with water, cures callosities." (*N.H.*, XXIV, LI, 88)

In tomb and temple illustrations, bundles of papyrus characterized by their bell-shaped tops and their gracile, long stems, represented the marshland of the West where Hathor received the deceased on their way to the Amenti, the eternal abode of the setting sun (Fig. 3.3). In temples, stone imitations of this plant built as a structural, albeit ornamental architectonic element (see p. 624) illustrate how artistic conservatism perpetuated its earlier utilization in an architecture built on wood.

It is significant, for example, that Imhotep's master work, the Saqqara complex he built for his master Zoser (*c.* 2700 B.C.), featured attached papyriform pilasters (Fig. 16.12). Later, pillars with capitals imitating papyrus buds supported the roofs of many temples, the most handsome being perhaps those of the temple of Luxor, built during the eighteenth to nineteenth dynasties (Fig. 16.13).

Medicinally, papyrus was used in external applications (*Eb.*, LXVII, 482), and the magic "Incantations for Mother and Child" recommended

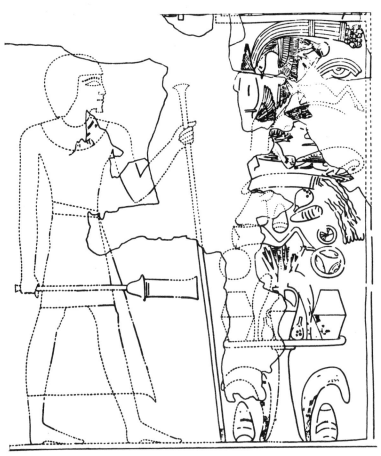

Fig. 16.14. Cyperus esculentus (in the middle of the offerings, to the right). Tomb of Mentuherkhepeshef. From Davies, 1918, plate V.

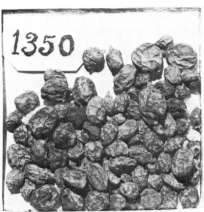

Fig. 16.15. Cyperus esculentus. Deir el Medineh. New Kingdom. Dokki Agricultural Museum, Cairo. No. 1350. photographed 1969

the uttering of one of its spells over papyrus stalks and carob (?) powdered in the "milk of a woman who had borne a male child" (*Zaub.*, I, 7, 3–5). In Pliny's time, as already stated, it was used in the same way as laminaria today and, after calcination, as a caustic remedy.

Sedges

Cyperus esculentus

Egyptian: see (k) (*Wb Dr.*, 536; *Fl.*, 27)
Arabic: *Hab'el ǎziz* (the precious grain, or the grain of the precious).

(k)

gyw

Cyperus esculentus is characterized by a system of hair-like fibrous roots bearing rounded or ovoid tubers, about half an inch in diameter. These tubers, at times wrongly called fruits or grains, are very nutritious, on account of their richness in carbohydrate, protein and fat.

C. esculentus has been known in Egypt at least since the fifth millenium B.C., in Tasian and Mostagedda times (Brunton, 1937); and Täckholm and Drar (*T.*, II, 61) believe that it was the most ancient foodstuff in Ancient Egypt, after emmer and barley. It is illustrated in many tombs (Fig. 16.14) and Netolitzki (1911, p. 42) even discovered it in the intestinal contents of pre-dynastic bodies. Specimens have been found in many sites (Schweinfurth, 1885, 1886, 1887), and are on show at the Agricultural Museum of Dokki, Cairo (Fig. 16.15). If the interpretation of the word *šny-t* be correct, it was one of the products that the Eloquent Peasant carried from his distant oasis to sell in the valley (Lefebvre, 1949, p. 48).

Egyptologists do not quite agree, however, on the Egyptian name of the plant. Whereas *gyw* is the usually accepted term designating it, the Ebers papyrus (*Eb.*, IX, 20) mentions a medicine it calls

"grains of *mnwh* also called *šnw-t* ".

Mnwḫ is a plural form of *mnh*, papyrus, or sedge, i.e. a *Cyperus*. As *Cyperus esculentus* develops long subterranean hair-like rhizomes on which grow globular tubercles, Loret (1935–1938) concluded that the identity of the "grains of *mnwḫ*" and, therefore, of earth's hair (*šnw-t*), was *C. esculentus*. Lefebvre agreed to this identification (1956, p. 122), while Ebbell proposed colocynth (*Eb.*, X, 28), and Dawson (1926), on the basis of the similarity of medical indications, favoured *Trigonella faenum graecum*.

Greek authors mentioned several plants that have been identified with *C. esculentus*. Thiselton-Dyer equated it with two distinct terms mentioned by Theophrastus; *malinathalle* (Theophrastus, 4, 8, 12) and *mnasion* (4, 8, 2 and 6) (see Hort 1916, p. 489). Pliny certainly took directly from him his description of anthalium that most classicists identify with *malinathalle* (*N.H.*, XXI, LII, 88; XXI, CII, 175). The equation of *anthalium* with *C. esculentus* has been obscured, however, by the resemblance of the first word to anthyllium (or anthyllum), the Cretan pitch-plant, *Cressa cretica*.

Whatever the correctness of these identifications, Theophrastus related that *malinathalle* was boiled in barley beer and then eaten as a sweetmeat (4, 8, 12); and Pliny, that *anthalium* was a food, but that he had been unable to find any other use for it (*N.H.*, XXI, CIII, 175).

Medically, the Ancient Egyptians prescribed it in various forms: in mixtures (*Eb.*, VI, 19; VII, 23; XIII, 83; *H.*, 46, 80); mouth "chews" (*Eb.*, XV, 101); enemata (*Eb.*, XCVI, 820); ophthalmic applications (*Eb.*, LX, 382); ointments (*Eb.*, LXXIII, 563; *H.*, 228); dressings (*Eb.*, LXVI, 472; *H.*, 232), or fumigations, to sweeten the smells of houses and clothes, together with myrrh, incense, etc. (*Eb.*, XCVIII, 852).

Persistence of the Cultivation of C. esculentus

The cultivation of this plant in Egypt has continued to the present day; and from Egypt, the Arabs spread its cultivation to North Africa, Sicily and Spain, where it is made into a refreshing drink, *orchata de chufa*. In Egypt as well as being directly consumed, especially at the *mowled* (birthday festival) of Sheikh el Badawi at Tanta, this tuber yields oil, and the residues are used as fodder.

Sari: Saripha

Another edible sedge may be the plant called by Theophrastus *sari* (4, 8, 5) and Pliny *saripha* (*N.H.*, XIII, XLV, 128). This plant has been tentatively identified as either *Cyperus fastigiatus* or *C. comosus* by Loret (*Fl.*, 30), and as *C. auricomus* by Thiselton-Dyer in his notes to the Theophrastus translation (Hort, 1916, Vol. II, p. 475).

Theophrastus wrote

"the *sari* grows in the water in the marshes and plains when the river has left them; it has a hard twisted root, and from it grow what they call the saria; these are about two cubits long and as thick as a man's thumb; this stalk too is three cornered like the papyrus and has similar foliage. This also they chew, spitting out the quid; and smiths use the root, for it makes most excellent charcoal, because the wood is hard . . ."

One can only be further amazed at Pliny (*N.H.*, XIII, XLV, 128)

"the saripha growing on the banks of the Nile also belongs to the shrub class: it is about three feet high and the thickness of a man's thumb; its foliage is that of the papyrus, and it is chewed in a similar manner. The root is highly rated in workshops for use as fuel, because of its hardness."

Notes: Chapter 16

1. Such decoration will be immediately visible to the reader in many of the figures in this work, e.g. Figs 3.3, 6.12, 6.13, 7.5, etc.
2. The result of a pun using *rmwt*, tears and *rmt*, mankind.
3. Though the same word *kyamos* is used, "our bean" is the Greek bean, *Vicia faba*.
4. An army leader from Cyrene in Libya.

5. Nowadays: Benghazi according to Rawlinson (1885, Vol. III, p. 145, n. 4).
6. A habit, similar to the present day custom of chewing peeled sugar cane.
7. This may have meant that burning papyrus was applied as a cautery. On the other hand, it is still believed in the Near East that cigarette ash added to alcoholic drinks, considerably strengthens their soporific action.

Chapter 17   *Vegetables and Legumes*

*"My Majesty made for him a garden
anew in order to present to him
vegetables and all beautiful flowers"*
Offerings of Thutmose III to Amon Ra (*A.R.*, II, 161)

"One hundred loaves . . . ten bundles of vegetables" (*A.R.*, III, 77).
These were the offerings of Rameses I to the gods, to thank them for
the victory they granted him, yet this was indeed a poor donation when
compared with Rameses III's munificence

". . . 2,170 measures of vegetables, 770,200 bundles of vegetables . . ."
(*A.R.*, IV, 243)

Such were the royal gifts to the gods. On an earthly level, an unusual
report attributed to King Horemheb (nineteenth dynasty, *c.* 1341–
1320 B.C.) tells of predecessors under whom the officials plundered the
poor, taking the best of their vegetables, allegedly as royal taxes (*A.R.*,
III, 59). Another reference to daily life credited Seti I with increasing
the daily allowance of the army to "vegetables without limit," providing
each man with two bundles of vegetables daily (*A.R.*, III, 207). Clearly,
vegetables were regarded as prestigious foods by the Ancients.

The Greek contrasted vegetables with "legumes". But their legumes
did not embrace all of the species included today under this category.
One thus sees the difficulty of being precise regarding the "legume-
taboo" mentioned in some texts, a type of problem discussed elsewhere
in this work. Two statements of Plutarch illustrate this puzzling in-
consistency. In one, he stated that in the month of Mesore (August–
September), legumes were brought to the god Harpocrates (*I. and O.*,
378, 68). In the other, that the priests abstained from most legumes
(*I. and O.*, 353, 5).

Legumes certainly were not avoided in Ptolemaic times. Around 70–50 B.C. a decree forbade, under penalty of death and under any pretext, carrying grain bought in Upper Egypt to Lower Egypt or to the Thebaid (*S.P.*, II, 209).

Nor was there any stigma attached to the production of legumes in Rome, where the names of the patrician families Fabius, Lenticulus and Cicero, stemmed from ancestors who produced the best crops of beans (*faba*), lentils (*lens*), and chick-peas (*cicer*) in their districts (*N.H.*, XVIII, III, 10); and this attitude would, no doubt, have prevailed with the Romans in Egypt. The following excerpt from a will of the Roman Period that includes legumes in the legacy confirms their acceptability

". . . whatever I may leave in the way of furniture . . . legumes . . ." (*S.P.*, I, 84)

From evidence available it appears, therefore that a blanket taboo was not applied to legumes in general, and that such avoidance as may have been practised was kept only at certain times of the year or periods of history, and concerned certain legumes only. We should therefore consider individually the vegetables and legumes.

Tuberous and Root Vegetables

Beet

There is no evidence that beat was grown in Ancient Egypt. Candolle, without giving any supporting citation, believed that its exploitation started three to four centuries before Christ. The sole reference to beet in antiquity that has come to our attention is in a papyrus of uncertain date, seemingly within the Greek era, that mentions beet being among vegetables grown in funerary gardens by Greek residents in Egypt (Lindsay, 1966 p. 298). In addition, Täckholm and Drar (*T.*, II, 374) thought that the *aron* of Pliny (*N.H.*, XIX, XXX, 3) possibly could be beet or turnip.

Colocasia antiquorum

Arabic: *qolqas*
Greek: ? *vingon, and aron*
Coptic: *pikorkasi*

> *Everything comes by chance, save qolqas, which requires tilling*
> *and watering*
> (Popular maxim)

To avoid confusion with the Egyptian bean discussed in Chapter 16 this plant is referred to in this section by its Arabic name *qolqas*. This aroid is known in temperate areas as the ornamental "elephant's-ear". A related aroid, *C. esculenta*, is grown in many tropical areas for its starchy root-stock and is widely termed *taro*.

Qolqas is a corm that probably originated in India from whence it spread . . . southeastward to Java, Ceylon, etc., and westward to Madagascar and East Africa (*T.*, II, 368). It must have reached Egypt through one of the two traditional routes of penetration of foreign plants into Egypt, Syria or Arabia. The former is the more likely because qolqas, as a vegetable, is only a recent newcomer to Arabia, whereas the Syriac language possesses a cognate word, *qalqas*, designating a plant.

Herodotus mentioned no plant that resembles qolqas. The only reference encountered in Greek literature may be a short discussion in Theophrastus (1, 6, 11) of a plant which, he said, was called in Egypt *uingon*

> "its leaves are large, and its shoots short, while the root is long and is, as it were, the fruit. It is an excellent thing and is eaten."

Despite the insufficiency of this characterization, Thiselton-Dyer translated *uingon* as colocasia (*in* Hort, 1916, p. 488).

On the other hand, Theophrastus described two kinds of *aron*, but these are usually referred to by botanists as aroids rather than qolqas. He did comment on an "edible aron" that had "no stem at all nor a flower". This seemed interesting to Täckholm and Drar (*T.*, II, 373) because of the failure of most varieties of qolqas to flower even under the best conditions. These authors added, however, that the two arons of Theophrastus both flower and set seed freely. As Theophrastus did not say where the sterile aron grew, they found his remark insufficient for an exact determination of its nature. Pliny described an aron (*N.H.*, XIX, XXX, 3) resembling qolqas, but Täckholm and Drar believed it to refer to beet or turnip (*T.*, II, 374).

On the other hand, the word *qolqas* is similar enough to *colocasion* to have been derived from it; but Täckholm (*T.*, II, 376) thought the derivation unlikely, seeing that the Greek writers could have known such a plant only from Egypt, and that still there is no evidence of its existence there.

Pliny's statement that "colocasia" leaves were plaited into vessels and goblets (*N.H.*, XXI, LI, 87) suggests the large broad leaves of that plant. Greiss (1957), in his extensive study of Ancient Egyptian baskets, mats and other straw work, could not identify any material derived from it. The provocative suggestion of Loret that *tekhi* was the name for qolqas has received no support (*T.*, II, 374).

Garlic (Allium sativum)

Ancient Egyptian: *khidjana* (?) *t ꜣ n ḥdw* (?)
Coptic: *shegen*
Greek: *skorodon*
Arabic: *thoum*

> *Whoever has eaten garlic knows its smell*
> (Popular saying)

In spite of the Biblical testimony to the existence of garlic in Ancient Egypt

"We remember the fish . . . the leek . . . and the garlic." (Numbers 11, 15)

the Ancient Egyptian name for garlic is debated. Loret (*Fl.*, 37) in 1892 stated that its Coptic name *shegen* had no cognate in Egyptian. Later

(1904), he announced that the name was *khidjana*, a word found in the Harris papyrus among a list of offerings presented by Rameses III, and in a demotic papyrus in Leyden. Lefebvre (1956, p. 102, n. 10), however, tentatively translated *t Ӡ n ḥḏw*, written in some medical papyri (*Eb.*, LXX, 519; *K.*, 28; *Carlsb.*, IV) as garlic. As to the present-day Arabic name, *thoum*, this is derived from Akkadian *shumu* (Campbell Thompson, 1949, pp. 52, 55).

Garlic has been found in its wild state in Egypt, and one might, therefore, conclude that it was introduced in early times, unless the peculiarities of the Egyptian garlic could stand for an autochthonous development. Egyptian garlic is smaller than its European counterpart; it often has as many as 45 pods; its taste is not so strong; and its bulbs are picked three months after planting. Sickenberger (1901, p. 295), the author of this description, singled it out under the name *Allium sativum L., B minus*. Dioscorides (II, 181) gave a similar description and added that it has a light purplish hue. It is remarkable that specimens of garlic from the Egyptian oases are very similar to this description of the pharaonic plant (Loret, 1904).

Presumptive evidence for the cultivation of garlic rather than its importation is the finding by Schiaparelli (Schweinfurth, 1886, p. 49) of long stems of garlic carrying leaves and the peduncles of flowers. It is obvious that, if garlic had been imported, its stems and leaves would not have been expeditioned with the pods.

Concerning this plant, one cannot fail to be impressed with the lasting belief in its therapeutic value. Pliny, who is otherwise strangely evasive on Egyptian garlic, cited several of its medicinal applications

". . . it keeps off serpents and scorpions by its smell . . . the ancient used also to give it raw to madmen . . . it relieves hoarseness if taken thus, or on gruel of peas or beans . . . when cooked in honey and vinegar it expels tape-worms and other parasites of the intestines[1] . . . its drawbacks are that it dulls the sight, causes flatulence, injures the stomach when taken too freely, and creates thirst . . ." (**XX, XXIII**, 50–57 selected)

More recent visitors to Egypt stated that garlic was imported from Syria (Sonnini, 1799, p. 69; Delile, 1813, p. 59), but there is little doubt that the plant was also grown there in antiquity. Herodotus (II, 125) even said that the costs of radish, onion and garlic provided for the builders of the pyramids were inscribed on their walls, although this is questionable since the Egyptians never inscribed on their monuments any accounting of costs.

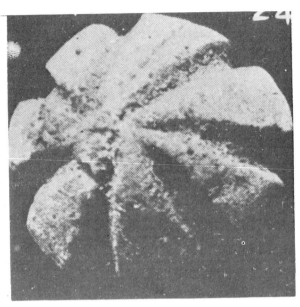

Fig. 17.1. Clay model of garlic found by Petrie at Naqada. Reproduced from Petrie (1920) plate 46, Fig. 24.

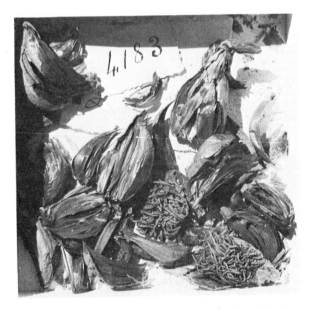

Fig. 17.2. Remains of garlic found at Deir el-Medineh. New Kingdom. Dokki Agricultural Museum, Cairo.

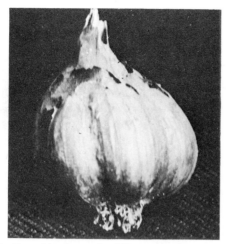

Fig. 17.3. Garlic. Found in the tomb of Tut-ankh-Amon. Cairo Museum.

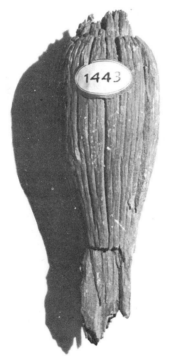

Fig. 17.4. Wooden model of onion. Found at Saqqara; probably late period. Dokki Agricultural Museum, Cairo. Photographed 1969.

Candolle (1886, p. 64) attempted to explain the absence of garlic from monuments by its being considered by the priests as unclean. Other writers stated it to be hallowed on the sole support of Pliny's remark that Egyptians took oaths on garlic and onions (*N.H.*, XIX, XXXII, 101), a habit that drove Juvenal to exclaim satirically.

"Oh, what holy folk whose gardens give birth to such gods." (Juvenal, 15)

But Loret (1904) explained that this Graeco-Roman fable was based on a false interpretation of ancient paintings. The Greeks, seeing tables loaded with victuals, including onions, being offered to the gods by the deceased, mistook the tables for altars and the vegetables for gods. On the other hand, the habit of swearing by onions could have been nothing more than the Mediterranean custom of swearing by food, e.g., by bread and salt, as a divine blessing to be forfeited if the oath was not kept.

Whatever be the case, if garlic were so highly considered, it could have been either in favour as a godly food, or respectfully avoided for the same reason.

Excavations do not substantiate the belief that garlic was regarded as impure. Clay models of this plant were found in the Pre-Dynastic cemetery of Al-Mahasna (Ayrton and Loat, 1911, plate XVI) and Naqada (Petrie, 1920, p. 43, plate 46, fig. 24) (see Fig. 17.1).

Bulbs of garlic were found in a New Kingdom tomb at Deir el-Medineh (Fig. 17.2). In Tut-ankh-Amon's tomb, a bulb called *A. cepa* by Lucas (1942) was later re-indentified by Täckholm and Drar (*T.*, III, 103) as *A. sativum*. Examination of the specimen, now in the Cairo Museum (Fig. 17.3) confirms this re-interpretation. Several additional finds have also been discussed by Täckholm and Drar.

Onion (Allium cepa)

(a)

♦ ⚓
| | | |
ḥḏw

Egyptian: see (a)
Coptic: *htit, emdjol* (Loret, 1904)

Like onions, mixed everywhere
(Popular saying)

The Ancient Egyptian name of the onion has been surmised to be *ḥdw* on the grounds that the word is written with the hieroglyph of a mace, which resembles an onion, read *ḥḏ*, followed by the determinative "herb" or "plant"—a view later accepted by Lefebvre (1956, pp. 97, 106), Ebbell (*Eb.*, LXXXIX, 751), and Faulkner (*F.*, 182), and confirmed by the cognate Coptic word *ḥtit*. On the other hand, Loret (*Fl.*, p. 37), having found a word, *badjar*, written beside a person carrying an onion, suggested that this word could be an alternative that gave rise to both Hebrew *bezel* and Arabic *basal*.

Carvings of onions appear on the inner walls of the pyramids of Unas (*c.* 2423 B.C.) and Pepi II (*c.* 2200 B.C.), in tombs of both the Old Kingdom (Fig. 6.19b) and New Kingdom (Fig. 16.14), although actual onions have not been found from earlier than the New Kingdom.

An apparent exception is the report by Ruffer (1919, pp. 74–76), although without any details, that onions were found with mummies as early as the thirteenth dynasty; this statement is contradicted by Elliot Smith and Dawson (1924, p. 165) who date the use of onions in embalming to the eighteenth dynasty.

New Kingdom and later finds of this bulb are common, however, and wooden models of onions were sometimes placed in tombs (Fig. 17.4). It is interesting that onion bulbs have often been found inserted in the bandages of mummies, or in their armpits, eye sockets, or body cavities (Elliot Smith and Dawson, 1924, p. 165) possibly, according to Sobhy and Meyerhof (1937), to stimulate the deceased to breathe, as is done with the living today on the day of Sham en-Nassim (see below).

Throughout Egyptian history onions appear with a dual quality, sometimes greatly revered and relished; at other times, or by certain groups, avoided or forbidden. Juvenal included onion with leek in his satire of their divine attribution (see pp. 660, 674), supported by Pliny (*N.H.*, XIX, XXXII, 101) who stated that oaths were taken on them; these statements do not, however, imply avoidance.

A common belief during the Roman Period that onions were unholy and unclean is extremely incredible and yet

". . . for the tale that Dictys, the nursling of Isis,[2] in reaching for a clump of onions fell into the river [Nile] and was drowned. But the priests keep themselves clear of onion and detest and are careful to avoid it, because it is the only plant that naturally thrives and flourishes in the waning of the moon. It is suitable for neither fasting nor festival, because in the one case it causes thirst, and in the other tears for those who partake of it" (*I. and O.*, 353, 8).

Thus, two reasons for avoidance are presented. One, by associating this vegetable with the waning of the moon, which symbolized the devouring of the "eye" of Horus by Seth, assimilated it to the Sethan animals; the other made of the avoidance a matter of convenience. It fitted with a Cairene proverb

"If your mother is an onion and your father garlic, how could your smell be sweet, poor chap!"

Such beliefs seem inconsistent with the previously quoted record of 12,712 measures of onion offered by Rameses III to the Nile god (*A.R.*, IV, 299) which indicates that, at least during that reign, there was no stigma attached to this plant. However, whatever the attitudes of the clergy and the nobility, onions were most certainly appreciated and enjoyed by common man. Herodotus (II, 125) related that the builders of the Pyramid of Cheops ate large quantities of onion, and the Israelites longed for the Egyptian onion (Numbers, 11, 5). Later, the epicure gastronomist Apicius added onion to Alexandrian fish sauces (10, 1, 6).

In Memphis, the rituals connected with the Sokaris festivals, held in connection with the winter solstice, prescribed wearing onions around the neck, and smelling them (Keimer, 1951). This was in keeping with the status of Sokaris as a funerary god associated with the continuous Osirian cycle of death and revival: as Ptah-Soker-Osiris, he was the inert form of Osiris awaiting the certainty of resurrection; and he also ruled the fourth and fifth hours of the night which the sun had to cross before re-appearing in the morning.

A similar tradition of eating onions and offering them to friends to smell is still observed in Egypt during the spring feast of Sham en-Nessim held on the Coptic Easter Monday. This is reminiscent of the springtime "ramp festivals" that continue to be marked in some parts of rural America. It is not certain, however, that the Sokar feast was identical with Sham el-Nessim, for it was celebrated at the beginning of the winter season. One may conclude, therefore, that the spring feast may have borrowed that custom from Antiquity, but it is impossible to ascertain the circumstances that gave rise to that habit.

The medical papyri contain many recipes for onions to be taken, orally (*Eb.*, XXXVII, 192b), or as vaginal douches (*Eb.*, XCVI, 828), or to be applied in ointments and dressings (*Eb.*, LXXIX, 634; *H.*, 237; *Ber.*, 54, etc.) Onion, translated as garlic by Lefebvre (1956, p. 102), was also used as a means of assessing female fertility. Introduced *per vaginam*, its smell could be perceived next day in the mouth of fertile, but not in that of sterile, women (*K.*, 28; *Carls.*, IV). This curious test, apparently based on the presumed patency of the genital tract, enjoyed lasting favour for over 4,000 years, for similar procedures were recommended by Hippocrates (Aphorisms, V, 54), Avicenna (Canon, III, 21, 9), and other Arab authors; and it persisted in European folk medicine.

As with garlic, Pliny, despite his evasiveness concerning onion cited, some general therapeutic uses for this plant

> ". . . onions, by the running caused by the mere smell, is a cure of feebleness of vision . . . used to induce sleep . . . chewed with bread heals sores in the mouth . . . with vinegar, honey, and wine [used against] dogbites . . . toothache. . . boiled onions given to eat to those affected by dysentery or lumbago . . ., eaten daily on an empty stomach [they] preserve a good state of health, loosen the bowels by putting the air in motion, disperse haemorrhoids when used as a suppository . . ." (*N.H.*, XX, XX, 39–43 selected)

Radish (Raphanus sativus)

Ancient Egyptian: *?smw* (*Wb.*, *Dr.*, 140); *?nwn* (*Fl.*, 108)
Coptic: *rapanon*; *pi-nouni* (*Fl.*, 108)
Greek: *raphanon*
Arabic: *figl*

> *Would that radish digest itself*
> (Popular saying)

The Ancient Egyptian name for radish is uncertain. *Swm* is a general word for herbs or weeds ("Kraut", *Wb. Dr.*, 140). In Coptic, however, *sim* means cabbage as well as radish, and it is possible that *smw* meant radish as well as herbs or weeds (*Wb. Dr.*, 440). In the Scalae,[3] radish is known in Coptic as *Pi-nouni*, probably corresponding to a plant *noun* often mentioned in hieroglyphic texts (*Fl.*, 108). Another name for it, also from the Scalae, is *rapanon*, obviously derived from Greek *raphanon*.

Apart from two radishes discovered in the twelfth dynasty necropolis of Illahoun by Petrie (1890, 1891), Täckholm identified leaves and a root of the specific Egyptian radish (Var. *aegyptiacus*). This variety differs from the red and black types in its colour, in its carrot-like shape, and in its glabrous leaves.

Otherwise, the evidence is purely literary. Pliny (XIX, XXVI, 84) is one of the few ancient writers who spoke of this vegetable in Egypt

> "In Egypt, where they are remarkable for sweetness they are sprinkled with soda"

The only other reference to it as a staple food is the statement of Herodotus (II, 125) that it was provided to the builders of the Giza pyramids. The Rawlinson and the Godley translations of Herodotus widely disagree, however, on the word *syrmaia*, used by Herodotus, the former translating it as "radish", and the latter as "purge"! The divergence may, however, be only apparent, the purge being possibly an extract of *syrmaia* (Barguet 1964, p. 1384).

It seems, however, that in antiquity the radish was more appreciated for its seed, which was processed into oil, than for its flesh:

> "In Egypt . . . the people are very fond of sowing radish seed if opportunity offers, because they make more profit from it than from corn [wheat] and have a smaller duty to pay on it, and because no plant there yields a larger supply of oil." (*N.H.*, XIX, XXVI, 80)

Radish juice was used to cure "Phtheiriasis", an unknown disease

> "They also say that radish juice is an essential specific for disease of the diaphragm in as much as in Egypt when the kings ordered post mortem dissections to be made for the purpose of research into the nature of diseases, it was discovered that this was the only dose that was capable of removing phthiriasis attacking the internal parts of the heart." (*N.H.*, XIX, XXVI, 86)

Regardless of the questionable effectiveness of radish as a therapeutic agent, this text reflects a remarkably modern notion of the value of autopsies in investigating the nature of disease. Finally, Herodotus (II, 88) reported that the cheapest method of embalming, the one that the poorer Egyptians could afford, was to clean their intestines with *syrmaia*, probably extract or oil of radish (see also under Oils, p. 785).

Turnip (Brassica rapa)

In the modern sense of the word, turnip is *brassica rapa*, but in antiquity "turnip" was a collective name including radish and other roots, exclusive of onion and leek. Loret does not mention it in his *Flore Pharaonique*, but Hunt (*S.P.*, I, 186) reported a list in a papyrus, dating from *c.* 1 A.D. where one of the vegetables is "turnips for pickling". In Thebes, turnips were found in tombs, but they cannot be dated (Fig. 17.5). Other finds from Kom Ouchim, now in the Dokki Museum, come from the Roman Period.

Unspecified Bulbs

Several writers mentioned other bulbs as foods in Egypt. Athenaeus (2, 64, B) stated

> ". . . The white and the Libyan kinds are like squills; poorest of all are the Egyptian . . ."

Pliny (XIX, XXX, 96, 97) presented his description of bulbs in a manner that suggests misidentification of arum for the Indian lotus, *Nelumbo nucifera*

> ". . . among the varieties of bulb there is also the one that in Egypt they call *arum*, which is very near to the squill in size and to the sorrel in foliage, with a straight stalk a yard long, of the thickness of a walking stick, and a root of softer substance, which can even be eaten raw."

Unfortunately, it is impossible to identify these bulbs or to ascertain how they were eaten.

Vegetables Cultivated for Their Stem, Leaf or Inflorescence

Agrostis (Cynodon dactylon)

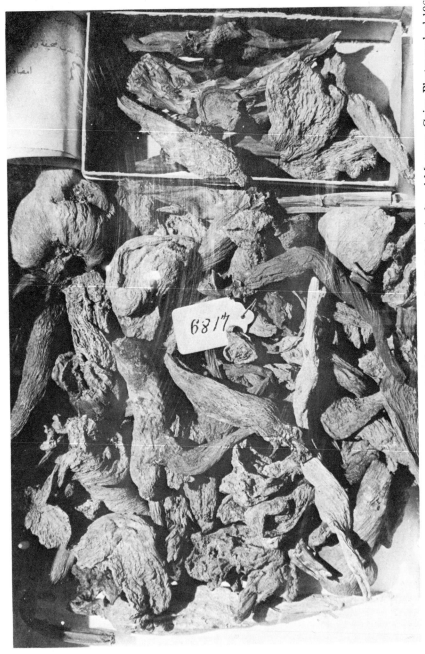

Fig. 17.5. Turnips. Uncertain origin, probably Thebes. Date uncertain. Dokki Agricultural Museum, Cairo. Photographed 1969.

Greek: *agrostis*
Arabic: *negil*
Other: "dogs' tooth grass"

This is one of the commonest weeds in Egypt. It is planted as lawn grass, its rhizomes are sold in the local herb market as a treatment of urinary lithiasis, as a diuretic, and as a deodorant; and its grass is a good fodder plant (*T.*, I, 383).

Gayet (*in* Bonnet, 1902) is said to have found a bunch of culms, and a garland that included them in a second to third century A.D. tomb at Antinoë, and Diodorus (1, 43, 1–2) related that it was one of the earliest foods of both man and his cattle in Egypt

". . . as for their means of living in primitive times, the Egyptians, they say, in the earliest period got their food from herbs and the stalks and roots of the plants which grew in the marshes, making trial of each one of them by tasting it, and the first one eaten by them and the most favoured was that called Angrostis, because it excelled the other in sweetness and supplied sufficient nutriment for the human body; for they observed that this plant was attractive to the natives, in remembrance of the usefulness of this plant, to this day, when approaching the gods, hold some of it in their hand as they pray to them; for they believe that man is a creature of swamp and marsh, basing this conclusion on the smoothness of his skin and his physical constitution, as well as the fact that he required a wet rather than a dry diet."

Artichoke (*Cynara scolymus, C. cardunculus var. sativa*)

According to Candolle (1886, p. 92) botanists long have held the view that the artichoke is a form obtained by cultivation from the wild cardoon and he fully agreed to that view. The cardoon was of course in favour with the early Mediterraneans, and Pliny commented on this habit by saying that it could not be mentioned without a feeling of shame

". . . since we turn even the monstrosities of the earth to purposes of gluttony. . ." (*N.H.*, XIX, XLII, 153)

On the indirect evidence of the lack of a Hebrew name for artichoke, Candolle (1886, p. 94) concluded that it was not cultivated in dynastic times. He questioned the identification of many tomb illustrations with this plant by Unger; but he offered no alternative. Loret, on the other hand, thought that these were pictures of lettuce (*Fl.*, 69).

The first reference to artichokes in Egypt is but indirectly related to it. This is a report cited by Athenaeus (*Deipnos.*, 2, 71, C) of Ptolemy IX (Evergetes II), composer of a treatise entitled *Commentaries*

> ". . . near Berenice, in Libya, there is a stream named Lethon . . . and in those regions grows an abundance of artichokes, which all the soldiers in our train picked and used as food, and they offered them to us, stripping off the prickles . . ."

Ptolemy's Egyptian soldiers may well have tasted this "new" edible out of curiosity, for there is little to suggest that the artichoke (today of ubiquitous use) was known in Egypt even in the Byzantine period.

Asparagus (Asparagus officinalis)

Attempts have been made to identify asparagus in tomb reliefs (Wönig, p. 208; and Unger, quoted by Loret, *Fl.*, 39). But these artifacts more probably illustrated bundles of reeds or of papyrus. There is indeed no known hieroglyphic word for the plant, and evidence that asparagus was grown in Egypt dates only to the Christian era, and only in areas impregnated with Hellenic culture. A papyrus found at Oxyrhynchus, written about the first year of our era, tells of a certain Antas who ate asparagus during the funeral feast of one of his friends (*S.P.*, I, 186). Another dated to *c.* 5 B.C. includes asparagus as one of several vegetables grown in Graeco-Egyptian funerary gardens. A third, found like the preceding two at Oxyrhynchus, and dated to the sixth or seventh century A.D., illustrated the nostalgic craving of persons living away from their native land. A Greek named Victor, working or stationed in Oxyrhynchus or in its vicinity for some time, wrote asking for asparagus to be sent to him day by day, for the vegetables there, he said, were rotten and disgusting (*S.P.*, I, 169).

It must be noted, however, that according to Galen, Greeks included under the term "asparagus" all stems growing upwards and various kinds of edible buds (de alim. fac. II, 58, quoted by Desrousseaux, 1956, p. 201).

Cabbage (Brassica oleracea)

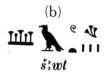

(b)

šȝwt

Ancient Egyptian: *ʔšȝt* see (b) (*Fe.*, 108)
Coptic: *krambi, shlodj, pi-htit, pi-shshiou* (*Fl.*, 108)
Greek: *kramby*
Arabic: *koromb*

> *Like a patch of cabbage, all heads*
> (Said of a vain person)

According to Candolle, cabbage was introduced into Egypt and the Middle East from Europe sometime after initial contacts had been made by the Greeks. This is an error if we accept Breasted's translation of a record of 620 measures of "cabbage" offered to the God Amon by Rameses III (*A.R.*, IV, 240). In this passage, Breasted translated the Egyptian word *šȝwt* as cabbage. This translation, however, is not universally accepted by Egyptologists.

From the Greek era, according to Loret (*Fl.*, 108), Petrie found cabbage in the tombs of Hawara. Especially noted by Greek visitors was the inferior flavour of cabbage grown in Egypt when compared with the quality produced in Asia Minor or the Greek islands

> ". . . the cabbage which grows in Cyme[4] is very good and sweet, but in Alexandria it is bitter. Seed brought from Rhodes to Alexandria produces a cabbage which is sweet for the first year but after that period it becomes acclimatized [bitter?][5] . . ." (*Deipnos.*, 9, 369, F)

Cabbage was especially prized by wine-bibbers because of its supposed prevention of the effects of excessive drinking as already indicated in Chapter 14.

670   *Food: The Gift of Osiris*

Celery (*Apium graveolens*)

The Ancient Egyptian word for celery was *m꜒tt* (see Lefebvre, 1956, p. 149, note 6). Dioscorides (III, 64) gave its Egyptian name as *mith* which is very close to its Coptic designation *mit* (Crum, 1962). Dawson (1933), however, proposed for this same word the translation "mandrake", an interpretation recorded with reservation by Faulkner (*F.*, 103).

There are recorded four kinds of *matet*, of which celery is thought to be the "northern matet" and parsley, the "desert matet" (see Parsley, p. 681). Daumas (1957), however, called attention to a plant called *matjet* and determined by the sign of a tree. This is mentioned in funerary texts as being the doorkeeper to heaven. Certain identification seemed to this author difficult, but he tentatively proposed *Calotropis procera* which was well known to Ancient Egypt (*Gpfl.*, 26) and was medically used by the Arabs. This, he believed, invited a revision of current identifications of its close homonym *matet*.

Celery was frequently found by Schweinfurth (1885) in garlands adorning mummies, and this author likened the custom to a comparable Greek tradition that gave rise in Greek to the expression "he needs celery for he is dying". Celery seeds from an Egyptian tomb are exhibited in the Firenze museum, but with no details of date or location (*Gpfl.*, 49). The Dokki Agricultural Museum in Cairo also possesses a few remains from the New Kingdom found at Abdel Qurna, Thebes (G.C. 3329 and 3330).

The only evidence of dietary use, however, is a short notice by Apicius (10, 1, 6) stating that the seeds were incorporated in sauces for grilled fish.

Medically, it was prescribed for the mysterious *âaâ* (see Chapter 2, and Ghalioungui, 1962). It was also given to retain urine (*Eb.*, L, 282), and it was applied externally to wounds (*Eb.*, LXVIII, 487) and stiff joints (*Eb.*, LXXX, 634).

Corchorus olitorius

Arabic: *melukhiya*

> *Melukhiya and soft bread ruined the barber*
> (Popular saying)

This is currently a popular leaf plant in Egypt and the Near East. It is usually eaten finely hashed, spiced with fried garlic and coriander and made into a soup with broth of rabbit, chicken, mutton or goose. The latter preparation is the object of the street cry

"Eaten with geese, my melukhiya."

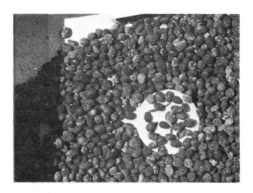

Fig. 17.6. Seeds of *Corchorus olitorius*. Found at Kom Ouchim. Roman Period. Dokki Agriculture Museum. Photographed 1969.

The fond partiality for this traditional dish is at the origin of its name, melukhiya or the royal, because it enjoyed the favour of kings, especially Moawia, the founder of the Umeyyad Dynasty. But it suffered a historical setback when the Fatimid El-Hakim (997–1021 A.D.) prohibited it together with cress, lupine and some sea-shells out of hatred for the Umeyyads (Maqrizi, 1958, Vol. III, pp. 177–188). The evidence that it was grown in Ancient Egypt is, however, inconclusive. Maspero defended that view (1901, p. 65) but gave as supportive evidence only Theophrastus and Pliny. Examination of these citations illustrates how tenuous is the identification

". . . corchorum[6] is a plant eaten at Alexandria. It has rolled up leaves, like those of the mulberry, and is beneficial, they say, to the hypochondria, for mange, and for freckles. I find also that scab in cattle is very quickly healed by it, and that according to Nicander[7] the bites of snakes also, if gathered before it blossoms . . ." (*N.H.*, XXI, CVI, 183)

Theophrastus only gave an ambiguous description

". . . there is also another plant which comes up of its own accord among the wheat; this, when the harvest is cleared they crush slightly and lay during the winter on moist ground; when it shoots, they cut and dry it and give this also to the cattle and horses and beasts of burden with the fruit which forms on it. The fruit in size is as large as sesame, but round and green in colour, and exceedingly good . . ." (Theophrastus 4, 8, 14)

Grains of this plant from the Graeco-Roman Period, may be seen at the Dokki Museum (Fig. 17.6). Schweinfurth (1873b) thought that this plant, along with others he mentioned, may be the remains of the vegetation that once covered all the valley and that is found now in Egypt only in the cultivated state.

Cress (Lepidium sativum L.)

Loret (*Fl.*, 110), on the assumption that *pi-ghleimi*, the Coptic name of this plant that grows in Egypt nowadays, sounds Egyptian concluded that *Lepidium sativum* was known to Ancient Egyptians; and he added that a few grains of that species are kept in the museum of Firenze under no. 3624.

Endive (Cichorium endivia)

Rawlinson (1881, Vol. 1, pp. 31, 84) wrote that endive was grown in Ancient Egypt, without citing the authority for his statement, but whether endive as we recognize it today was used in Ancient Egypt is difficult to ascertain. The confusion stems from Pliny's identification (or mis-identification)

". . . there is a wild endive called in Egypt succory . . ." (*N.H.*, XIX, XXXIX, 29)

but in another passage he wrote

".. . in Egypt they call the wild kind [of endive] cichorium; the cultivated they call *seris*, a variety which is smaller and has more veins . . ." (*N.H.*, XX, XXIX, 73).

In yet another passage he turns to a third form

".. . in Egypt, next in esteem after colocasia comes chicory, which I have spoken of as wild endive . . . it has a tough root, so that it is even used to make binding ropes . . ." (*N.H.*, XXI, LII, 88)

Regardless of their exact identity, it is evident that one or more leafy plants translated as "endive" were known and used at that time in Ancient Egypt. It is an interesting coincidence that *seris* which, according to Pliny was the local name of cultivated *cichorium* (see above), is now the Arabic name of wild chicory or succory (*cichorium intybus*) that is relished, cooked or raw, by fellaheen and city-dwellers alike, in both its wild and cultivated forms.

Pliny (XX, XXIX, 73) further discussed the medicinal value of endive

".. . their juice with rose oil and vinegar relieves headache; moreover, drunk with wine, pains of the liver and bladder . . ."

The lack of material evidence, however, led Candolle (1886, p. 98) to write

".. . no positive proof is found in ancient authors of the use of this plant by the Greeks and Romans; but it is probable that they made use of it and several other Chicoria . . ."

Leek (Salad leek, Allium kurrat)

(c)

i3kt

Egyptian: see (c) also meaning vegetables in general
(*Wb. Dr.*, 12; *F.*, 9; Lefebvre, 1956, p. 66)
Coptic: *ege, edji*
Greek: *prason*
Roman: *porrum*
Arabic: *kurrat*

Cheaper than kurrat [*leek*]
(Popular saying)

According to Täckholm (*T.*, III, 86) many early records, and some recent "flora" referring to *A. porruw* or *A. schoenoprasuw*, concern the plant known in Egypt as *A. kurrat*. But *A. porrum*, the European leek, now called in Egypt *kurrat roumi* or *kurrat abu shusha* has never been found in Ancient Egypt. Leaves, at first stated to belong to *A. ampeloprasum* (Schweinfurth, 1886) but later identified as *A. sativum*, have been found in a tomb excavated by Schiaparelli at Dra ʿAbul Naga, dating either to the twentieth to twenty-sixth dynasty or to the Greek Period. Undated seeds of kurrat found at Thebes, and now on exhibit at the Cairo Agricultural Museum, were found by Täckholm (*T.*, III, 104) to be slightly different from the seeds of modern kurrat.

But there are abundant Ancient Egyptian references to leek as food

> "fix his allowance at a thousand loaves of bread, a hundred jars of beer, one ox, and a hundred bunches of leeks." (Erman, 1966, p. 44)

A poem in praise of a new city, Per-Rameses, the precursor to the Graeco-Roman city of Pelusium, tells of the food consumed in the city and grown in the surrounding country

> "its granaries are full of barley and wheat, and they reach into the sky. Garlic and leek for victuals [are there] and lettuce, pomegranates, apples and olives." (Erman, 1966, p. 206)

Known for their freshness, Egyptian leeks were dreamed of by the Jews led by Moses (Numbers, 11, 5).

A popular school text-book, obviously written to extol school education, tells of the plight of the farmer and contrasts his occupation and life with those of scribes

> "the gardener bringeth loads, and his arm and neck ache beneath them. At morn, he waters the leek, and at evening the vines . . . it also goeth more ill with him than any calling." (Erman, 1966, p. 69)

Such evidence that the leek was commonly raised indicates that it was relished. Yet, there are late literary passages that cast an aversion to eating it, possibly on religious grounds

> ". . . no one worships Diana, but they (The Egyptians) have a taboo about biting into a leek or an onion; this they think is unseemly." (Juvenal, 15)

and we have seen (pp. 660, 661) similar literary allusions to onions.

Wilkinson (1854, Vol. I, p. 323), on the evidence of the biting quip of the Roman satirist, concluded that leeks were forbidden to the priests of Egypt, although he did not marshal any other supporting evidence. In opposition to Juvenal, a papyrus from the Greek Period told of leek served at a meal (*S.P.*, I, 180); and Pliny (*N.H.*, XIX, XXXIII, 110) wrote that the most esteemed leek came from Egypt. In another much longer passage (*N.H.*, XX, XXI, XXII, 44–49 select), he discussed in great detail the medicinal value of the leek

". . . [bleeding] after miscarriage is arrested by drinking the juice with woman's milk . . . the bites of beasts are treated by leek in vinegar as are those of serpents and other poisonous creatures . . . the juice also is drunk with wine to counteract the bites of serpents and of scorpions . . . it is applied to wounds, is an aphrodisiac, quenches thirst, serves as a pick-me-up after drunkenness, but is said to dim the eyesight and to cause flatulence which do no harm, however, to the stomach but relax the bowels . . ."

The medical use of leek is confirmed by the papyri that prescribed it for wounds and for diseases of the limbs (*metw*) (*H.*, 237); to darken burn scars (*Eb.*, LXIX, 501); or as applications to human bites (*Eb.*, LXIV, 432).

Lettuce (Lactuca sativa)

Egyptian: see (d) or (e)
Coptic: *pi-ob*

(d)

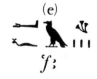

ibw

Who came with but a gift of lettuce,
neither came nor even glanced
(Popular saying)

(e)

ꜥfꜣ

The lettuce grown in Egypt is characterized by its straight vertical surge that may reach one metre in height. Loret (*Fl.*, 69), by a comparison of Coptic *pi-ob* for the plant, suggested that the hieroglyphic plant *ibw* designated it, but this identification did not appear acceptable to

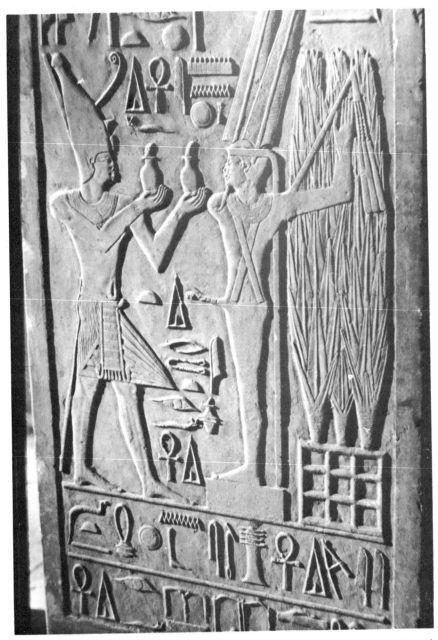

Fig. 17.7. Senusret I offering milk to the god Min. Behind the god three lettuce. Chapel of Senusret I. Karnak, Middle Kingdom. Photographed 1969

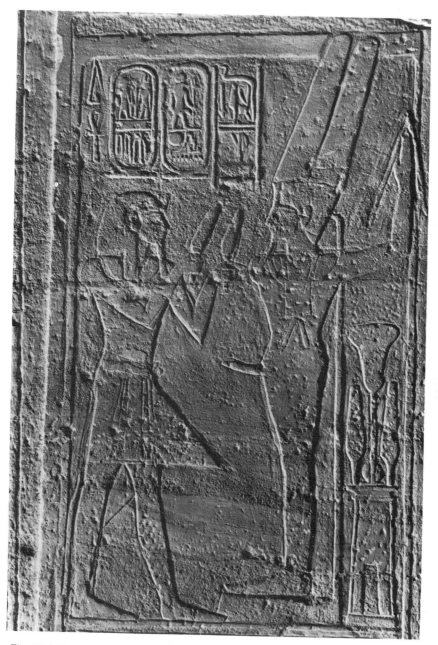

Fig. 17.8. Rameses II offering lettuce to Min. Temple of Abu Simbel. Documentation Centre, Cairo.

Keimer (*Gpfl.*, 126), and von Deines and Grapow consider *ibw* an as yet undetermined plant (*Wb. Dr.*, 21). The Egyptian name for lettuce is now known to be ʿ*bw*, translated by Erman and Grapow in their Aegyptisches Handwörterbuch as "an aphrodisiac" (1961, p. 24), and in their Wörterbuch der aegyptischen Sprache (Vol. 1, p. 176) as (1) lettuce, (2) an offering to the ithyphallic Min and Amon and (3) a large bunch of flowers. Actually, the vast majority of Egyptologists accept the first identification (Keimer, 1924a, b).

Either because of its proud vertical growth, of its verdure, or, as Keimer suggested, because it is the only Egyptian plant to exude a milky juice when squeezed, it was believed to be an aphrodisiac and to be somehow associated with the reproductive function. This belief persists in Upper Egypt. On the other hand, Athenaeus (*Deipnos.*, II, 69) believed it to cause impotence, and it is still prescribed in European folk medicine as a sedative.

Whatever the origin of these beliefs, the plant was early associated with Min, the god of vegetation and procreation. One of the main attributes of this god was a botanical motif drawn behind him that has received various interpretations. This is made of one or several vertical, more or less conical plants, set on a square structure or on the very socle on which the god stands.

In earlier illustrations, the details of the leafage are clearly drawn (Fig. 17.7), and the square base seems to be a schematic rendition of the field on which the plant is growing. After the eighteenth dynasty, however, the treatment was often so stylized that the true nature of the whole motif escaped the artist, as happened to many artifacts in the history of Egyptian art (Fig. 17.8). The plant was variously seen as a cypress, a sycamore, a persea, a fig tree, a palm, an acacia (see Gauthier, 1931, pp. 164, 165); and the square structure took the shape of a chest, a stool, or, finally, a gate. There is, however, now a near consensus that the plant is a lettuce.

In some illustrations in which Pharaoh is seen presenting one or two of these leafy vegetables to the god (Fig. 17.8), the legend often clearly states that the aim of the oblation is to have the god perform the act of procreation (Gauthier, 1931, p. 166).

Apart from these religious or ritual illustrations, lettuce appears among offerings in many tombs, and, often previously taken for artichoke or pine cones, its true nature is now recognized (Fig. 6.19b).

Seeds of lettuce have been reported by Keimer, on the authority of Braun, to have been in the Berlin Museum (*Gpfl.*, p. 290), and a number of seeds (Fig. 17.9) found in a Roman pottery vase are on exhibit at the Agricultural Museum of Dokki.

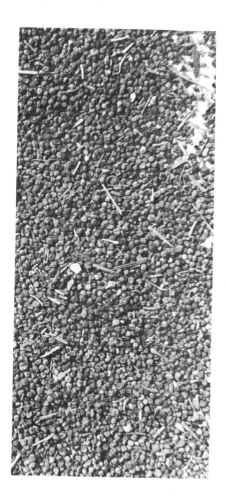

Fig. 17.9. Lettuce seeds. Roman Period. Found in a Roman pottery vase. Bought at Luxor. Dokki Agricultural Museum, Cairo. (2700). Photographed 1969.

From *ibw*, bread was made (*Wb. Dr.*, p. 21). Only *ibw*, not ʿ*bw* was used medicinally, either internally or externally. Internally, its use seems to have been restricted to the enigmatic *âââ* (*Eb.*, XLVI, 239). Its seeds (*Eb.*, XXVI, 111; *Eb.*, LXXXI, 650), its "hair" (*H.*, 136), and its oil (*Eb.*, XLIII, 253) were utilized in ointments to soften the *mtw* (limbs) and to relieve headache. At times, northern *ibw* (*Eb.*, LXXXIII, 663), at others, southern *ibw* (*Eb.*, L, 282) were specified.

In view of the claimed influence of lettuce on sexual function, it is interesting to find it, in Ebers's translation, recommended to cure impotence (LXXXIII, 663) and, in popular belief, it is often regarded still as an aphrodisiac.

Mallow (Malva parviflora)

Arabic: *khubbeza, khubbaz*

> *Mallow at noon, beans at night*
> (Said of a poor man)

Now a favourite component of a stew cooked with rice and chick-peas, mallow was recorded by Täckholm among the vegetable remains of the Coptic monastery of Phaebamon (1961, p. 26). It is nowadays used also for its astringent properties in an infusion as a gargle.

(f)

mȝtt

Parsley (Petroselinum crispum)

Egyptian: *matet, mȝt . t ḫȝšt* and *mȝt . t mḥy . t*, see (f)
Arabic: *baqdounes*

> *Like parsley, grown in dung and thrust into shish kebab*
> (Said of a social climber)

Of the four varieties of *mȝt . t* mentioned in ancient Egyptian texts, the northern variety, *mȝt . t mḥy . t* has been identified by Loret (1894) with parsley. Lefebvre (1956, p. 149) was of opinion, however, that parsley was *mꜣt . t ḫꜣš . t* (desert or mountain parsley). He based his translation on the resemblance of this word to Greek for parsley, *petroselinum* (desert or rock parsley or celery) an analogy with the Greek derivation of *petroleum* (rock oil) and with Egyptian *pr ḥr ḫꜣšt . f* (that which comes from its mountain) for mineral oil. He further pointed to the resemblance of *mꜣt . t* to Greek *mith* (selinon according to Dioscorides (III, 64)). The extent of its use as a foodstuff in Ancient Egypt is not evident, but Keimer (*Gpfl.*, 39) accepted that it was cultivated in Ancient Egypt since it is still being sold in Egyptian herb markets.

Medically "desert matet" was prescribed against urinary incontinence (*Eb.*, I, 282), to treat an "obstacle in the right side" (*Eb.*, XLIII, 209) and "the right side" (?hemiplegia) (*Eb.*, XC, 758).

Pliny (XX, XLVI, 117) described two kinds of parsley which could confirm the meaning of the word "desert" or "mountain mꜣtt" . . . mountain parsley (XX, XLVI, 117) beneficial to the urine and menses, and rock parsley especially good for abscesses (XX, XLVII, 118].

Purslane (Portulaca oleracea)

Arabic: *regla*

This vegetable, now commonly eaten as a salad or in stews, is called in Coptic *mehmouhi*. According to Loret the related word *makhmakhai* was discovered by Maspero in an Ancient Egyptian text, and Apulaeus gave it the Egyptian name *mothmutin* (*Fl.*, 72, 73).

Other Vegetables

Many other plants were said by Pliny to be eaten by Egyptians: *oetum, arachidne, chondrylla, hypochoeris, caucalis, enthryscum, scandix* (goat's beard, or *tragopogon*), *saffron, parthenium, trychnum, aphace, achynox, epipetron* (*N.H.*, XXI, LII, 89), *tribulus* (water-chestnut, *trapa natans*) (*N.H.*,

XXI, LVIII, 98). A few unidentified ones have also been mentioned among offerings, like *yufiti* (*A.R.*, IV, 234), *samu* (*A.R.*, IV 392) and *beny* (*A.R.*, IV, 380).

Legumes

Beans (Vicia faba)

iwryt

Ancient Egyptian: see (g)
Coptic: ?*fel* (Keimer, 1929) *pi-ouro*
Arabic: *foul*

The *Vicia faba* bean, a staple today in Egypt, was certainly known to Ancient Egyptians. Samples were found by Schweinfurth in the fifth dynasty funerary temple of Sahure (unpublished findings reported by Keimer, 1929a), and in tombs at Dra ʿAbul Naga (1884, 1885), but his dating of the latter to the twelfth dynasty has been questioned (Keimer, 1929a). They were also reported by Newberry in Hawara and Illahoun (1890), although the single seed found was smaller than the variety now cultivated, pointing to Asia Minor as its place of origin; and, from the Roman Period, a number were found at Kom Ouchim (Fig. 17.10). The name in Egyptian is believed to be *iwryt*, although Keimer (1929a) translated this word *Vigna sinensis* Endl. (Old name: *Dolichos lubia* Forsk) and believed *Vicia faba* to have been called *pr* in Egyptian, and *fel* in Coptic.

The term "bean meal", so commonly encountered in the medical papyri, must, however, remain non-specific, as it could equally apply to *Vicia faba*, to the so-called Egyptian bean, or to any of several other varieties existing in Egypt such as *vetch, Vicia sativa*, gesse *V. sinensis*, "*Lathyrus sativus*", *Lathyrus hirsutus, L. aphaca, Vicia lutea*, which have all been found in ancient tombs. In fact, this medicinal bean-meal could have been the pilos of Theophrastus (4, 8, 7) who stated that it was prepared from ground *Kuamos*, a term that, in his time, was confusingly applied to both *Vicia faba* and Egyptian bean. Indeed, the "bean" used by the medical profession might not have been a "bean" at all. Consider, for example, the present application of this word to coffee beans, strychnos bean, Calabar bean, none of which is a bean, except in shape.

It is interesting, in this connection, to note that the Arabic name of stewed *Vicia faba*, *foul medammes*, is quite close to an Ancient Egyptian word preserved in Coptic, *metmes*, and that Arabic *bessara*, a special bean purée, has a Coptic parallel, *pesouro* (Sobhy, 1921).

Another culinary preparation, fried balls of spiced purée of germinated beans called *taamiya*, is an extremely popular dish in the whole Middle East. It has given origin to the proverb "Who tastes of taamiya would sell his bonnet for it."

Much has been written about taboos attached to beans, but the crux of the matter lies in identifying the prohibited plant.

We have already discussed this ban in several sections.

The first mention of a restriction is found in the teachings attributed to Pythagoras who, as a young man, was trained for some time with Egyptian priests. Pythagoras, it was believed, based this rule on the belief that beans were produced from the same matter as man. Other ancient writers mentioned this taboo, but they advanced other reasons. Diodorus (1, 89, 4) observed that priests abstained also from other foods, like lentils, and viewed the avoidance as a manifestation of self-denial, for if they

> "all ate of everything the supply of no article of consumption would hold out."

Pliny thought that beans were shunned because they caused sleeplessness and dulled the senses; while he cited the Pythagorean view and the consequent custom of employing beans in memorial sacrifices, as well as other current beliefs: that certain letters of gloomy omen are inscribed on bean flowers; that it brings luck to carry home from the harvest a "harvest-home bean" or to include a bean in lots offered at auction sales; that when beans are grazed down they fill out again by the waxing moon; or that they cannot be boiled in sea or salted water (a Sethian element) (*N.H.*, XVIII, XXX, 118–119). Plutarch, on the other hand, found that the Egyptian priests avoided legumes because of their superfluity (*I. and O.*, 353, 5).

Royal decrees or records seem to indicate, however, that this legume was appreciated by the people, and agreeable to the gods. Thus Rameses II wished to show his concern for his people

> ". . . Upper Egypt continually conveys for you to Lower Egypt, and Lower

Egypt conveys for you to Upper Egypt, barley . . . and beans in immense quantity"

and Rameses III offered to the Nile god, on one occasion, 11,998 jars of "shelled beans" and, on another, 2398 jars (*A.R.*, IV, 301 and 350).

Rawlinson, paradoxically, substantiated his belief that beans (*Vicia faba*) were grown on the statement of Herodotus to the effect that

"priests would not even endure to look on them"

by noting his doubt that beans could grow in Egypt without being sowed (*Her.*, II, 37, note 6), believing that the mere mention of the avoidance indicated their cultivation. But examination of these sources indicates a shift of the discussion from *Vicia faba* to another bean, the Egyptian bean (see Chapter 16). This is immediately clear when the citation from Theophrastus (4, 8, 7–8), is examined

". . . [its] head, which is like a round wasp's nest, and in each of the cells is a bean [*kuamos*]"!

The confusion comes from the Greek word *kuamos* as was explained in Chapter 16.

Wilkinson (1854, Vol. I, p. 323), commenting on this avoidance believed that it was restricted to the upper classes, and did not apply to the peasant

". . . this aversion, which originated in a supposed sanitary regulation, and which was afterwards so scrupulously adopted by Pythagoras, did not prevent their cultivation; nor were the people obliged to abstain from them; and they were allowed to eat them in common with other pulse and vegetables which abound in Egypt . . ."

He did not, however, cite supporting evidence for this general thesis, other than the probability that the poor had little to lose religiously by breaking the taboo, while the nobility and priesthood were under close religious scrutiny.

Avoidance was thus variously attributed to esoteric or trivial motives; and it may be concluded from the variety of offered reasons that the prohibition was probably allegorical and that its true explanation was kept secret by its originators.

Medically, beans (*iwryt*) were at times used internally (*K.*, 10). Externally, they were ingredients in mouth rinses (*Eb.*, LXXXVI, 704), dressings (Eb., LXXI, 534), applications to "soften" stiff limbs (*Eb.*, LXXX, 640), and fumigations (*Ber.*, 78). Bean meal made into a paste with oil and honey was applied to a prolapsed rectum (*Ch.B.*, 5, 7–8); and cooked (toasted?) beans, mixed with oil, were applied to the penis to "regularize" urine (*Eb.*, XLIX, 270).

Cretan beans are mentioned in the Ebers papyrus where an unknown plant *gngnt*, translated as "senna" by Ebbell (IX=28), is compared to them.

"Castor" beans will be discussed in Chapter 19.

Chick Pea (Cicer arietinum)

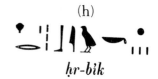

(h)

ḥr-bik

Ancient Egyptian: see (h)
Arabic: *ḥommos* (the green plant is *malana*)
Coptic: *arsha* (*Fl.*, 92)

The linguistic proof of the existence of chick peas in Ancient Egypt is, at present, stronger than the archaeologic. This has been obtained from the name of a plant *ḥr-bik* hawk's face, cited in a twentieth dynasty list. Keimer (1929b), who called attention to the resemblance of the chick-pea to the face of the hawk, added that no other Egyptian bean possesses that appearance; that in Magyar chick pea is called "owl's head"; and that one of its main names in Hebrew is "small nose", because of the beak-like prominence on that legume. According to Montet (1958, pp. 80–81) this would have been no reason against eating it, except possibly on particular occasions, or in certain places.

The only positive reference to the chick pea that has come to our attention is rather late; it dates to *c.* 255 B.C.

". . . as a token of goodwill I have sent you from Sosus 2 artabae of chick-peas bought at 5 drachmae each and if there are any at Naucratis, I will try to buy you about 20 artabae more and bring them up to you myself." (*S.P.*, I, 92)

There are finds of chick peas, however, dating to *c.* 1400 B.C. (Fig. 17.11) and to the second to third century A.D. (Newberry, 1889, pp. 49, 53). Their hieroglyph proves that they were grown at least since the New Kingdom, while the small faenza models said to come from a Middle Kingdom tomb at Matariya (Keimer, 1929a) would date their history earlier.

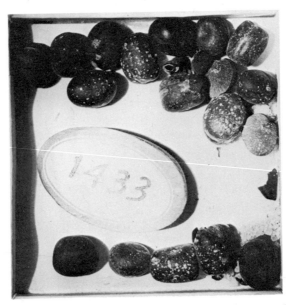

Fig. 17.10 Broad beans (*Vicia faba*). From Kom Ouchim. Roman Period. Dokki Agricultural Museum, Cairo. Photographed 1969.

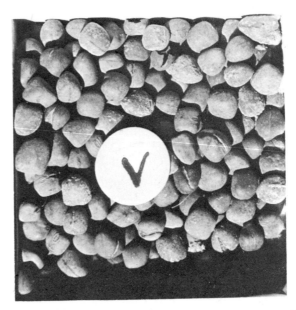

Fig. 17.11. Chick peas (*Cicer arietinum*). Deir el-Medineh. About 1400 B.C. Dokki Agricultural Museum, Cairo. Photographed 1969.

Today, they are eaten dry, either salted or sugar-coated. They are made into a dip with oil and condiments. Green, they are called *malana* (the full) and are cried in streets

"Like almonds, my malana"

and their ballooned, nearly empty shell serves as a pejorative comparison for empty-headed boastful persons

"Like malana, puffed up on nothing".

Lentils (Ervum lens)

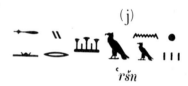

(i)

ʿȝrš

Egyptian: see (i) and (j)
Coptic: *arshin*
Greek: *phacos*
Latin: *lens*
Arabic: ʿads

(j)

ʿršn

Scorn not the case of the Egyptian lens
(Virgil, Georgics L., 228)

Lentils have been found in Pre-Dynastic tombs (Brunton, 1948), in the underground stores of Zoser's pyramid (Lauer *et al.*, 1951), among funeral offerings at DraʿAbul Naga and Deir el Bahari (Schweinfurth, 1885) and at sites of all epochs, down to the Coptic era, in Phaebamon's Monastery (Täckholm, 1961, p. 19). A painting in the tomb of Rameses III shows a servant preparing a meal interpreted as a dish of lentils; and the literature confirms the wide use of this vegetable in Egypt. The "Tale of Wen-amon" (*c.* 1085 B.C.) relates that Egyptian lentils were bartered for Lebanese cedar wood (*A.R.*, IV, 582), and a late text indicates that they were offered to gods

"they bring to him [Harpocrates] as an offering the first fruits of grown lentils" (*I. and O.*, 377, 65)

a custom stemming from the belief that Isis gave birth to Harpocrates

". . . imperfect and immature, amid the early flowers and shoots." (*I. and O.*, 377, 65)

Strabo (17, 1, 34), during his visit to Egypt, observed a peculiar sight in front of the Giza pyramids. These were heaps of stone chips, among which some were like lentils both in form and size, and other winnowings of half-peeled grains. He was told that these were the petrified remains of the food of the workmen who built the pyramids; and he thought that this was not improbable.

It is more probable, however, that these "fossilized lentils" were the small shells of marine protozoans, the *nummulites* that are found by the millions throughout the geologic formations on which the Giza pyramids were built. Indeed, the Sphinx itself is carved from this fossiliferous bedrock.

During the Alexandrian era, lentils were associated with Alexandria. Athenaeus (4, 158, D) wrote

"... yet, you men of Alexandria, have been brought up on lentil food and your entire city is full of lentil dishes . . ."

The association was current all through Mediaeval times and appeared even in the writings of St Augustine as quoted by Walker (1957, p. 112)

"... lentils are used as food in Egypt, for the plant grows abundantly in that country, which renders the lentils of Alexandria so valuable that they are brought thence to us as if we grew none . . ."

Another northern Egyptian site famous for lentils was Pelusium in northern Sinai. Martial (*Epigrams*, 13, 9) wrote

"receive lentils of Nile, a present from Pelusium; they are cheaper than spelt, dearer than beans . . ."[8]

If this truly indicated the relative value of the lentil, it had decidedly declined between the Ptolemaic Period and the time of Martial (A.D. 40–102), for a papyrus dated to 113 B.C. informs us that the price of lentils in relation to wheat was 1:1 (*S.P.*,II, 398 and 516 A).

Pliny (*N.H.*, XVIII, XXXI, 123) described two kinds of Egyptian lentils

"... one rounder and blacker, the other normal in shape . . ."

In addition, he said that a lentil diet was conducive to an equal temper. The Romans believed that lentils were a cure for many diseases, particularly diarrhoea and sores; but lentils were also believed to dull eyesight, to injure the lungs, and to hinder sleep (*N.H.*, XXII, LXX, 142–144).

Nevertheless in spite of the favour they enjoyed, lentils were sometimes displaced by other foods. An amusing papyrus illustrates the plight of an unfortunate lentil-cook in the face of such a competition

". . . to Philiscus, greeting from Harentotes, lentil cook of Philadelphia. I give the product of 35 artabae a month and do my best to pay the tax every month in order that you may have no complaint against me. Now the folk in the town are roasting pumpkins. For that reason, then, nobody buys lentils from me at the present time. I beg and beseech you then, if you think fit, to be allowed more time, just as has been done in Crocodilopolis, for paying the tax to the king. For in the morning they straightaway sit down beside the lentils selling their pumpkins, and give me no chance to sell my lentils." (*S.P.*, II, 266)

This poor cook could have suffered from any of the taboos attached to lentils, such as the restriction mentioned by Dioscorides (1, 89, 4); this, however, seems to have been one of self-denial rather than of impurity. This is the only reference to such a restriction, and the overwhelming evidence is that this legume was widely eaten by poor and rich alike, appreciated and enjoyed throughout most of Dynastic, Greek and Roman Periods.

Lupine (Lupinus albus, L. termis Forsk.)

Coptic: *tharmos*
Arabic: *termis*

When he called his lupine sweeter than almonds, he was answered
"a deceit only fit for children"
(Popular saying)

Lupines are now widely consumed in Egypt. Sonnini (1799, Vol. 3, p. 17) heard them cried in the streets of Embabeh near Cairo, possibly as they are today

"Delicious and salted fruits of gardens"

and he added that one saw in the streets nothing but people peeling them.

On the slim argument that Hebrew has no name for this plant, Candolle (1886, p. 327) concluded that it could have been introduced into Egypt only after the Exodus. But Unger mentioned it among cultivated plants in Ancient Egypt (1860, p. 65). Wilkinson (1878, Vol. II, p. 143) stated that lupines have been found in tombs and he, elsewhere, wrote, apparently on the authority of Columella (see Chapter 13, p. 543) that it was added to beer for flavour (1854, Vol. I, p. 54). Maspero, likewise, mentioned that it was found in tombs (1901, p. 65), but none of these authors presented any evidence in support of his statement.

According to Täckholm (1961, p. 20), the only species represented in Pharaonic Egypt is *L. digitatus*; this has been found twice, once at Abusir, from the Middle Kingdom, and again at Hawara from Graeco-Roman times.

Schweinfurth (1886, p. 256) found empty husks in a tomb at Draᶜ Abul Naga, but he was careful to point out that they were recent. Nevertheless, because of the existence of a Coptic name for it, he considered that it was known to the Ancient Egyptians. Lupine beans from the Roman Period are found in the collection of the Dokki Agricultural Museum (Fig. 17.12).

Pea (Pisum sativum)

(k)

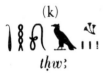

*thw*ꜣ

Egyptian: see (k)
Coptic: ? *Tilakonthe* (Fl. 93); ?*sabsae* (Keimer, 1929a)
Arabic: *besella, basel*

He used to eat peas, but luck failed him
(Popular saying)

The ancient name of this plant was identified as *thw*ꜣ by Dawson (1935) and Lefebvre supported his view (1956, p. 130). Both Montet (1958, p. 80) and Rawlinson (1881, Vol. I, pp. 31, 84) wrote that peas

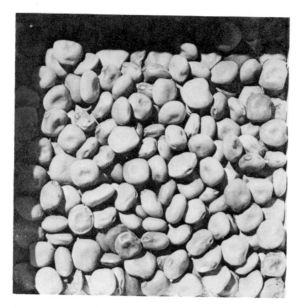

Fig. 17.12. Lupine *Lupinus termis*. Roman Period. Dokki Agricultural Museum, Cairo. Photographed 1969.

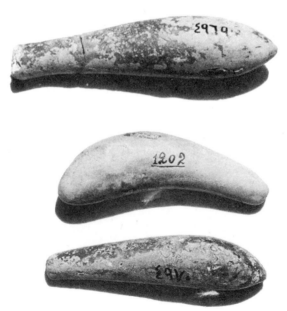

Fig. 17.13. Models of *Cucumis melo*. New Kingdom. Dokki Agricultural Museum, Cairo. Photographed 1969.

were known but, as usual, did not give any documentation. Candolle (1886) however, wrote that there was no indication proving their culture. Nevertheless, peas were found in abundance in the cemeteries of both Hawara (Newberry, 1889, pp. 49, 53) and Kahun (Newberry, 1890), the latter proving that they were grown ever since the twelfth dynasty.

Medically, they were prescribed internally with other ingredients for a condition that may have been angina pectoris (*Eb.*, XXXVII, 191), for ? paresis (*Eb.*, LXXVII, 607); and, externally, to "cool" the members (*Eb.*, LXXXV, 693), and to induce maturation in inflamed glands (*Eb.*, CIV, 859; *Eb.*, CV, 860).

Other Legumes

Vigna sinensis (Arabic: *Lubia*) was identified in an unpublished note by Schweinfurth in fifth dynasty offerings. Keimer, who cites this note (1929a), described small faenza models of this plant, the identification being confirmed by Loret on account of the characteristic black spot on the seed. Keimer further added that this bean was the bean *par excellence* of Ancient Egypt.

Vetch (Lathyrus sativus)

Arabic: *Gilban*

This legume grows wild nowadays all over Egypt, and is used as fodder. It is documented in Egypt throughout its history, from Neolithic (Brunton and Caton-Thompson, 1928) through the Pharaonic and Coptic eras (Schweinfurth, 1886; Newberry, 1889; Keimer, 1929a; Täckholm, 1961). The plant that Greek authors frequently mention under the name *aracos* (*N.H.*, XXI, LII, 89) may be identical with this bean (Jones, 1951, Vol. 7, p. 491).

In addition, Loret (*Fl.*, 94), on the grounds that fragments of *Vicia sativa* were found in a brick of the Dashur pyramid by Unger (1862) concluded that its culture in Ancient Egypt is thereby proved.

Vegetables Cultivated for their Fruits

In this section we discuss food articles that are essentially fruits but which, on account of their lack of sweetness, are regarded as vegetables in the culinary sense.

Gourds, Cucumber, Pumpkin

We differentiate today with great precision between cucumbers, gourds, squash, pumpkins (Figs 6.20, 17.13) and similar plants but, in antiquity, some of these distinctions were not always made or, if they were, they did not always correspond with ours. At least in Graeco-Roman times, gourd was clearly distinguished from cucumber, for a papyrus from *c.* 141 A.D. lists

". . . 20 gourds, 40 cucumbers." (Lindsay, 1966, p. 286)

This vegetable was eaten stuffed. A recipe of Apicius (3, 4, 3) details its preparation in the "Alexandrian" fashion.

Part of the uncertainty lies in the English connotation of the word gourd, particularly as used in the southwestern United States, where it is the common name of a very astringent, unwholesome arid land plant that is carefully avoided. In the translation of the papyrus quoted above, it is not clear whether "gourd" is used in the sense of squash, pumpkin or vegetable marrow; but it is certainly contrasted with the cucumber.

Distinction between squash and pumpkin is also unclear, for even botanists call them by the same name *cucurbita pepo* which stems from the Latin name for gourd.

Cucumber (Cucumis sativus, C. chate)

Arabic: *khiar*

Erman (1966, p. 212), in his translation of a letter from an Egyptian student(?) to his teacher, used the word "cucumber"

"... I will plant for thee acres ... with cucumbers and [?] as the sand for multitude."

In contrast, Candolle [1886, p. 266] believed that cucumbers were not found in Ancient Egypt and, on the basis of etymological studies of Hebrew and Egyptian texts, stated that the

"cucumber for which the Israelites longed [Numbers, 11, 5] was indeed a 'mistranslation'."

Loret (*Fl.*, 74) interpreted some mural illustrations previously thought by Unger to represent *Cucumis chate* as cucumber (*C. sativus*). He further speculated that *chate* was a poor transcription of Arabic *qatta*; and that this word's cognate in Ancient Egyptian, *qadi* ($k\bar{\jmath} d . t$), which designates a creeping plant (literally "on its belly") that grows a flower resembling the lotus (*Eb.*, LI, 294) could only be *C. chate*.

However, Loret's translation was rejected by Keimer (*Gpfl.*, 132), who thought that $k \ d . t$ was a general term for *cucurbitaceae* and probably for other fruits as well.

Loret noted, in addition, that Arabic *qassa*, *qatta* and Hebrew *qissouaim*, are names of *C. chate* as well as *C. sativum*, and that three Coptic words for cucumber, *banti*, *tighe* and *shope* are translated in the Scalae, *qatta*, except the last which is translated *faqqous* and, in a single instance, "water melon" (*Fl*, p. 75). Both *qatta* and *faqqous* are varieties of cucumber.

Shope is very close to *šbt*, the Egyptian name of a plant utilized by physicians, and translated by von Deines and Grapow (*Wb. Dr.*, 486), "a kind of cucumber or melon" (Gurken oder Melonenart), by Lefebvre "melon" (1956, p. 172), and left untranslated by Ebbell (*Eb.*, XCVIII, 852).

Still another word is thought to indicate cucumber. This is *šsp* (*Eb.*, XLIV, 219, 220; *Wb. Dr.*, 505; Lefebvre, 1956, p. 146), although Keimer (*Gpfl.*, 130) translated it *C. melo*.

According to Ebbell's translation, this plant was used medicinally, either internally (*Eb.*, L, 278), against polyuria or urinary frequency; or externally, against

"all afflictions caused by a god or a goddess" (*Eb.*, XLVI, 246)

or to relieve the

"members of a toe" [?] (*Eb.*, LXXXI, 647)

Okra (Hibiscus esculentus)

Arabic: *bamia*

> *When the okra merchant was beaten, the merchant of melukhiya ran screaming "Calamity befalls greengrocers".*
> (Said of unjustified mass panic)

The evidence is meagre for the existence of this plant in Ancient Egypt. A fruit called *banu*, which is fairly close to the Arabic *bamia*, is said to be mentioned in the Harris papyrus without any description (Ruffer, 1919, p. 78). The plant is most probably of African origin (Candolle, 1886, p. 190), but it is found in Egypt only in the cultivated state.

The only historical references to okra are Rosellini's interpretation of a drawing, which was rejected by others; a similar interpretation of a Beni Hassan illustration by Wönig (1886, p. 219) which does not seem to be better founded; and a find of this vegetable reported by Maspero (1901, p. 65) without any details.

Notes: Chapter 17

1. Garlic is still used in folk medicine against tape-worm, and we can testify to its value (P.G.).

2. Graves discusses the equation of Dictys with Horus and believes that this is an allusion to Persaeus (1961, 73, 4).
3. Scalae were Coptic-Arabic lexicons.
4. Greek city in Asia Minor located in the district of Aeolia south of Troy.
5. Statement attributed to Diphilus, a Greek writer of the fourth century B.C.
6. There is no evidence that the corchorum cited in this passage is *Corchorus olitorius*.
7. Nicander of Colophon, born in this famous city of Asia Minor, was famed as both a physician and poet. He flourished *c.* 137 B.C.
8. At present, lentils grow exclusively in Upper Egypt. But, to foreigners, Alexandria or Pelusium may have meant simply Egypt in general, i.e. the port of embarkation and of exports. This identification of Alexandria with Egypt is still current among Greeks.

Chapter 18   *Fruit*

As in any ancient country, the fruit crops of Egypt have been continuously changed through the centuries by new additions. Some fruits were indigenous or, at least, there is proof that they have been known since the earliest ages, others are documented only from Graeco-Roman times, while still others were introduced much later, either with the Arab conquest from Asia, or even later after the discovery of the New World.

In many cases, interest in some fruits, long known but neglected, was re-awakened in response to international needs. Thus, Mohamed Aly, in his search for new sources of revenue, in 1813 ordered the planting of 30,000 olive trees in the Fayoum to satisfy the soap industry of Marseilles and, in 1815, the planting of a million mulberry trees to meet the needs of the Lyons silk factories.

The uncertainty of some translations of the names of fruits from ancient literary sources is apparent and must be recognized. But even on the surer grounds of actual finds, the earliest documented date for a given fruit must be taken—unless proof to the contrary be available—as the latest possible date for its introduction, since negative evidence at earlier dates cannot be considered conclusive, and the appearance of a fruit in sizeable quantities must have been sometime after its introduction.

Table 1 summarizes the earliest dates of evidence for each fruit, leaving details and references to be discussed in the text.

Principal Fruits Mentioned in the Literature

(a)

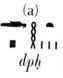

dph

Apple (Malus sylvestris)

(b)

dph

Ancient Egyptian: apple (a), apple tree (b)
Coptic: *djepeh*
Arabic: *toffah*

697

Table 1

The earliest evidence of the existence of different fruits in Egypt

Fruit	Earliest record	Nature of evidence	Reference
Apple	nineteenth dynasty	Literary	*A.R.*, IV, 301
Carob	? first dynasty [wꜥḥ]	Literary	Emery and Saad (1938)
	twelfth dynasty	Find	Newberry (1890)
Cherry	5 B.C.	Literary	Lindsay (1966)
Christ's thorn	first dynasty	Find	Emery and Saad (1938)
Citron	second century A.D.	Literary	*S.P.*, 1, 18
Egyptian plum	eighteenth dynasty	Find	Dokki museum
Fig	second dynasty	Schist vessel	Cairo museum 6280
Grapes	third dynasty	Find	Lauer *et al.* (1951)
Hegelig	third dynasty	Find	Lauer *et al.* (1951)
Juniper	Pre-Dynastic	Find	Brunton (1937)
Olive	eighteenth dynasty	Find	Schweinfurth (1886)
Palm, Argun	fifth dynasty	Find	*T.*, II, 299–300
Palm, Date	Pre-Dynastic	Find	*MAE*, 119
Palm, Doum	Pre-Dynastic	Find	Brunton *et al.* (1928)
Peach	Graeco-Roman	Find	Newberry (1889)
Pear	Graeco-Roman	Find	Newberry (1889)
Persea	third dynasty	Find	Lauer *et al.* (1951)
Pomegranate	twelfth dynasty	Find	Schweinfurth (1886)
Sycamore fig	Pre-Dynastic	Find	*MAE*, 119
Water melon	New Kingdom	Find	*Fl.*, 73

The Hebrew (*tappoukh*), Coptic (*djepeh*), and Arabic (*toffah*) names of this fruit are all extremely close to *dph*, its presumed Egyptian name. In view of the ancient usage of the term golden-apple in relation to oranges, and to a claimed difficulty of growing apples outside temperate zones, it was suggested that these three words should be translated "orange". This objection does not stand, however, seeing that the orange tree was introduced in Egypt only after the Christian era, and that the apple tree grows in the Nile valley nowadays. The apples, however, are inferior in quality and size to foreign grown ones. Really good apples are scarce, usually imported, and thus justify the proverb applied to ignorant pretentious upstarts

"What does a fellah know about apples?"

There are only two Ancient Egyptian references to apples, both dated to the nineteenth dynasty: one states that Rameses II planted apples in his Delta gardens (*Fl.*, 82); and the other that Rameses III offered 848 baskets of *dpht* to the Nile God (*A.R.*, IV, 301). Nevertheless, knowledgeable historical botanists consider all records of apple from Pharaonic times extremely uncertain (Täckholm, personal communication).

Carob (Ceratonia siliqua)

Arabic: *kharroub*

> *Like carob, a ton of wood for a drachm of sugar*
> (Popular saying)

Three words have been proposed by Loret (*Fl.*, 87, and 1893) as the Ancient Egyptian name of the carob: *w ʿḥ*, *ḏꜣrt*, and *nḏm*.

The first, *w ʿḥ*, literally means moon-shaped, and was thought by Loret to designate the dry pod. Lefebvre agreed, but only provisionally (1956, p. 65). Ebbell translated this word "manna" (*Eb.*, VII, 22). But Keimer (1943) did not accept this latter interpretation, and von Deines and Grapow (*Wb. Dr.*, 134) considered the meaning unclear. *W ʿḥ* was found inscribed on two pottery jars in a first dynasty tomb of Hemaka at Saqqara (Emery and Saad, 1938, p. 51). It was incorporated in oral medicines (*Eb.*, VII, 22; XIV, 43, etc.); it was chewed (*Eb.*, LIV, 314), administered in enemas (*Eb.*, XCVI, 819), fumigations (*Ber.*, 77), or dressings (*Eb.*, LXVIII, 482d). But in none of these indications is there any clue as to its nature.

The second name, *ḏꜣrt*, was stated by Loret to define the *fresh* fruit, on the ground of its closeness to its name in Coptic, *djiri* (*Fl.*, 145) in Arabic, *girat*, and in southern French *carouge*. Keimer (1931) judged this suggestion worthy of attention. Lefebvre (1956, p. 51), however, agreed with Dawson (1934) on translating this word "colocynth".

The third name, *nḏm*, read by Loret *noutem* (*Fl.*, 88) was written with the sign of a pod (? of *Acacia nilotica*) *nḏm*(c) which could also be read

(c)

nḏm

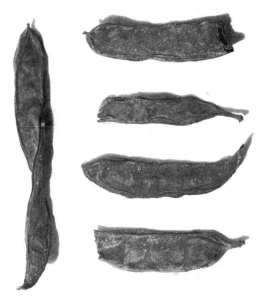

Fig. 18.1. Carob pods. Coptic period. Dokki Agricultural Museum, Cairo. No. 4216.
Photographed 1969.

"sweet". Loret therefore concluded that since carob was the only sweet-
tasting pod known in Egypt, *ndm* must have been the name of that plant.
De Buck (1967, p. 175), Faulkner (*F.*, 144), and Erman and Grapow
(1961, p. 91) read this sign ideographically "carob tree". On the other
hand, Gardiner (1950, p. 483, no. 29, n. 2) questioned this interpretation
and read it simply "pod from some sweet smelling tree"; while Ebbell
(*Eb.*, XXII, 80) translated it without presenting any grounds,
"moringa", a tree previously recognized by Loret (*Fl.*, 86) and Keimer
(1929c) in Ancient Egyptian *bꜣḳ*.

Pods and grains of carob have been identified by Newberry in a
twelfth dynasty find at El-Lahun (1890), and in a Graeco-Roman
cemetery at Hawara (1889). Fruits were also found in an eighteenth
dynasty tomb at Deir el-Medineh (Bruèyre, 1937, p. 108); a bow of
carob wood is said by Harris (1962, p. 443) to be kept in The Kew
Botanical Garden; and a few pods are shown at the Dokki Agricultural
Museum (Fig. 18.1).

Regarding its use, Rawlinson (1881, Vol. 1, p. 28) and Wilkinson
(1854, Vol. 1, p. 57) both listed the tree as the most important fruit
tree in Egypt, but neither of them gave any evidence to support his

statement. Maspero (1901, p. 30) wrote that it was called both *dunraga* and *tenraka*, without any references, and Breasted (*A.R.*, IV, 301) quoted a gift of 106,000 measures of carob-pods offered by Rameses III to the Nile-God Hapi.

On the other hand, the Greek botanist, Theophrastus (4, 2, 4), denied the existence of the carob in Egypt

". . . the fruit is in a pod; some call it the Egyptian fig erroneously; for it does not occur at all in Egypt, but in Syria and Ionia . . ."

Four centuries later, Pliny (XIII, XVI, 59) drew upon this same statement of Theophrastus, and wrote

". . . another tree is the one called by the Ionians the ceronia, which also buds from the trunk, the fruit being a pod, which has consequently been called by some the Egyptian fig. But this is clearly a mistake, as it does not grow in Egypt but in Syria and Ionia . . ."

Should one re-interpret the old tradition relating that St John lived in the desert on the "locust-bean" (translated carob), as meaning that he actually ate locusts, a traditional Arab relish?

Today carob trees are rather scarce in Egypt and are restricted to a thin strip on the northern coast. Their curious shape gave rise to the frequently heard threat

"I'll make of your life a carob: black and twisted."

Cherry (Prunus avium, Prunus cerasus)

Coptic: *tamaskion, pi-tamaskinos* (*Fl.*, 84)
Arabic: *kereiz*

In a papyrus dated to the year 5 B.C., the terms of lease of a garden land in Alexandria stipulated that the workers were to hand over the gardens, doors, and shadufs[1] in good working condition and

". . . in addition, 200 transplanted plants of the winter cherry. . ." (Lindsay, 1966, p. 298)

Montet (1958, p. 81) stated that cherries were not grown in Egypt prior to the Roman Period, and this evidence is seemingly supported by Pliny (*N.H.*, XV, XXX, 102)

". . . down to 74 B.C., there were no cherry trees in Italy. Lucullus first imported them from Pontus, and in 120 years they have crossed the ocean and got as far as Britain, but all the same no attention has succeeded in getting them to grow in Egypt. . ."

Two hundred "transplanted plants" growing in Alexandria during 5 B.C. may not by themselves substantiate establishment of the cherry in Egypt before this date, but the term "winter cherry" could be inter- preted as being different from another variety that grew perhaps in summer; and if year-round production of the cherry was indeed a reality in 5 B.C., this would indicate introduction of the fruit into Egypt in Pre-Roman times. In any case, the evidence at present does not indi- cate that cherries were known to the Ancient Egyptians, though in later history they were indeed part of the total food picture of the country. Their Coptic name *tamaskiou*, *pi-tamaskenos*, suggests that they were already widely cultivated in Damascus at the time when they were imported in Egypt (*Loret, Fl.*, 84).

Christ's Thorn or Jujube (Zizyphus spina-Christi)

(d)

nbs

Ancient Egyptian: see (d) (*F.*, 130)
Coptic: *kinari* (*Fl.*, 133)
Arabic: *nabq*

The early one ate the jujube
(i.e. The early bird ate the worm)

Christ's thorn or jujube is a very popular fruit nowadays in Egypt, and was, no doubt, a genuine Egyptian product. Today it grows naturally in Africa, but in former times it covered all the Nile Valley (Schwein- furth, 1873b). It has been discovered in the tomb of Hemaka (first dynasty) by Emery and Saad (1938), in the underground galleries of the Zoser complex at Saqqara (Lauer *et al.*, 1951) that date back to the third dynasty, in tombs of the twelfth dynasty at El Lahoun (Newberry,

1890), in twentieth dynasty Theban tombs (Schweinfurth, 1885, 1886) and in many other sites.

Its name *nbs*, rather close to Arabic *nabq*, recurs in funeral offerings of all epochs. Its fruits, leaves, meal and paste were widely used medicinally, internally (*Eb.*, XLIII, 210), in enemas (*Eb.*, XXXIII, 159), and externally (*Eb.*, XLIX, 272).

Later writers wrote of its popularity. Theophrastus (4, 3, 3) described it in great detail

". . . the Egyptian Christ's thorn [sic] is more shrubby than the lotus; it has a leaf like the tree of the same name of our country, but the fruit is different; for it is not flat, but round and red, and in size as large as the fruit of the prickly cedar or a little larger; it has a stone which is not eaten with the fruit, as in the case of the pomegranate, but the fruit is sweet, and if one pours wine over it, they say that it becomes sweeter and that it makes the wine sweeter . . ."

Pliny (XIII, XXXIII, 111) did not discuss a separate "Egyptian" variety of Christ's thorn, but he stated that the plant is widely found in Cyrenaica, where the kernel was also eaten.

Citron (Citrus medica)

Arabic: *naffash, kabbed, trong*

Pliny (*N.H.*, XIII, XXX, 102) wrote that the finest citron fruit was to be found in the vicinity of the temple of Hammon[2] and that it also grew in the interior of Cyrenaica. The earliest reference to consumption of this fruit to come to our attention is a second century A.D. papyrus

". . . we undertake to lease for one year the produce of all the date palms and fruit trees which are in the old vineyard for which we will pay as a special rent $1\frac{1}{2}$ artabae of fresh dates, $1\frac{1}{2}$ artabae of pressed dates, $1\frac{1}{4}$ artabae of walnut dates, $\frac{1}{2}$ artaba of black olives, 500 selected peaches, 15 citrons, and 400 summer figs . . ." (*S.P.*, I, 18)

Perhaps because of its appearance, there has been much mysticism surrounding the citron. Asclepiades, in the 60th book of his *Egyptian History*, no longer extant, wrote that Ge (the earth) brought it forth in honour of the "nuptials" of Zeus and Hera (Athenaeus, 3, 83, C).

Pliny (XII, VII, 15–16) recorded that the citron tree "refuses" to grow anywhere except in Persia and Media where it was highly valued for its medicinal properties. Both Theophrastus (4, 4, 2) and Pliny (XXIII, CVI, 105) discuss the citron as an antidote to poisons, and the former even lists the citron as a "breath-sweetener".

Athenaeus (3, 84, D–F) has indicated awareness of the mystical/ medicinal properties attributed to this plant when he wrote

". . . I am well aware, too, that when the citron is eaten before any food, dry or liquid, it is an antidote to every poisonous ingredient; I learned this from a townsman of mine who was entrusted with the governorship of Egypt. He had sentenced some convicted criminals to be devoured by wild beasts, and they were to be thrown among the creatures called asps. As they were entering the theatre assigned for the punishment of the robbers, a peddler-woman in the street gave them in pity some of the citron which she was holding in both hands and which she was eating. They took it and ate, and when, after a short time, they were thrown among those cruel and monstruous creatures, the asps, they received no injury when bitten. Perplexity seized the magistrate, and finally he questioned the soldier who guarded them to see whether they had eaten or drunk anything; when he learned that the citron had been given to them, he ordered next day that a piece of citron should be given, exactly as before to one convict, but not to the other, and the one who ate suffered no injury when bitten by the reptiles, but the other died the moment he was struck . . ."

Such beliefs have survived. Citrons are still believed today to drive away the "evil eye". Since counting is held to attract the evil eye, there is a saying

"Counting calls for lemons."

As to the existence of lemon in Ancient Egypt, Loret claimed that its Coptic names *Ketri, Kithri*, etc., are certainly derived from an Ancient Egyptian word and that, therefore, the words citron, cedrat, etc. originated in Egypt (*Fl.*, 101, 102). A fruit of the Passalacqua collection from Thebes, first identified as a Citrus was found later by Braun (1879) to be a sycamore fig. Another, of unknown origin and date, preserved in the Louvre Museum, was identified by Loret and Poisson (1895) as a *C. cedra* (a synonym?) which was known to the Hebrews under the name *hadar*. The Dokki Agricultural Museum at Cairo also contains several specimens (Fig. 18.2), from the Graeco-Roman times. Leaves of the plant were found by M. Gayet in burial equipment at the ancient necropolis of Antinoë which dates to the Greek Period (Bonnet, 1905).

Other Citrus Fruits Recently Introduced in Egypt

Citrus lemon is now cultivated in two varieties, sour lemon (Arabic: *lemoun adaliya*), and sweet lemon (*Lemoun helw*). It is of late introduction and probably came from Italy or Syria.

The small very scented lemon, *Citrus aurantifolia* (Arabic: *lemoun baladi* or *benzeheir*), was introduced about the tenth century A.D., probably via Palestine. These lemons are highly appreciated and recommended to clarify the blood and ease sick stomachs. Hence the saying

"He thinks himself a lemon in a nauseated town."

Grapefruit (*Citrus paradisi*) is also of recent introduction. It is a favourite component of weight-reducing diets. *Citrus aurantium*, sour orange (Arabic: *narang*), is of recent introduction. It is used in marmalade; its flowers are used in perfumery, and the tree is utilized as a stock on which to graft sweet oranges.

Citrus sinensis, sweet orange (Arabic: *bortoqal*), was introduced into Europe from China during the fifteenth century. Later, when the Portuguese traded with the Orient, they transported it into Italy, where it acquired the name Bortogallo.

Citrus reticulata, tangerine, mandarine (Arabic: *yusuf effendi* or *Yussafandi*, from the name of Yusuf Effendi, an Egyptian who studied agriculture at Grignon in France and on his way back to Egypt, in 1830, acquired from Malta a plant that he gave to Mohamed Aly). The first tree was planted at Shubra, a suburb of Cairo, and was then propagated on a large scale.

Fortunella margarita (Arabic: *kumqat*), a small orange no larger than a grape, is of quite recent introduction.

Egyptian Plum (Cordia myxa)

Ancient Egyptian: see (e)
Other: "Sebesten"
Arabic: *mokheit*

(e)

išd

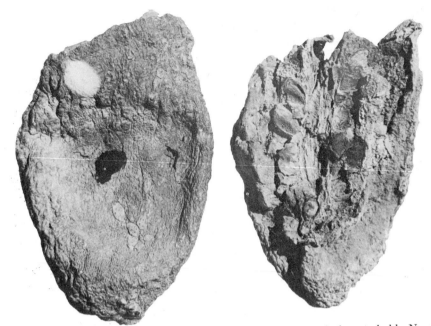

Fig. 18.2. Rests of fruit of *Citrus medica*. Luxor. Period uncertain but probably New Kingdom. Dokki Agricultural Museum, Cairo. No. 4200. Photographed 1969.

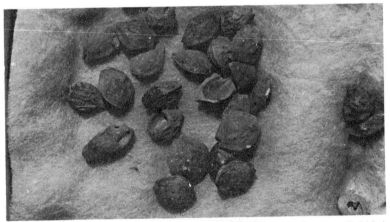

Fig. 18.3. Seeds of *Cordia myxa*. Deir El Medineh. Eighteenth dynasty. Dokki Agricultural Museum, Cairo. No. 1541. Photographed 1969

There is considerable confusion about the fruit called by ancient authors the "Egyptian plum".

Plum, as discussed by Theophrastus (4, 2, 10), has been identified as the sebesten (*Cordia myxa*), a tropical species flourishing today in India, which has been found in many Egyptian tombs (Newberry, 1889), and of which Ancient Egyptian specimens are exhibited at the Dokki Agricultural Museum (Fig. 18.3). This is the text of Theophrastus

> ". . . there is another tree, the Egyptian plum which is of great size, and the character of its fruit is like the medlar which it resembles in size, except that it has a round stone. It begins to flower in the month of Pyanepsion [October], and ripens its fruit about the winter solstice and it is evergreen. The inhabitants of the Thebaid, because of the abundance of the tree, dry the fruit; they take out the stones, bruise it, and make cakes of it . . ."

Pliny, however, seemed to have confused the issues, although he apparently differentiated between *Prunus domestica* and *Sebesten*. In one passage (*N.H.*, XIII, XIX, 64) he draws exclusively on the description of the sebesten, as given above by Theophrastus, only using the Latin word *prunus* rather than *myxa*, the Latin equivalent of sebesten

> ". . . this region [in the neighbourhood of Thebes] also contains the Egyptian plum [prunus] tree, which is not unlike the thorn last mentioned; its fruit resembles a medlar, and ripens in the winter, and the tree is an evergreen. The fruit contains a large stone, but the fleshy part, owing to its nature and to the abundance in which it grows, provides the natives with quite a harvest, as after cleaning it they crush it and make it into cakes for storage . . ."

Elsewhere, however, he distinguished between his *prunus* and the sebesten, calling the latter by its proper name *myxa*

> ". . . in Egypt the myxa is also used for making wine . . ." (*N.H.*, XIII, X, 51)

and

> ". . . the sebesten also, according to more learned authorities, was not introduced from Persia for punitive purposes, but was planted at Memphis by Perseus, and it was for that reason that Alexander, in order to do honour to his ancestor, established the custom of using wreaths of it for crowning victors in the games at Memphis. It always has leaves and fruit upon it, fresh ones sprouting immediately after the others . . ." (XV, XIII, 46)

This last passage is at variance with the description of sebesten given by Theophrastus (4, 2, 10); but is nearly identical with that of the persea given by that author (4, 2, 5).

Again, in his description of the peach, the persea and the sebesten, Pliny differentiated the first from the latter two, then wrote that the sebesten and the persea are nearly alike (*N.H.*, XV, XIII, 45). Thus it seems that he found little difference between the sebesten and the persea, while Theophrastus did. In fact, the fruits of these species are indeed similar.

Other sources of information concerning the "plum" are the various papyri of the Greek and Roman Period. Lindsay (1966, p. 298) cited a letter dated to *c.* 5 B.C. where 2,000 wild "plums" were used as partial payment for the lease of a garden at Alexandria. Another lease, dated to A.D. 141, listed $\frac{1}{4}$ artabae, 2 choiniks of dried sebesten as partial payment (Lindsay, 1966, p. 286).

In the various medical papyri, a fruit called *išd* has been translated by Loret (*Fl.*, 64, 103) and, after him, by Ebbell (*Eb.*, XII, 36; XXII, 79, etc.) as sebesten, *Cordia myxa*. Loret, however, seems later to have changed his opinion. This identification has also been refuted by both Keimer (1929c) and Lefebvre (1956, p. 106, n. 11).

(f)

dȝb

Fig (Ficus carica)

Ancient Egyptian: see (f) (*F.*, 309)
Arabic: *tin*

Agamiya [Honey confection] ye figs!
(Cairo street cry)

Very few finds of figs have been reported, most of the archaeological material consisting of sycamore figs: a fruit of the Passalacqua collection in the Berlin Museum (Braun *et al.*, 1877), some fruits from Deir el Medina (eighteenth dynasty) (Bruyère, 1937), and others from more recent times. Small faenza models of figs, probably of the Middle Kingdom, were described by Keimer (1926a), and a schist vessel in the shape of a fig leaf (second dynasty) was found at Saqqara and is now in the Cairo Museum (No. 6280).

Literature, however, is more instructive.

One of the earliest records of figs in Ancient Egypt is in the interesting biography of a third dynasty noble, Methen

> ". . . a house 200 cubits long and 200 cubits wide, built and equipped; fine trees were set out, a very large lake was made therein, figs and vines were set out . . ." (*A.R.*, 1, 173)

Figs are also mentioned among divine foods in the Pyramid Texts (Utterance 440). Indeed, figs are one of the most common fruits depicted in tomb reliefs and paintings (Figs 6.19, 18.4), some of which humorously illustrate monkeys among the branches, throwing with one hand figs in the baskets held by the peasants, and greedily helping themselves with the other.

King Rameses III offered 15,500 measures of figs to the God Amon-Ra at Thedes (*A.R.*, IV, 240), and one recalls the longings of the Israelite exiles as they wandered in Sinai

> ". . . and wherefore have ye made us to come up out of Egypt, to bring us in unto this evil place? It is no place of seed or of figs . . ." (Numbers, 20, 5)

Many other references to this fruit survive in Greek and Roman writings. Herodotus related that figs were among the ingredients with which sacrificial animals were stuffed prior to being burnt (II, 40). In the fourth century B.C., Theophrastus wrote of the curious properties of figs and grapes in Egypt

> ". . . they say that in the district of Elephantine neither vines nor figs lose their leaves"

an intriguing statement, strengthened, however, by the mention in a papyrus dated to A.D. 280 of "summer figs before the inundation" and "winter figs" (*S.P.*, I, 18). Plutarch (*I. and O.*, 378, 68) reported on what seems to be ritual eating of figs during certain festivals

> ". . . on the nineteenth day of the first month, when they are holding festival in honour of Hermes [Thot] they eat honey and a fig; and as they eat they say, 'a sweet thing is truth' . . ."

Pliny (XV, XIX, 70) described a black variety of fig grown in the region of Alexandria

> ". . . also among black figs the Alexandrian is named from its country of origin . . . it has a cleft of a whitish colour, and it called the 'luxury-fig'. . ."

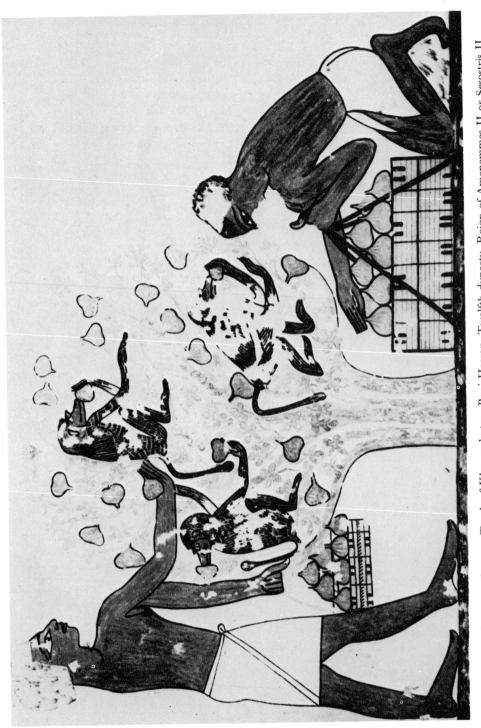

Fig. 18.4. Monkeys in a fig tree. Tomb of Khnum-hotep. Beni Hassan. Twelfth dynasty. Reign of Amenemmes II or Sesostris II. 1920–1900 B.C. From Davies (1936) Vol. I, plate VII.

It may be noted that this designation of the black Alexandrian fig is still applicable today, for the northern coast of Egypt is well known for its splendid production of both white and black figs. The above quotation is Pliny's sole mention of the fig, *Ficus carica*: elsewhere, his mention of "Egyptian fig" refers to *Ficus sycomorus* (e.g. *N.H.*, XIII, XIV, 56).

According to Athenaeus (4, 149, F) dried figs were eaten in banquets at Naucratis where he was born, and a nearly contemporary papyrus rebuked somebody who sent a rather "poor present of figs"

"... from Appianus. When one dispatches even the smallest load, he ought to send it with a letter stating what has been sent and by what carrier. And the goods which you dispatched were not so many as to require a man and a donkey to leave their work for them, only four baskets of rotten figs. And it was evident from the poorness and dryness and parched appearance of the figs that the estate has been neglected. But about this we shall have an account to settle between ourselves . . ." (*S.P.*, I, 141)

In Roman times figs were desired even in after life, since pottery models of this fruit were found in excavations of that period (Fig. 18.5).

Among the uses of figs other than in direct consumption one might add to their utilization in stuffing sacrificial beasts (see above), the production of some kind of wine from their juice (see Chapter 15) and their manifold medical prescription in mixtures (*Eb.*, XXIII, 92; XLV, 227), in enemas (*Ch.B.*, 32), in suppositories (*Eb.*, XXXI, 141), and in wound dressings (*Sm.*, 9).

(g)

wnšy

Grape (Vitis vinifera)

(h)

i̓rr·t

Ancient Egyptian: grapes or raisins (g) (*Wb.Dr.*, 136, 137)
vine (h) (*F.*, 9)
grapes (i) (*F.*, 9)

Arabic: ʿ *enab*

(i)

i̓rr·t

In summer eat grapes; in winter sugar cane
(Popular saying)

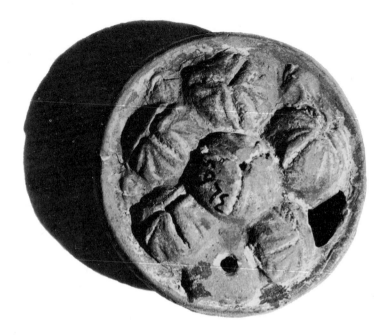

Fig. 18.5. Pottery model of figs. Roman. Dokki Agricultural Museum, Cairo. Photographed 1969.

Throughout history the primary use of grapes has been the production of wine (discussed in Chapters 14 and 15). However, grapes, as a fruit, were much appreciated by Egyptians. Today, as in antiquity, the western Delta lands are centres of grape production, and the description of Athenaeus (1, 33, D) is still valid

> ". . . the wine is abundant in this region and its grapes are very good to eat . . ."

Scenes of viticulture often appear in tombs (Fig. 14.1) where the various stages of cultivation, harvesting and production are recorded. All New Kingdom illustrations depict vines growing on arbors, although Pliny wrote

> ". . . and the greater part of the world lets its vintage grapes lie on the ground inasmuch as this custom prevails both in Africa and in Egypt and Syria . . ." (*N.H.*, XVII, XXXV, 185)

Such a difference might indicate that a change in techniques had supervened between the New Kingdom and Roman Period.

Seeds of varieties of wild vine have been found in prehistoric sites. According to Helback (1966), the earliest evidence of grapes comes from El-Omari.

The most ancient tombs contained grapes among the funeral offerings (Schweinfurth, 1884, 1885; Lauer *et al.*, 1951; Newberry, 1889), and these or models of these are on show in practically all museums (*Fl.*, 99; Keimer, 1929b, and Figs 18.6 and 18.7). In spite of their many varieties, having been variously classified as Damascus grapes, Corinthian grapes, or *V. vinifera*, var. *monopyrena* (although these contained three stones each), all the preserved specimens are black (Fig. 18.6), with a thick skin, and the vine leaves are covered with white hairs on their inner surfaces.

The Greek authors confirmed that numerous varieties of *Vitis vinifera* were developed in Egypt

". . . the vine is as abundant in the Nile Valley as its waters are copious, and the peculiar differences of the wines are many, varying with colour and taste . . ." (*Deipnos.*, 1, 33, E)

Moreover, some kinds were imported and seemed to do well in the new land. Among these foreign varieties, Pliny listed the Thasian, the "soot" and the pine tree grapes (*N.H.*, XIV, IX, 74).

A papyrus from the Greek Period, *c.* 210 B.C., tells of a robbery that took place in a Fayoum village

". . . Theophilus, son of Dositheus Philiston, son of [?], and Timaeus, son of Telouphis, raided the fruit garden of the aforesaid Pitholaeus, which is in the bounds of the aforesaid village [Apollonias,] and stripped the grapes from ten vines, and when Horus, the guard, ran out against them, they maltreated him and struck him on any part of the body that offered; and they carried off a vinedresser's pruning-hook . . ." (*S.P.*, II, 334)

Even the everyday method of care and cultivation of the vine was the subject of a papyrus dated to A.D. 280

". . . concerning the vineyard . . . layering as many vine-shoots as are necessary, digging, scooping hollows round the vines and trenching . . . keeping the vines well tended, giving space to the growths, cutting back, needful thinnings of foliage . . ." (*S.P.*, I, 18)

Biblical literature contains several references to the vine. Describing

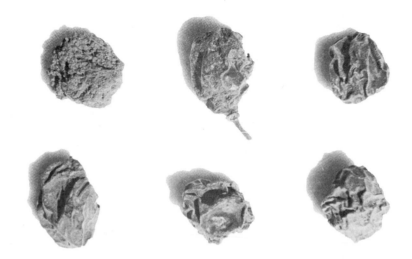

Fig. 18.6. Raisins. Deir el Medineh. New Kingdom. Dokki Agricultural Museum, Cairo. No. 1407. Photographed 1969.

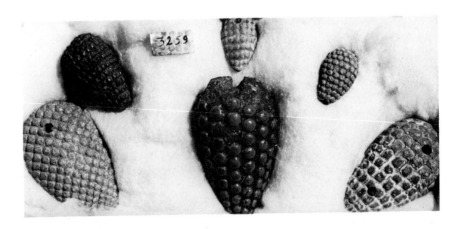

Fig. 18.7. Faience bunches of grapes. New Kingdom. Dokki Agricultural Museum, Cairo. No. 3259. Photographed 1969.

to Biblical Joseph a dream that puzzled him, Pharaoh's Chief Butler narrated

". . . behold, a vine was before me, and in the vine were three branches; and it was as though it budded, and her blossoms shot forth, and the clusters thereof brought forth ripe grapes . . ." (Genesis, 40, 9–10)

and the Egyptian grapes were among the fruits and foods desired by the Israelites (Numbers, 20, 5).

Raisins (Fig. 18.6)

> *The blows from the beloved are as sweet as raisins*
> (Popular saying)

Grapes were preserved by drying in the sun; in "raisin" form, they were much in favour. One need only recall an offering of "11,872 jars of raisins", made by Rameses III (*A.R.*, IV, 301). They were included in lists of spices, and seemed to be somewhat set apart from other fruits. Heredotus (II, 40) reported that raisins, along with other spices and fruits, were packed into the cleaned carcases of sacrificial animals; they were also included in the famed ointment, *Kyphi* (see Chapter 9, p. 435).

During the Roman Period raisins were used in cooking. Apicius (10, 1, 6–8) recommended their addition to several recipes attributed to Alexandrian "chefs"; and this is still the custom in all the Near East, whether raisins be cooked with rice, or added to stuffing.

Medically, both grapes and raisins had many uses, one sometimes being substituted for the other in alternative recipes, e.g. *Eb.*, LXXXIX, 631

". . . figs, sebesten, grapes, *isw*, wine, *inst*, juniper, *swt*, *dhwty*, frankincense, cumen, *ḏꜣrt*, yellow ochre . . ."

and *Eb.*, LXXIX, 632

". . . [another] figs, sebesten, raisin, *ḏꜣrt*, *inst*, yellow ochre, . . . frankincense . . ."

They were incorporated into mixtures, enemas, external applications and inhalations (*Eb.*, XXIII, 99; XXX, 132; XXXIV, 172; XLIV, 223; LXXIII, 566; XC, 759; *Ber.* 77; *Ch.B.*, 25, 32, etc.

Hegelig (Balanites aegyptiaca)

Arabic: *hegelig*
English: thorn tree, Egyptian balsam, Zachum oil tree

The earliest find of balanites is a kernel from Saqqara dated to the third dynasty (Lauer *et al.*, 1951). Täckholm (1961, Vol. III, p. 23) noted that almost all balanites kernels from Ancient Egypt were perforated (Fig. 19.9), probably to obtain the inner almond that yielded its precious oil (see Chapter 19); and from analysis of ancient honey which contained abundant balanites pollen, she concluded that it must have been widely cultivated.

More recently, P. Belon du Mans (A.D. 1547) found it in Sinai used as a source of oil (Sauneron, 1970, p. 129 b). Nowadays, the tree is confined to the oases, Upper Egypt, and the Sudan.

Juniper (Oxycedrus macrocarpa)

Arabic: ʿar ʿar

Fruits of juniper have been found from epochs spanning the Pre-Dynastic period (Brunton, 1937) to the seventh century A.D. (Winlock and Crum, 1926).

The tree, however, was never indigenous to Egypt, but berries were probably imported from Greece or the Near Eastern countries. The fruits were utilized in making perfumes, and their oil was probably the one, wrongly called cedar oil, used in anointing the dead body (Lucas, 1962, p. 309).

Melons (Cucurbitaceae)

I. Melon: General Varieties (Cucumis melo)

Egyptian Arabic: *shammam*

Artistic representations of melons or gourds (see Chapter 17, pp. 693–695) are occasionally seen in tombs (Figs 6.19b, 6.20, 17.13); but it is impossible to identify them with certainty. Schweinfurth (1885) identified material found by Schiaparelli at Dra ʿ Abul Naga as melons, but he pointed out that this particular tomb may have recently served as a storehouse. From the Graeco-Roman period Newberry (1889) found specimens of *Cucumis melo* at Hawara (Fig. 17.13).

The first literary evidence of existence of melons in Egypt is the Biblical passage telling of the longings of Israelites on their way out of Egypt (Numbers, 11, 5). A very much later report (A.D. 280) tells of four large white melons paid as partial settlement of the lease of a vineyard (*S.P.*, I, 18).

II. Water Melon (Citrullus vulgaris)

(j)

bddw-kꜣ

Ancient Egyptian: see (j)
Coptic: *pi-betuke, pi-betikhe* (*Fl.*, 73)
Hebrew: *abbattikhim* (Numbers, 11, 5)
Egyptian Arabic: *battikh*

Fill up your stomach with a summer water melon
(Popular saying for: Don't worry)

The identification of *bddw-kꜣ* with water melon seems justified by the relation of the Arabic, Coptic and Hebrew names for this plant.

Leaves of water melon were found in the coffin of Nebseni (New Kingdom) at Deir el-Bahari (*Fl.*, 73), and seeds are exhibited in the Dokki Agricultural Museum (Fig. 18.8).

Keimer, however, did not accept it (*Gpfl.*, 18, 33). In some Scalae (Coptic–Arabic dictionaries), Coptic *betuke* or *batikhe* is translated otherwise, *bâdingan barri* (wild egg-plant or aubergine, *Solanum melongena*). Loret, who cites this translation (*Fl.*, 73), hesitated, therefore, between water melon and egg-plant. The latter originated in Southeast Asia and was introduced into Egypt at an unknown date. The oldest reference we found to it is Nabulsi's description of the flora of the Fayoum in the fourteenth century A.D. (Salmon, 1901). It was not mentioned in the twelfth century relation of Abdullatif al-Baghdady (1965); but Pierre Belon du Mans (1547, see Sauneron, 1970, p. 112a) saw it cultivated later.

Curiously, egg-plant is associated in Egyptian dialect with madness or foolishness. To call a man *bâdingan* is to call him a senseless fool. One tenuous explanation is that pellagra—and consequent insanity—flourish in the autumn when egg-plant is reaped.

Bddw-k? was utilized in medicine: internally (*Ber.*, 111), in suppositories (*Eb.*, XXX, 139), in ointments (*Ber.*, 83), and in an obstetric prognostic test

"If *bddw-k*? and sycamore fruits are mixed with the milk of a woman who has borne a male child and are given to be swallowed; if she vomits she will bear children, if she passes wind she will never bear." (*Ber.*, 193, 194)

Olive (Olea europea)

Ancient Egyptian: *djedet*? (Loret 1886)
Coptic: *djeit*
Arabic: *zeitun* and: *zeit*, oil

Nowadays, olives are grown only in the Fayoum for pickling, and in Siwa and the West coast for oil. There is considerable difference in opinion, however, about the date of the first cultivation of the olive in Ancient Egypt. An early translation of the Pyramid Texts referred to a sacred olive tree in Heliopolis (Speleers, 1923–1924); but this was a mistranslation of *b*?*k . t* as olive (Speleers, 1923–1924, Vol. II, p. 32). On the other hand, Newberry (quoted by Harris, 1962, p. 35) stated

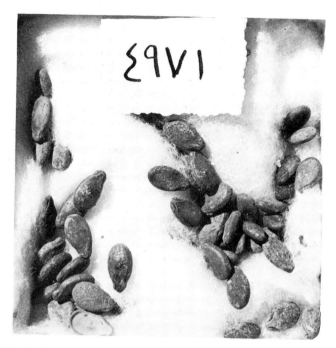

Fig. 18.8. Seeds of water melon. Thebes. New Kingdom. Dokki Agricultural Museum. Photographed 1969.

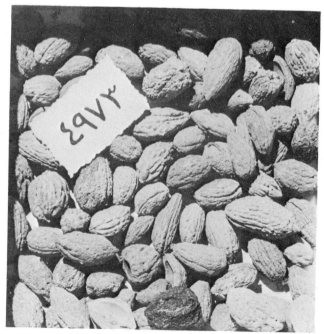

Fig. 18.9. Olive stones. Site unknown. New Kingdom. Dokki Agricultural Museum. Photographed 1969.

that the original home of the olive tree and of the olive oil trade was probably the region adjoining the west of the Nile Delta, which would be in keeping with the known abundance of olive trees in Siwa and North African countries west of Egypt. At present, according to Fakhry (1973, Vol. I, p. 27) there are some 25,000 olive trees in Siwa, some of them very old. As we mentioned in Chapter 18, 30,000 olive trees were planted in 1813 in the Fayoum by order of Mohamed Aly.

Montet (1958, p. 82) held, however, that the olive tree was introduced during the Second Intermediate Period by the Hyksos (*c.* 1730–1580). Kees (1961, p. 81) believed that it was not found in Ancient Egypt, though he admitted that cultivation was attempted by Rameses III and accepted Strabo's statement (17, 1, 35) that olives were found only in the Fayoum and Alexandria. Theophrastus (4, 2, 9), however, wrote almost three hundred years before Strabo

". . . for the olive also grows in that district [Thebaid], though it is not watered by the river, being more than 300 furlongs distant from it, but by brooks; for there are many springs. The oil produced is not inferior to that of our country, except that it has a less pleasing smell, because it has not a sufficient natural supply of salt . . ."

Pliny (XIII, XIX, 63) wrote in addition

". . . in the neighbourhood of Thebes, where oak, persea, and olive are also found . . ."

With this previous information, and with the knowledge that Strabo travelled widely inside Egypt, indeed to the latitude of Asswan if not further, it is difficult to understand how he could have overlooked the obvious, unless he paid only special attention to the Fayoum

". . . this nome [Arsinoite] is the most noteworthy."

Actual finds of olive tree material date to the eighteenth dynasty (Schweinfurth, 1886; Newberry, 1890), and olive stones are preserved in many museums, e.g. in the Dokki Agricultural Museum at Cairo (Fig. 18.9), but these are very few, and illustrations of the olive tree on monuments are unknown; the few published ones are of extremely doubtful significance (*Gpfl.*, p. 29). However, during and after the New Kingdom, garlands and wreaths made of various plants often included olive twigs (Schweinfurth, 1886; Loret, 1886), and its leaves are prominent in the "crown of justification" that was placed on Tut-ankh-Amon's head (Desroches-Noblecourt, 1963, p. 241 and Fig. 146), and in Roman garlands (Fig. 18.10). (See also under Fats, Chapter 19.)

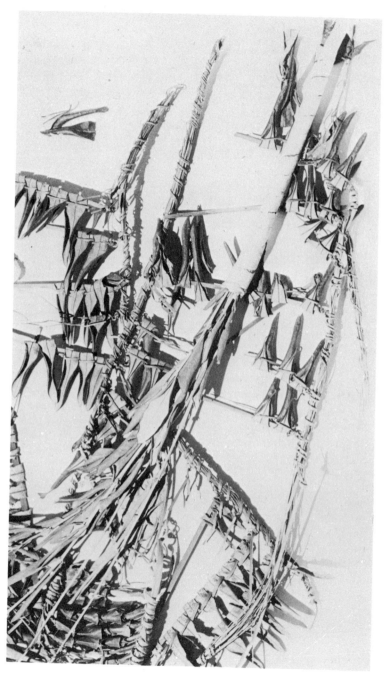

Fig. 18.10. Leaves of *Olea europea*. Roman period. Dokki Agricultural Museum, Cairo. Photographed 1969.

Palm Trees

(k)

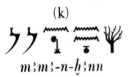

mꜣmꜣ-n-ḫꜣnn

I. The Argun Palm (Medemia argun)

Ancient Egyptian: see (k) (stone-doum)
Arabic: *argun, dom el dulla, dullakh*

The argun palm was quite a common tree in Egyptian gardens. Ten of these unusual trees were growing in Anna's garden at Thebes and were illustrated in his tomb (Boussac, 1896). Its fruits have been found in tombs of all epochs, from the fifth dynasty onwards (Fig. 18.11), and an extensive list may be found in Täckholm and Drar's monumental work (*T.,* II, 299–300). As picked from the tree, the fruit is edible but in Nubia it is first buried for some time, whereupon it acquires a sweet taste, said to resemble that of the coconut (*T.,* II, 298).

Nowadays, the depredations of camel drivers who pluck out its fan-shaped foliage to make camel beds have led to its disappearance, save from some remote desert spots in Nubia along the old caravan road from Upper Nubia to Meroe, and from the Dunkul oasis and Nakhila near Kurkur where it was recently rediscovered.

(l)

bni

II. Date Palm (Phoenix dactylifera)

(m)

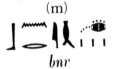

bnr

Ancient Egyptian: see (l) and (m) (*F.,* 83), date juice (n)
                                    (*F.,* 83)

Greek: *phoenix*
Arabic: *balah, tamr*

(n)

bniw

If you give my son a date, my stomach will taste its sweetness
                                                    (Popular saying)

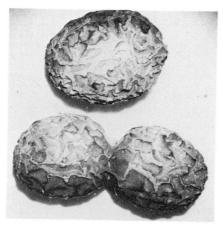

Fig. 18.11. Argun palm *Medemia argun.* Luxor. Dokki Agricultural Museum, Cairo. No. 374. Photographed 1969.

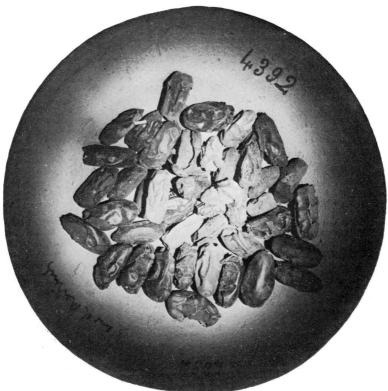

Fig. 18.12. Dried dates. Deir el Medineh. New Kingdom. Dokki Agricultural Museum, Cairo. No. 4392. Photographed 1969.

The date palm is one of the most important botanical species of the whole Near East. As Candolle defined it, its geographic distribution forms a broad zone stretching from Senegal to India, between the 15th and 30th parallels. In all of that area the thousands of relatively isolated palm groves that dot the caravan routes are evidence of the ease of transport of dates, and of the quick germination of their stones (Candolle, 1886, pp. 301–304).

Egypt, which lies in the middle of this zone, now grows about 40 varieties (*T.*, II, 188); the latest official census estimated the date palm production at 5,083,400 trees (*T.*, II, 169), and their production at about 400,000 tons (*T.*, II, 170).

Schweinfurth (1891) thought that it was a descendant of *P. reclinata*, now found only in South Africa, but of which some specimens from Ancient Egypt exist in the Museum of Florence, according to Migliarini (*Fl.*, 35). Others believe it to have originated in that part of Africa to which the Canary Islands were originally connected (Beauverie, 1930).

It is even possible that it originated in Egypt. Stones of *P. reclinata*, at first thought to belong to *P. sylvestris* (date sugar palm), both now unknown in Egypt, have been found in an upper palaeolithic site at Kharga by Caton-Thompson and Gardner (1934, p. 84). This plant is widely distributed today in the savannah regions of Tropical Africa, and this discovery might mean that this tree, which requires a humid climate, once grew wild in Africa, and that the date palm could have originated in the continent but later disappeared under the influence of climatic change.

Dates are very rich in carbohydrates and proteins. Taken along with milk as in present day Bedouin diets, they constitute a complete nourishment. One is not surprised, therefore, to learn that date stones were found even in Pre-Dynastic sites (MAE, 119). Nevertheless, Täckholm and Drar doubt that the early Egyptians could have known artificial pollination, which is necessary to the propagation of palm tree (*T.*, II, 218), and they reckon as genuine only one Pre-Dynastic specimen, found at El-Omari by Debono (1948); the others they regard as dubious. It is known, however, that the Egyptians distinguished male from female trees (*Fl.*, 35) and they may, therefore, have practised artificial pollination.

Genuine dynastic finds of dates and date-cakes are countless. Täckholm and Drar (*T.*, II, 219–233), Keimer (1924a) and others, give extensive lists of these, and fruits as well as models are exhibited at the Dokki Agricultural Museum (Figs 18.12, 18.13, 18.14).

Equally numerous are literary references from the eighteenth dynasty (*A.R.*, II, 159) onwards, of which the most munificent is a gift of Rameses III

"65,480 dates to Re at Helopolis" (*A.R.*, IV, 215, 244)

One cannot fail to be impressed also by the palmiform columns of temples (Fig. 18.15) and the numerous illustrations of date palms in reliefs, frescoes, and decorative panels, particularly under and after the New Kingdom.

From the Greek and Roman Periods many more descriptions of the tree, its fruit, and its preparations have survived; but historians were not in agreement on the merits of the Egyptian dates, although they agreed that the best came from Siwa (Theophrastus, 4, 3, 1; Pliny, *N.H.*, XIII, XXIII, 111–112). Plutarch (*Table Talk*, 8, 4, 732, C–D) spoke out in its favour

"If the Greek date palm were like that of Syria or Egypt, there would be no other tree to compare it with . . ."

a statement at variance with Strabo's opinion (17, 1, 51)

". . . throughout the whole of Aegypt, the palm tree is not of a good species; and in the region of the Delta and Alexandria it produces fruit that is not good to eat; but the palm tree in the Thebaid is better than any of the rest . . ."

Pliny (*N.H.*, XIII, IX, 47), who praised the dates of Siwa, also found fault with those of Upper Egypt

". . . all over the Thebaid and Arabia the dates are dry and small with a shrivelled body, and as they are scorched by the continual heat their covering is more truly a rind than a skin . . ."

In another passage (*N.H.*, XIII, IX, 48), he further discussed the dates of Upper Egypt

". . . the date of the Thebaid is packed into casks at once before it has lost the aroma of its natural heat; if this is not done, it quickly loses its freshness and dries up unless it is warmed up again in an oven."

And he added that they were then used to fatten pigs (*N.H.*, XIII, IX, 48, 49).

This statement would generally correspond to that of Theophrastus (2, 6, 8)

". . . the only dates that will keep, they say, are those which grow in the

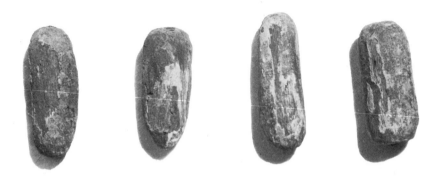

Fig. 18.13. Wooden dates. Thebes. New Kingdom. Dokki Agricultural Museum, Cairo. Photographed 1969.

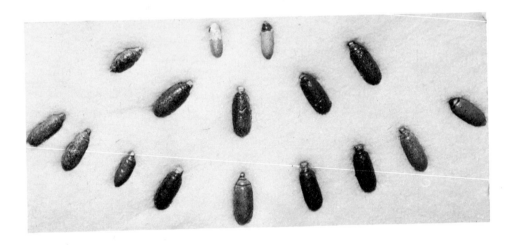

Fig. 18.14. Faience necklace of dates. New Kingdom. Dokki Agricultural Museum, Cairo. No. 1900. Photographed 1969.

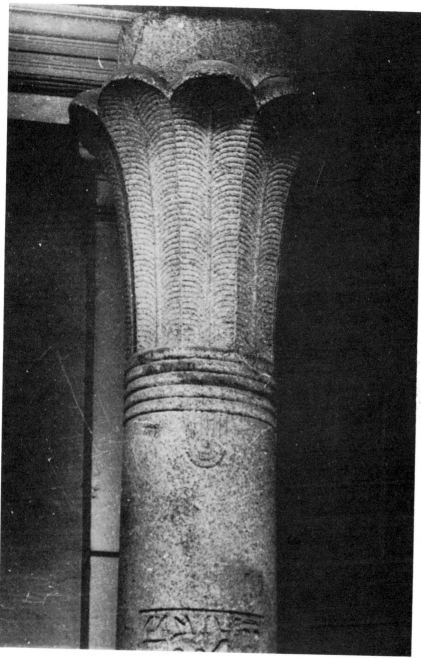

Fig. 18.15. Palmiform capital from the temple of Sahure. Sixth dynasty. Abusir. Now in the Cairo Museum. Used with permission.

valley of Syria, while those that grow in Egypt, Cyprus, and elsewhere are used when fresh . . ."

Petronius, however, in his account of a dinner with Trimalchio praised both Syrian and dried Theban dates

"Then the servants came up . . . A great dish and on it lay a wild boar of the largest possible size . . . from its tusks dangled two baskets woven from palm leaves, one full of fresh Syrian dates, the other of dried Theban dates." Trimalchio added 'And have a look at the delicious acorns our pig in the wood has been eating'. Young slaves promptly went to the baskets and gave the guests a share of the two kinds of date." (Petronius, *The Satyricon and The Fragments* p. 54)

These different judgments probably reflected experience either with the poorer qualities of dates, or with dried dates out of season. Indeed, dates were so popular that an Egyptian soldier stationed far from his home country could not keep from recording his sentimental longing for them

". . . I reside in Kenkentaui and I am without equipment. I pass the night under trees that bear no fruit to eat. Where are their dates?" (Erman 1966, p. 204)

In fact the word for dates, *bnr*, came to mean "sweet" and to be extended to all the various meanings of "agreeable" or "sweet": *bnr mrw . t*, beloved; *bnr-ib* good hearted; *bnr ns . t*, speaking well, sweet tongue, etc. (Wallert, 1962, p. 47).

The enthusiastic partiality to this juicy fruit, general in all the Near East, is manifest in the fond cries of street vendors

"You, child of the tall mother, your stones are almonds"

Significance and Importance of the Palm Tree

The importance of the palm tree in Egyptian lore was even more vividly reflected in the halo of sacredness that surrounded it. Its name *bnr* or *bni* was very close to *bennu*, the name of the phoenix (see Volume 1, Chapter 6). The Greeks called that miraculous bird by the same name they gave to the fruit (phoenix), which is not derived, as has been sometimes stated, from the Phoenicians, alleged to have distributed it around the Mediterranean.

Because it was supposed to grow a palm every lunar month, this tree was associated with the counting of the flow of time, and with control of the span of life (Fig. 1.1) (van de Walle and Vergote, 1943). In hieroglyphs the stripped rib of the palm meant "year", and this sign was often associated since the first dynasty with the *heb-sed* jubilee of life-renewal (Wallert, 1962).

It was even one of the plants drawn as a symbol of Upper Egypt (Wallert, 1962, p. 76) and its various parts were imitated in amulets, jewels, shrines, furniture and sacred architecture, from Archaic to Greek times. Palm trees appear in rock drawings of the Egyptian desert (Winkler, 1938–1939, Vol. 1, p. 11), in proto-historic palettes like Narmer's palette (Legge, 1900) and other slates. Palmiform columns support the heavy roof of Sahure's temple (fifth dynasty) (Fig. 18.15); and like the *doum palm* (see below) it had special significance in drawings of gardens and tombs, where it was often drawn with monkeys seated on its branches, as in Rekh-mi-Re's tomb (Davies, 1943, Vol. 1, p. 78, plate 110) where this important vizier is illustrated while receiving dates from the hands of a priest.

Even now the tree is surrounded by an aura of sacredness. Brides' chairs, and graves are ornamented with palms. According to Täckholm and Drar, bridegrooms, the day after their wedding, strip a palm leaf, slit it at the point and touch their friends with it for good luck (*T.*, II, 188). In common language the custom of celebrating a victory with palms has given rise to the phrase "the palm of victory," and to "palms" in military decorations. Christian traditions still recall Christ's entry into Jerusalem carrying palms and on the anniversary of that day, "Palm Sunday", Egyptian Christians carry palms which they weave and plait into all kinds of shapes.

Uses of Dates Other than in Food

Apart from being directly consumed as fruit or as date-cakes of which Beauverie (1930) described a specimen, date-juice served to make a type of wine (Chapter 15), and to flavour beer (Chapter 13).

Medically, dates were used internally in medications designed to purge (*Eb.*, VII, 22), to clear the enigmatic *wḥdw* (*Eb.*, XXIV, 98), or to regulate the urine (*Eb.*, XLIX, 263). In vaginal pessaries, with other ingredients, they enhanced fertility (*Eb.*, XCIII, 783). And they entered into various fumigations (*K.*, 20), bandages to the belly (*Eb.*, XXXV, 177), ointments (*Eb.*, XC, 762), and in an Asiatic ophthalmic prescription (*Eb.*, LXIII, 422).

Date-meal, date juice either fresh or fermented, date stones and pressed dates were utilized in the same ways (*Wb.Dr.*, 172–179). Pliny (XXIII, LI, 97) described several medicinal uses of dates and of concoctions made from them

> "They relieve a cough and are flesh-forming food. The juice of boiled dates used to be given by the ancients to invalids instead of hydromel to restore their strength and to assuage thirst; for this purpose they used to prefer Thebaic dates, which are also useful, especially in food, for the spitting of blood. The dates called caryotae are applied with quinces, wax, and saffran to the stomach, bladder, belly and intestines. They heal bruises. The kernels of dates, if they are burnt, take the place of spodium . . . are an ingredient of eye-salves."

Comparison of the Ebers papyrus with the above-mentioned prescriptions reveals curious coincidences.

Nowadays, there is no part of the tree that is not utilized, and country-people ingest its pollen to enhance fertility.

III. Doum Palm (Hyphaene thebaica)

(o)

𓍯𓍯𓆰

mꜣmꜣ

Ancient Egyptian: (o) (doum tree) (*F.*, 103)
(p) (doum fruit) (*Fl.*, 83)
Arabic: *doum*
Berber: *kwkw* (Loret, 1935–1938)

(p)

kwkw

The Doum palm has characteristics of its own. Even to the lay traveller, the large terminal crown of leaves on its branches, its spadix over one metre long, and its repeatedly forked trunk, are immediately recognizable (Fig. 18.16). Its fruit is about 7–8 cm long, 7 cm broad, irregular, bumpy, brown-glossy, punctate, with a stone about 4 cm long, 2·5 cm broad with a narrow cavity (*T.*, II, 274).

As with the palm tree, all of its parts are used in Egypt—its timber, leaves, stalks, fruit, and even its stones which serve as vegetable ivory to make buttons, rings, beads and the like.

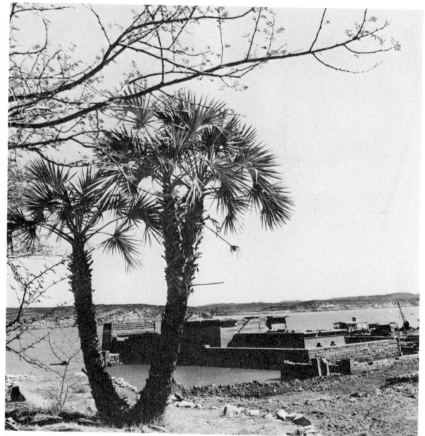

Fig. 18.16. Doum palm. Kalabsha. Nubia. Documentation Centre, Cairo.

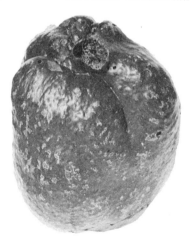

Fig. 18.17. Fruit of the doum palm. Tomb of Tut-ankh-Amon. Dokki Agricultural Museum, Cairo. Photographed 1969.

The fruit is eaten either raw, after being soaked in water, or made into a syrupy decoction.

Today, this palm, one of the landmark trees of Upper Egypt, is found almost exclusively south of Qena within the Nile Valley; its northern ecologic boundary in the eastern desert is, however, the much visited group of stately branching palms situated at the mouth of Wadi Doum (The Doum Valley), approximately 35 miles south of Suez, along the Red Sea.

In Ancient Egypt it was cultivated since the remotest antiquity. Täckholm and Drar went so far as to state that there is no period of Egyptian history from which finds of doum have not been reported (*T.*, II, 282–289). They were found as early as in Badarian settlements (Brunton and Caton-Thompson, 1928), and fruits were deposited in Tut-ankh-Amon's tomb (Fig. 18.17). The primary use of the tree, however, was not as a provider of food. Fragments of doum fibres were identified in mats (Greiss, 1957, p. 41) and its wood and stone were useful building materials and served to make small objects of daily use.

Its fruit, however, was held in high regard. Rameses III offered 449,500 measures to Amon-Ra at Thebes (*A.R.*, IV, 241), and we know of a prayer that was addressed to it, possibly by travellers lost in the wilderness and in need of sustenance

"... thou, great doum palm, that is sixty cubits in height, whereon are fruits, stones are in the fruits, and water is in the stone ..." (Erman 1966, p. 306)

For it was indeed sacred, more especially to Thot who, in his personification as a baboon, was often pictured with it on ostraca (Fig. 18.18) on jewels, and in the many paintings of the gardens that the deceased wished to visit after his death, to enjoy the cool shade of its leaves and the tasty fruits that he liked (Davies, 1927, plate 16, p. 23; Keimer, 1939; Wallert, 1962, pp. 86, 87).

Theophrastus called the tree *koukiophoron*, a word evidently derived from Egyptian *kuku*. He gave a good description of the fruit, and contrasted it with that of the date palm

"... it has a peculiar fruit, very different from that of the date palm in size, form and taste; for in size, it is nearly big enough to fill the hand, but it is round rather than long; the colour is yellowish, the flavour sweet and palatable. It does not grow bunched together like the fruit of the palm, but each fruit grows separately; it has a large and very hard stone." (2, 6, 9)

The most obvious difference between the doum and the date palm, however, is the branching of the former (Fig. 18.16). This was underlined by both Theophrastus

". . . the palm, speaking generally, has a single and simple stem; however, there are some with two stems, as in Egypt . . ." (2, 6, 9)

and by Pliny who described the tree as having branches spread out like arms (*N.H.*, XIII, XVIII, 62).

Regarding its uses, Theophrastus (2, 6, 10) wrote that in Ethiopia and Upper Egypt, its fruit was used to make a variety of bread, and both he and Pliny even noted that "curtain rings" were made out of its stones (Theophrastus, 4, 2, 7; Pliny, *N.H.*, XIII, XVIII, 62).

Nevertheless, Täckholm and Drar wrote regarding the Greek statements

". . . the often repeated statement that Strabo and Pliny both described the doum palm under the name of Thebaic palm is erroneous for, whereas Strabo praised the Thebaic date as the best, Pliny despised it as the worst date grown in Egypt. It is probable that the two authors meant two other different fruits, but not doum . . ." (*T.*, II, 281)

Montet (1958, p. 81) stated that the fruit was commonly used in Ancient Egyptian medicine, but the only mention of anything remotely like it in the medical papyri is a prescription in the Rameses papyrus V, recommending *maa*, a fruit, that Dawson thought could be a variant of *mama* (*mꜣmꜣ*), or a copying mistake (*Wb. Dr.*, 212). Nowadays, the fruit is ground and prepared into a drink recommended in gastro-intestinal disturbances, which is not surprising, in view of its astringency. According to Beadnell and Llewellyn (1909, pp. XIV, 248)

"the spongy internal portions of the nut forms an important article of food in some parts of the Sahara and, when mixed with an infusion of dates, constitutes a cooling drink much valued in febrile disturbances . . ."

Peach (Prunus persica)

Egyptian Arabic: *khokh*

Peaches were found in the Graeco-Roman necropolis of Hawara (Newberry, 1889), and in four other sites, all from the Roman or

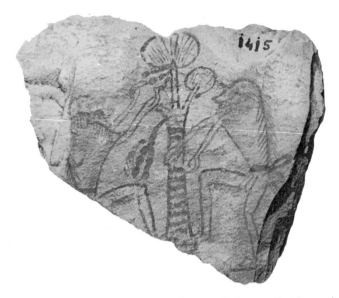

Fig. 18.18. Ostraca of limestone representing two baboons climbing a doum palm Thebes. *c.* 1400 B.C. Cairo Museum. Used with permission.

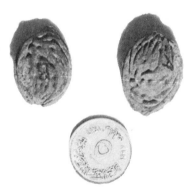

Fig. 18.19. Two peach stones. Saqqara. Late period. Dokki Agricultural Museum, Cairo. Photographed 1969.

Coptic period (see Täckholm, 1961, Vol. III, pp. 15–16). Theophrastus did not mention them in his history of plants, so that they were probably unknown in Egypt before the fourth century B.C. Pliny (*N.H.*, XV, XIII, 45), however, related that they came to Italy from Egypt, through Rhodes, shortly before his time, and added

> "It is not true that the peach grown in Persia is poisonous and causes torturing pain, and that, when it had been transplanted into Egypt by the kings to use as a punishment, the nature of the soil caused it to lose its dangerous properties . . ."

Of the Greek Period, similarly, a papyrus dated to A.D. 280 records a payment of 500 selected peaches as partial settlement for the lease of a vineyard (*S.P.*, I, 18). This evidence, added to the discovery of peach kernels from the late period at Saqqara (Fig. 18.19), opens to question Montet's opinion that it was not grown in Egypt before Roman times (1958, p. 81).

Pear (Pyrus communis)

Arabic: *kommethra*

To our knowledge, the only literary reference to pears in Egypt sheds little light on the time of its introduction

> ". . . pears having the name of their place of origin are the Amerian, the latest of all kinds, the Picentine, the Numantine, the Alexandrian, the Numidian, and the Greek . . ." (*N.H.*, XV, XV, 55)

This single reference is confirmed, however, by the discovery of specimens of this fruit in the Graeco-Roman necropolis of Hawara (Newberry, 1889), and by its Coptic names, *kortholos apidia*, and *apios*, which sound more Greek than Egyptian (*Fl.*, 83).

Nevertheless, in Grecian and Roman Europe, it was a common fruit. There are in Theophrastus about forty passages describing this fruit, and Pliny devoted to it a large section, especially when compared to the single above mentioned reference to the Alexandrian variety. With this information, it is apparent that pears were grown in Egypt in pre-Roman times, although Montet (1958, p. 81) believed that the pear was not grown in Egypt prior to that period.

Candolle (1886, p. 230) did not mention its existence in Egypt during dynastic times, and wrote that there is no Hebrew or Aramaic name for the pear, an index that he uses throughout his text as a proof to the introduction of various foods into Egypt as "Post-Exodus" in date. He did write, however, that pears do not flourish in hot climates, although the variety grown near Alexandria today is quite good.

(q)

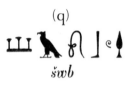

šwb

Persea (Mimusops schimperi)

Ancient Egyptian: see (q) (*Gpfl.*, 31, 144; *Fl.*, 263)
Arabic: *lebakh*

Fruits of a species of Mimusops have been found in many tombs: e.g. by Petrie (1889) at Illahoun (twelfth dynasty); by Schweinfurth at Gebelein (1886) and in the wreaths around the mummy of Rameses II (1883); by Lauer *et al.* at Saqqara (1951) (third dynasty); and in the tomb of Tut-ankh-Amon (Fig. 18.20). There has been originally some argument about the exact species involved, *M. elengi* or *M. kummel* (*Fl.*, 61) but the consensus of opinion seems to identify it as *M. schimperi.*

M. schimperi is generally taken to be the persea of antiquity, of which one of the best descriptions was written by Theophrastus (4, 2, 5)

". . . in Egypt, there is another tree called the persea which, in appearance is large and fair, and it most resembles the pear in leaves, flowers, branches, and general form, but it is evergreen, while the other is deciduous. It bears abundant fruit and at every season, for the new fruit always over-takes that of last year. It ripens its fruit at the season of the etesian winds; the other fruit they gather somewhat unripe and store it. In size it is as large as a pear, but in shape it is oblong, almond-shaped, and its colour is grass green. It has inside a stone like the plum, but much smaller and softer; the flesh is sweet and luscious and easily digested; for it does not hurt if one eats it in quantity."

Pliny, as usual, appears guilty of plagiarism

"Egypt also possesses a tree of a peculiar kind called the persea, which resembles a pear but is an evergreen. It bears fruit without intermission, as when it is plucked a fresh crop sprouts the next day, but its season for ripening is when the midsummer winds are blowing. The fruit is longer than a pear, and is enclosed in a shell like an almond and a rind the colour of grass, but where the almond has a kernel this has a plum, which differs from an almond kernel in being short and soft, and although temptingly sweet and luscious, is quite wholesome . . ." (*N.H.*, XIII, XVII, 60–62)

Strabo (17, 2, 4) believed the persea to be unique to Egypt and Ethiopia. Other authors hold that it had been imported in mythological times, its name being allegedly derived from the hero Persaeus who was said to have planted it in Egypt.[3] Diodorus, however, seemed to imply that he adopted another etymology

"There are also many kinds of trees, of which that called persea, which was introduced from Ethiopia by the Persians when Cambyses conquered those regions."

Pliny (*N.H.*, XIII, 45) compared the persea to red myxa (sebesten) and stated that it refuses to grow anywhere except in the "east". In the same passage, he added that

"careful writers indicate that the persea, as originally grown in Persia, was poisonous; causing torturing pain, but upon introduction into Egypt the strange nature of the soil caused it to lose its dangerous properties."

This may have been the source of Abdul Latif al-Baghdady, who wrote in the twelfth century A.D.

"Aristotle and other writers say that the labakh [identified now as the persea] was in Persia a mortal poison, but having been transported to Egypt, became a food." (1965, pp. 33–35)

Examination of these passages reveals the kind of inconsistencies with which historical botanists have to contend. How could this tree be sacred to Isis and (or) Osiris if it were introduced only in the Persian Period? Was it indigenous in Egypt or not?

The confusion has been compounded by the various identifications of modern writers. Rawlinson (1881, Vol. 1, p. 28) thought the persea was *Balanites aegyptiaca*, a tree bearing a fruit completely different from that of *Mimusops schimperi*, and his description of the fruit of what he calls persea applies quite clearly to the latter

"the persea which is now rare in the Nile Valley but is met with in the Ababdeh desert and grows in great profusion on the road from Coptos to Berenice, is a bushy tree or shrub, which attains the height of 18 or 20 feet

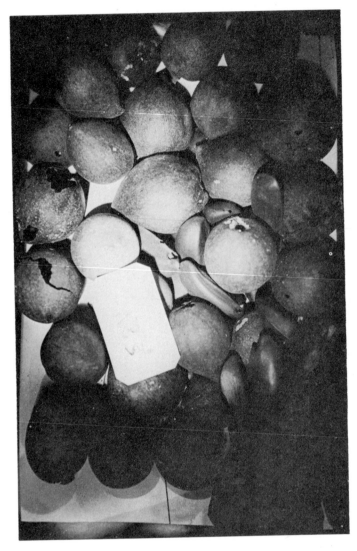

Fig. 18.20. Persea, *Mimusops schimperi* found in Tut-ankh-Amon's tomb. Dokki Agricultural Museum, Cairo. No. 4472. Photographed 1969.

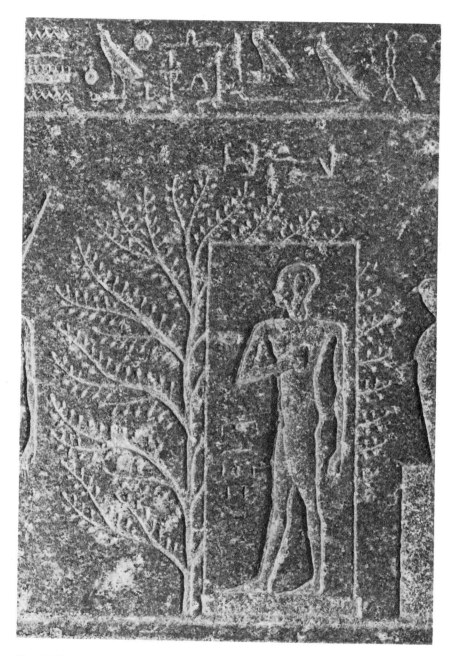

Fig. 18.21. Nectanebu inside the foliage of a Persea tree. Coffin of the Pharaoh Nectanebu. Cairo Museum. Used with permission.

under favourable circumstances. The bark is whitish, the branches gracefully curved, the foliage of an ashy grey, more especially on its under
surface. The lower branches are thickly garnished with long thorns, but
the upper ones are thornless. The fruit, which grows chiefly on the upper
boughs, and which the Arabs call 'lalob' is about the size of a small date,
and resembles the date in general character. Its exterior is a pulpy substance of a subacid flavour; the stone inside is large in proportion to the
size of the fruit, and contains a kernel of a yellowish-white colour, oily, and
bitter. Both the external envelope and the kernel are eaten by the
natives . . ."

For some mystic reason the tree was regarded as sacred, and kings
were often depicted protected by its foliage, or emerging from it (Fig.
18.21). Plutarch, after saying that it was sacred to Osiris (*I. and O.*,
359, 20), stated that the persea was especially consecrated to Isis, because
its fruit resembles a heart and its leaf a tongue (*I. and O.*, 378, 68),
referring to the Egyptian teaching that creation was an act of the will
(represented by the heart), effected through the utterance of the word
(the tongue), an explanation that recalls Biblical memories

> And God said, let there be light; and there was light." (Genesis, 1, 3)
>
> "By the word of the Lord were the heavens made and all the host of them
> by the breath of his mouth." (Psalms, 33, 6)

Another tradition identified the oval "cartouche" in which royal
names were inscribed as a persea leaf (Figs 1.20 and 6.45), for it was
on a leaf of this tree that the god Thot wrote the kings' names on their
accession to the throne (Fig. 18.22).

That it enjoyed prestigious regard, at least in Roman times, is confirmed by a law passed under Emperor Arcadius, forbidding under
penalty of a fine to uproot or to sell any persea tree in Egypt (Codex
Iustiniani, XI, 78); and, as a concluding point of mythologic hearsay,
one might quote Aelian (10, 21) who wrote that crocodiles were hung
from persea trees then flogged as they wept "crocodile tears".

(r)

inhmn

(s)

nhym

Pomegranate (Punica granatum)

(t)

nhym

Ancient Egyptian: tree (r) (*F.*, 24) and (s) (*Fl.*, 137)
fruit (t) (*Gpfl.*, 151)

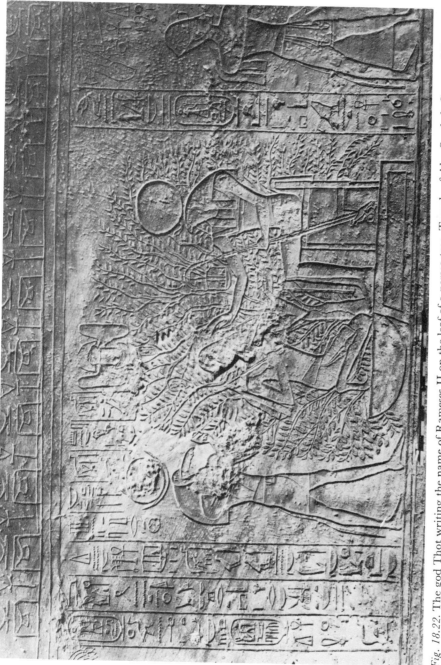

Fig. 18.22. The god Thot writing the name of Rameses II on the leaf of a persea tree. Temple of Abu Sembel. Centre of Documentation, Cairo.

Coptic: *erman*
Hebrew: *rimmoun*
Arabic: *orman, romman*

Her breasts are two pomegranates
(Popular comparison)
Eat a pomegranate and visit a bath, your
youth will haste back
(Popular saying)

Because of its distinctive shape, archaeologists and botanists can identify the pomegranate with certainty in many of the reliefs and frescoes on the walls of Ancient Egyptian tombs (Fig. 18.23).

The name of this tree *inhm, nhym,* was written in the hieroglyphic script in several different ways, which would indicate, according to Loret (*Fl.*, 76), that the plant was not indigenous to the country, but that it was imported into Egypt where it kept its original name. Its Coptic name was the related word: *erman* or *herman,* cognate with Hebrew *rimmoun,* Arabic *orman* and Berber *armoun,* thus confirming a single foreign origin, probably from Persia, but possibly, as one of its Latin names *Malum punicum* suggests, from Northwest Africa.

The oldest Egyptian text mentioning this tree was found at Thebes in the tomb of Ani (or Anna), who lived under Thutmose I, where it is cited among the trees he planted in his funerary park (Boussac, 1896). It was, therefore, introduced before that period and, in fact, Schweinfurth identified it among vegetable remnants from the twelfth dynasty at Dra'Abul Naga (1886), and other authors reported to have found it in tombs of the following periods (*Gpfl.*, 47, 104) right through the Christian era (second to third centuries) (Newberry, 1889) (see Fig. 18.24).

The oldest illustration of pomegranates dates to the reign of Thutmose III, when this king is shown at Karnak receiving an offering of this fruit (*Gpfl.*, 47), and the fruits and trees appear very often in illustrations of gardens from the twentieth dynasty onwards.

The first literary record of its use in Egypt occurs in the medical papyri (see later). Otherwise, it is first cited under the nineteenth dynasty, during the reign of King Rameses III

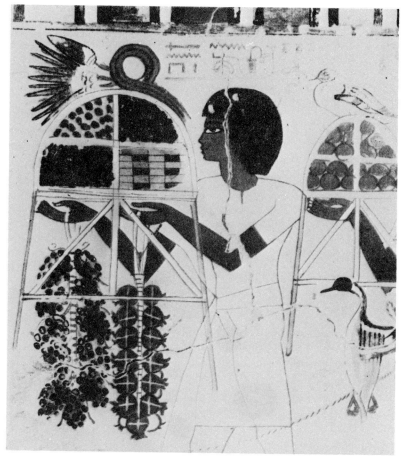

Fig. 18.23. Offering bearer carrying pomegranates, grapes, and lotus flowers. Tomb of Sebkhotep. Thebes. New Kingdom. From Davies (1936), Vol. I, plate XLIV.

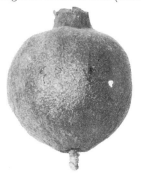

Fig. 18.24. Pomegranate. Kom Ouchim. Roman Period. Dokki Agricultural Museum, Cairo. Photographed 1969.

". . . 15,500 measures of pomegranates offered to Ammon-Ra . . ."
(*A.R.*, IV, 241)

This fruit was also one of those that the Israelite exiles craved during the Exodus (Numbers, 20, 5).

Theophrastus, in his treatise on plants, discussed the changes certain species, like pomegranates, undergo when transplanted in countries where soil and climatic conditions are different from those prevailing in their previous environment

> ". . . a few kinds in some few places seem to undergo a change, so that wild seed gives a cultivated form, or a poor form one actually better. We have heard that this occurs, but only with the pomegranate, in Egypt and Cilicia; in Egypt a tree of the acid kind both from seeds and from cuttings produces one whose fruit has a sort of sweet taste . . ." (2, 2, 7)

Pliny (*N.H.*, XIII, XXXIV, 113) likewise discussed the pomegranate in Egypt

> ". . . these apples have a special structure resembling the cells in a honeycomb, which is common to all that have a kernel. Of these, there are five kinds, the sweet, the sour, the mixed, the acid, and the vinous; those of Samos and of Egypt are divided into the red-leaved and the white-leaved varieties . . ."

Achillus Tatius (3, 6, 1) wrote that Zeus, in his temple at Pelusium, was sculptured holding a pomegranate in one hand as a mystical symbol. He did not elaborate further, unfortunately, on the significance of this fruit.

Medically, parts of the pomegranate tree were prescribed as a vermifuge (*Eb.*, XVI, 50; XIX, 63; *Ber.*, 6, 10). This was certainly very effective, because of the pelletierine in the bark. Pomegranates probably entered, too, in the fabrication of the highly praised *shedeh* wine (see Chapter 15).

As usual with fruits that kept well, the fruits served as objects of barter and payment. They are mentioned in a papyrus dated to A.D. 141 as partial payment for a lease (Lindsay, 1966, p. 286).

(u)

kꜣw

Sycamore Fig (Ficus sycomorus)

(v)

nht

Ancient Egyptian: the fruit (u) (*F.*, 283)
the tree and tree in general (v) (*F.*, 135)

Arabic: *gemmeiz*
Synonyms: Egyptian fig, Egyptian mulberry, fig mulberry
Greek: *sykon* (fig) and *moron* (mulberry)

Shaken by the wind, half a penny a measure,
like honey my sycamore figs
(Street cry)

". . . then answered Amos, and said to Amaziah, I was no prophet, neither was I a prophet's son; but I was a herdman, and a gatherer of sycamore fruit . . ." (Amos, 7 ,14)

The sycamore fig (Fig. 18.25), sometimes called Egyptian mulberry by ancient authors, is a tree completely different from the typical sycamores and mulberries found in the southern parts of the United States. The best descriptions of this tree occur in the Greek and Roman texts whose writers were amazed at the quality and manner of growth of this Egyptian fruit. Though the sycamore fig is of only secondary importance in Egypt today, witness the popular saying

"Eat sycamore fruit until figs come into season"

their delicate fragrance is still appreciated by all Egyptians.

The love that the Ancient Egyptian bore for the sycamore, however,—a tree so popular and such an integral part of his familiar landscape that he called all trees after it, *nht*—meant much more to him than mere fondness of its fruit; it was a deep filial cult.

The Memphite nome in the north, and the Letopolite in the south, were both called "The Land of the Sycamore"; no doubt an allusion, not only to the abundance of the tree, but also to the cherished myth that it incarnated the "doubles" of two beloved goddesses, Hathor and Nut. One of the titles of Hathor "Lady of the Sycamore", and the profusion of paintings of both goddesses as sycamores receiving offerings (Fig. 18.26) or suckling the king, attest to the holiness and maternal status of this tree.

The archaeological history of the sycamore fig dates to Omarian times, from which identifiable remains have been found (*MAE*, p. 119), through the Dynastic Period (Schweinfurth, 1885, 1886; Lauer *et al.*, 1951). So abundant were the finds that Loret (*Fl.*, 46) thought it justifiable to write that the sycamore is one of the Egyptian trees of which the

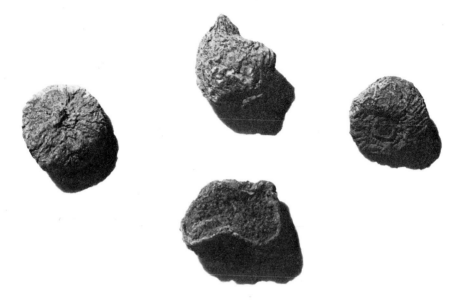

Fig. 18.25. Sycamore fig, *Ficus sycomoris*. Saqqara. Third dynasty. Dokki Agricultural Museum, Cairo. No. 1368. Photographed 1969.

greatest quantity of dry remains were found in tombs, sometimes filling whole baskets.

Medically, sycamore figs were prescribed against the mysterious "blood-eater" (?scurvy?) (*Eb.*, LXXXIX, 749). It was part of a drink designed to distinguish fertile from sterile woman (*Ber.*, 193), and of medicinal mixtures (*Eb.*, XLII, 207 b–c; *Eb.*, LXVII, 477). Its leaves were applied to hippopotamus bites (*H.*, 243), and its latex was used to darken scars (*Eb.*, LXIX, 501).

From the Greek period records concerning the fruit (called Egyptian fig and mulberry) are numerous. Theophrastus (4, 2, 1) reported

". . . now the sycamore to a certain extent resembles the tree which bears that name in our country [the mulberry *morus nigra*]; its leaf is similar, its size, and its general appearance; but it bears its fruit in quite peculiar manner, as was said at the very outset; it is borne not on the shoots or branches, but on the stem; in size it is as large as a fig, which it resembles also in appearance, but in flavour and sweetness it is like the 'immature-figs,' except that it is much sweeter and contains absolutely no seeds, and it is produced in large numbers. It cannot ripen unless it is scraped; but they scrape it with iron claws; the fruits thus ripen in four days. If these are

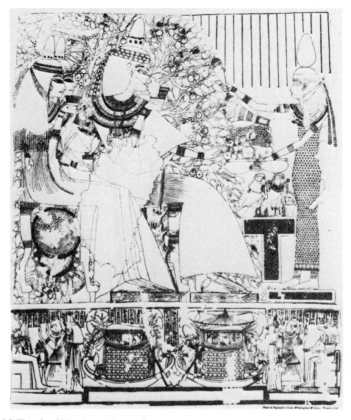

Fig. 18.26. Tomb of Userhet. Thebes. New Kingdom. Userhet, his wife, and his mother, receiving food and drink from the goddess of the sycamore, so indicated by the tree on her head. In the lower register, the voyage of the dead to Abydos and his return. From Davies (1927) plate IX.

removed, others again grow from exactly the same point, and this some say occurs three times over, others say it can happen more times than that."

Diodorus Siculus (1, 34, 8) discussed the value of this tree as a source of food for the poor

". . . while of the fig-mulberry trees one kind bears the black mulberry and another a fruit resembling the fig; and since the latter produces throughout almost the whole year, the result is that the poor have a ready source to turn to in their need . . ."

Strabo, however, (17, 2, 4) cursorily passed over it with the remark that it was not prized for its taste.

Pliny (*N.H.*, XIII, XIV, 56–57) neglected to identify his source, but it is easy to see that it was Theophrastus

". . . Egypt also has many kinds of trees not found anywhere else, before all a fig, which is consequently called the Egyptian fig. The tree resembles a mulberry in foliage, size and appearance; it bears its fruit not on the branches but on the trunk itself, and this is an exceedingly sweet fig without seeds inside it. There is an extremely prolific yield, but only if incisions are made in the fruit with iron hooks, otherwise it does not ripen; but when this is done, it can be plucked three days later, another fig forming in its place, the tree thus scoring seven crops of extremely juicy figs in a summer. Even if the incisions are not made new fruit forms under the old and drives out its predecessor before it is ripe four times in a summer."

Elsewhere, Pliny (*N.H.*, XXIII, LXX, 134) discussed the medicinal value of the "Egyptian mulberry"

". . . in Egypt and Cyprus are mulberries of a unique sort, as I have already said. If the outer rind be peeled off they stream with copious juice, a deeper cut, so wonderful is their nature, finds them dry. The juice counteracts the poison of snakes, is good for dysentery, disperses superficial abscesses, and all kinds of gatherings . . ."

Athenaeus (2, 51, B–C) also ascribed therapeutic value to the syca-more fig

". . . in these, the natives make a slight incision with a knife, and leave them on the tree. Fanned by the breeze, they grow ripe and fragrant in three days, especially when the winds are from the west, and they are then edible; so much so that the mild coolness they contain makes them fit to be made into a poultice with oil of roses and applied to the stomachs of fever patients, affording no little comfort to the ailing. But this fruit is produced on the Egyptian mulberry directly from the wood, and not from fruit stalks . . ."

Miscellaneous Fruits and Nuts with Limited References and Citations

Fruits

Many more fruits existed in Egyptian orchards and appeared on Egyptian tables, but they are difficult to identify. Some of them, used medicinally, could have been edible items in addition to being of pharmacological usefulness, like the numerous unexplained or still unread fruit names cited in the Ebers and other papyri.

Apricot (Prunus armenica)

Arabic: *meshmesh*

Originally from China, apricots have been cultivated in Egypt from Graeco-Roman times onwards. The short time they are in season, their quick disappearance from markets after their first appearances give rise to a common joke

"Tomorrow with the apricots"

which is equivalent to saying "never".

Blackberry (Rubus spp. ?)

Diodorus Siculus (1, 34, 9) writes of this fruit

". . . the fruit called the blackberry is picked at the time the river is receding and by reason of its natural sweetness is eaten as a dessert . . ."

It cannot be determined from this single citation whether the "blackberry" of Diodorus Siculus was indeed *Rubus* spp., the modern terminology for the blackberry, or if this designation only implied a colour, which would have fit a wide variety of genera and species.

Dates (Species Unknown)

Lichtheim (1957) translated an ostracon dated to the Roman Period, found at Medinet Habu, which lists a tax imposed on the *Itm*-palm; a variety mentioned only, so far, in this document.

Mulberry (Morus nigra and M. alba)

Arabic: *tut aswad*

Who refuses mulberries will accept their syrup
(Popular saying)

There exists confusion between this species and the "Egyptian mulberry" (the sycamore fig). Athenaeus (2, 51, E) cursorily remarked that people in Alexandria call the mulberry tree, *morea*. It was apparently introduced into Egypt in Roman times. Since 1920, it has been ravaged by the mealy bug and most of its varieties have disappeared, except the Arandali Variety (Täckholm, personal communication).

Morus alba, the white mulberry, however, was introduced only with the silkworm in the early Islamic Period.

Plums (Prunus domestica)

Egyptian Arabic: *barquq*

Originating in southwest Asia, this fruit was planted in Egypt since Roman times.

Prickly Pear (Opuntia ficus-indica)

Arabic: *tin shoky* (prickly fig)

Rawlinson (1881, Vol. 1, p. 28) lists this fruit as one with a "high degree of probability" of having been cultivated and eaten in the times of the "pharaohs". But Candolle (1886, pp. 274–275) was more correct in his statement that the prickly pear is a North American species and could not have been introduced into Europe or Africa prior to the Spanish Conquest. He added that it has been called the "Indian fig", a somewhat confusing but rather general appellation seeing its name in Arabic "spiny fig" or "prickly fig" (*tin shoky*), and in French "Barbary fig" (*figue de Barbarie*).

Today, the carts loaded with prickly pears that the vendors sell, peel and offer for immediate consumption are one of the picturesque sights of Egyptian summer nights.

Snb

Snb berries are mentioned among the gifts of Rameses III

"11,872 jars to the Nile god."

However, the word has not been translated yet.

Nuts

> *Like nuts, yields only to cracking*
> (of a stubborn person)

Almonds (Amygdalus communis)

Arabic: *lôz*

Confusion exists over the antiquity of the almond tree in Egypt. Candolle (1886, pp. 219, 221) wrote that it was indigenous in the eastern Mediterranean and western Asia. Wilkinson was of the opinion that it was one of the principal trees of Ancient Egypt (1854, Vol. 1, p. 57), but

Montet stated that it was unknown there before the Roman Period (1958, p. 81) Indeed, no ancient Egyptian name for the almond is known. Its Coptic name, *leuke* or *peukinon* (leukinon?) seemed to Loret (*Fl.*, 83) to be of Greek origin.

Earlier, Theophrastus, who wrote of the fruit-bearing trees in Egypt, did not mention it in the *Enquiry into Plants* (1916); while Pliny (*N.H.*, XIII, II, 8) indicated that, in his time, the tree was already established in Egypt, although it was used primarily as a source of oil (see Chapter 19), a use likewise cited by Athenaeus (*Deipnos.*, 15, 688, F).

The weight of evidence, however, indicates that the almond tree has never been widely grown in the Nile Valley. Very few finds are known, the earliest being a few remains in an eighteenth dynasty tomb excavated by Schiaparelli, described by Mattirolo (1926); about 30 almonds found in the tomb of Tut-ankh-Amon (Lucas, 1942); and the handle of a walking-stick made of almond wood kept in the museum of the Royal Botanical Gardens at Kew (Lucas, 1962, p. 330). In addition, four specimens were found in the Ptolemaic cemetery of Hawara (Newberry, 1890).

In Graeco-Roman times nuts, particularly almonds, were eaten as appetisers and, like cabbage (pp. 669 and 586), they were thought to neutralize alcohol

> "almonds induce sleep and increase the appetite . . . it is said that if about five of these almonds are taken before a carouse, drinkers do not become intoxicated." (*N.H.*, XXIII, LXXV, 144, 145)

Pliny recorded also their medicinal use in combating jaundice (*N.H.*, XXIII, LXXVI, 146).

Recently, their cultivation has received increased attention in the Mariut district and the Western coast, and their name in Arabic (*lôz*) has become synonymous with ease, sweetness, pleasure giving.

Hazel nut (*Coryllus avena*)

Arabic: *bondoq*

The hazel nut is only imported.

Pine nut (Pinus pinea)

Pine nuts were probably imported into Egypt from Libya and the Lebanon, for their cultivation in Egypt is very limited. Two cones were found by Mariette in a tomb at Dra ʿ Abul Naga attributed to the twelfth dynasty (Schweinfurth, 1884); a few others were found by Newberry at Hawara (1889), and some, of an unknown date, were discovered at Saqqara (Fig. 18.27). If the Egyptian name of the pine-cone, *ab*, be confirmed, these might have played an important role in solar mythology (*Fl.*, 42).

Evidence of the consumption of pine nuts is late. It consists in recipes of Alexandrian cuisine given by Apicius (3, 4, 3).

Medically a plant, *pr . t šny*, said to come from Byblos is often mentioned in the Ebers papyri. This has been interpreted by Ebbell (*Eb.*, LVIII, 361, etc.) and Lefebvre (1956, p. 39) as pine nuts. But von Deines and Grapow (*Wb. Dr.*, 201) think that the word is, as yet, untranslatable. They comment that the use of *pr . t šny* in medicine is so broad that it does not seem to have any special indication in any particular domain. It might have served, therefore, as a flavouring agent.

Walnut (Juglans regia)

This is also called *Nux persica, n. juglans, n. basilica, persicum, karyon,* and other names. Such taxonomic variations usually indicate a long and involved history. Evidently, the walnut was not known in Egypt prior to initial contacts with Persia, for there are no records of its existence in Egypt before the Ptolemies. A letter is known, dating to about 205 B.C. (*S.P.*, 1, 180) asking for shoots of walnut trees; and several specimens from the Roman Period are kept at the Dokki Agricultural Museum (Fig. 18.28). Today, the tree is found only in a few gardens. *Carya illinoensis* (Pecan nut), however, has recently been more extensively grown and seems to succeed better.

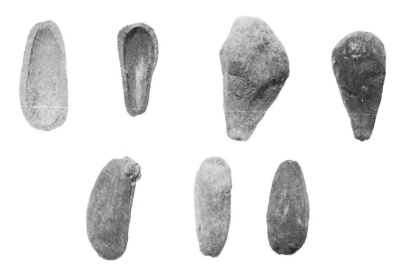

Fig. 18.27. Pine nuts (*Pinus pinea*). Saqqara. Date unknown. Dokki Agricultural Museum, Cairo. No. 404. Photographed 1969.

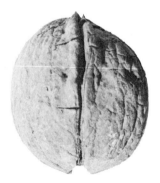

Fig. 18.28. Walnut. Kom Ouchim. Roman. Dokki Agricultural Museum, Cairo. No. 279. Photographed 1969.

Notes on Some Fruits recently Introduced in Egypt

Avocado Pear (*Persea americana*, Arabic: *zibdiya*) has only very recently been introduced from Latin America, but still is uncommon.

Banana (*Musa nana*, Arabic: *moz hindi* and *M. sapientum*, Arabic: *moz balaaı*), is called in Arabic *moz* after Antonio Musa, physician to Augustus; but, curiously, the European name etymologically stems from Arabic *banan* finger. The oldest Egyptian find is a leaf from the fifth century A.D. found in a vase.

Custard apple (*Annona squamosa*, Arabic: *qishta baladi* and *A. cherimola*, Arabic: *qishta hindi*), a recently introduced fruit, originating in Latin America, has deserved, on account of its fleshy syncarp, the Arabic name *qishta* (cream).

Guava (*Psidium guajava*, Arabic: *gawafa*), a native of tropical America, introduced only lately in Egypt, has become one of the most popular fruits.

Kaki or Japanese persimmon (*Diospyrus kaki*, Arabic: *kaki*) originated in Japan and China. Several varieties have been successfully grown in Egypt in the last 30 years.

Mango (*Mangifera indica*, Arabic: *manga*) from India, Burma and Malaya, was introduced by Mohamed Aly and first planted in his Shubra palace (in a Cairo suburb). Its cultivation has received attentive care and several superb varieties have been developed in Egypt. In spite of its high cost, it is considered the king of fruits in Egypt and has come to qualify spicy feminine beauty.

Medlar (*Eriobotrya japonica*, Arabic: *bashmala*), a native of China that grows especially well in the Lebanon where it is called *ikidunya*, is only of recent introduction.

Papaya (*Carica papaya*, Arabic: *babaz*) from tropical America is, likewise, a recently cultivated fruit, albeit on a small scale.

Peanuts (*Arachis hypogaea*, Arabic: *ful sudani*) is nowadays the only nut cultivated on a large scale in Egypt. But it is a recent culture.

Pistaccio (*Pistacia vera*, Arabic: *fustuq*) is a recent introduction from the Near East, as an experiment at Borg el-Arab on the western Mediterranean coast.

Quince (*Cydonia vulgaris*, Arabic: *safargal*) is a native of Iran and Turkestan. Lately cultivated especially around Ismailia, it serves to make jellies and jams.

Notes: Chapter 18

1. Hand-worked lifts utilized to raise water.
2. Another spelling of Amon.
3. Persaeus entered the Egyptian Pantheon through one of those *après-coup* etymologies with which the Greeks were fond of identifying Egyptian gods with theirs: at Chemmis (modern Akhmim) the Egyptian god Min was called *wrshy*, "The Guardian". Preceded by an article, this word becomes *pa-wrshy*, probably was pronounced *p-orseus* or *p-orses* (Barguet, 1964, p. 1384). Hence the identification.

Chapter 19   *Fats and Dairy Products*

Fats in General

The results of the analyses of specimens of Ancient Egyptian fats carried out by various chemists have been ably reviewed by Harris (1962, pp. 327–329). In most cases, the material consisted largely of palmitic or stearic acid with, in some instances, small proportions of oleic, myristic, azelaic and nonoic acids, indicating an animal origin. The specimens that Harris, himself, examined were mostly solid fatty acids. Thirteen presented as elastic brown or orange-red solid material, probably altered drying oils. He concluded that it was not possible to distinguish whether these were of animal or vegetable origin.

It is, nevertheless, certain that fat from both sources was utilized, although some degree of indefiniteness blurs our interpretation of the Ancient Egyptian words for fats, as it sometimes does nowadays when the words "grease", "fat", "lard" and "oil", are indiscriminately interchanged.

Two words designating fatty material constantly recur in the texts: Ꜥd and mrḥt. In a detailed analysis of their contexts, von Deines and Grapow (*Wb. Dr.*, 116–121 and 250–279) could show that Ꜥd was the word used in designating cattle, ibex, or goose fat; and that it was applied to a vegetable product only in connection with fir-oil (translated by Ebbell as turpentine: *Eb.*, XCIV, 806). They concluded that whenever Ꜥd is mentioned without indicating its source it meant animal fat; and, further, from the interchangeability of Ꜥd and Ꜥd of ox in many repetitious prescriptions, e.g. *Eb.*, LIII, 308 and 313, etc., that it meant ox fat.

Mḥrt, on the other hand, was mainly used for vegetable fats except, occasionally, in connection with hippopotamus, birds, reptiles, worms and fish. They concluded that *mrḥt* meant oil unless coupled with the name of an animal.

Considering, however, the near impossibility of obtaining adequate amounts of fat from some of the small animals often connected with *mrḥt*, and the frequent mention of the indications "to be cooked" or "to be boiled" (*Eb.*, 467, 469) in these recipes, von Deines and Grapow were inclined to think that the recipes meant, not the fat of the animal but the animal in fat, i.e. fried.

Fat in Cooking

The last contention leads us to discuss the role of fat in Ancient Egyptian cooking. Greek gourmets, of course, often dwelt on the merits of fried foods, but the lack of genuine culinary recipes in the available literature of the Ancient Egyptians seriously limits our knowledge of the part that fats played in their cuisine.

Nevertheless, and despite the limitation of the Ancient Egyptian kitchen vocabulary as known today to terms for boiling and roasting, one should not assume that meats or vegetables were never fried or sautéd, or that the fats and oils offered to temples or supplied to workmen and soldiers were served raw.

When Sinouhe told of his adventure in Retenu (Syria) he boasted that there was milk in every dish, meaning, according to Lefebvre (1949, p. 12, n. 39), that his food was cooked in milk or butter. Both these methods of cooking meats and vegetables are usual today among Moslems and Christians alike in the Near East. It is curious that one should find more relevant information in the medical papyri, of which many a recipe recommends cooking or boiling animal ingredients in oil, e.g. *Eb.*, LXVI, 469

"a black lizard pounded and boiled in oil"

or *Eb.*, LXVI, 467

"leg of hound . . . boiled thoroughly with oil"

Such instructions surely indicate a knowledge of frying.

Animal Fats

Positive information on animal fats is available in some tomb finds, like the ninety-one jars labelled ʿ*d* found in the temple of Amenophis

III by Hayes (1951) who, judging from the invariable determination of this word on the labels by a closed jar, stated that the material had been poured into these jars in a liquid state. The fat was described in almost every case as "fresh" or "sweet"; in one, it was called "fat of prime meat of the cattle stable"; in another, "fresh fat of goats"; and in fifteen, "fat of Meshwesh bulls" (a Libyan breed).

Next in sources are the lists of offerings. These, as listed in Breasted's *Ancient Records* (1906), were of four kinds: undefined fat, probably ox fat (*A.R.*, III, 208, 413; IV, 286, 344, etc.); goose fat (*A.R.*, IV, 322, 376); white fat (*A.R.*, IV, 233, 239, etc.); and a type that Breasted translated as butter (*A.R.*, IV, 233, 301, 376), and that Harris (1962, p. 330) surmised was molten butter (*Wb.* IV, 130, 1–5) which, on being melted, separated from the remaining components (water, casein, sugar) and resulted in a product which, like *ghee* or Arabic *masly* or *samna*, keeps better.

As examples of such donations, one might mention the ration of the King's Messenger and Standard-Bearer that we have often quoted (*A.R.*, III, 208), and Rameses III's endowment of the temple of Memphis

". . . bulls, cattle beyond limits, I have brought all their numbers in millions, as for the fat thereof, it has reached heaven, and the dwellers in heaven have received it". (*A.R.*, III, 413)

Medical Use

Medically, the fat of the following animals was utilized: antelope, ass, various birds, cat, crocodile, chaenopod worm, fish, goat, goose, hippopotamus, ibex, lion, mouse, ostrich, ox, pig, sheep and snake; with the reservation previously discussed that some of these may have been not the fat of the animal, but the animal cooked in fat.

It is remarkable that animal fat was predominantly used externally. The relatively few exceptions used internally were either unspecified fat (*Eb.*, XXII, 75), goose-fat (e.g. *Eb.*, XXIV, 97), or ox fat (*Eb.*, LXXXV, 698). Otherwise, animal fats were included in suppositories (*Eb.*, XXXI, 142, 144), ointments (*Eb.*, LXXXVI, 712a), dressings (*Eb.*, LXVIII, 495), inhalations (*Ber.*, 63), or eye preparations (*Eb.*, LXII, 401).

A prescription to improve the hair combined fat from six animals: lion, hippopotamus, crocodile, cat, snake and ibex (*Eb.*, LXVI, 465). One wonders whether apothecaries, if such existed, kept zoological gardens to satisfy prescribing physicians.

Milk

> "Whiter art thou come, my son, O King? . . . He is come to these his two mothers, the two vultures, they of the long hair and the pendulous breasts . . . They draw their breasts to his mouth, and never more do they wean him". (*Pyr.* No. 508; Erman, 1966, n.9)

The above Pyramid Text clothes with a poetic garb the belief, still current in many religions and lores, that milk as the very essence of the mother, is the vehicle through which she imparts her virtues and nature to her child. The Holy Koran (IV, 23) considers incestuous all marriages between a man and a woman who was his nurse, or between two persons suckled by the same woman. Of a bold and well-born man, Egyptians today say that he drank from his mother's milk and, of knowledge obtained at first hand, that it was drawn from the mother's breast. Other sayings assert the exclusive right of a child to its mother's milk, such as

> "nothing is more lawful than one's mother's milk"

or

> "a free woman would starve rather live off her breasts"

which is an expression that could receive more than one interpretation.

On practically every Ancient Egyptian monument, this motherly function is raised to divine levels: young princes assert their descent from gods by depicting themselves as being suckled by goddesses (Fig. 19.1); Isis, the paragon of mothers, gives her breast to Horus in the innumerable statuettes (Fig. 1.4) that might well have inspired the early Christian and Mediaeval motive of the *Virgo lactans*; Hathor, Lady of the Western Marshes (the world of the dead) admits pharaohs to eternal bliss by feeding them on her milk (Fig. 3.3).

Kings made ritual offerings of milk to the gods (Fig. 19.2). In Horemheb's tomb, a text prays the gods to grant milk to the Hereditary Prince

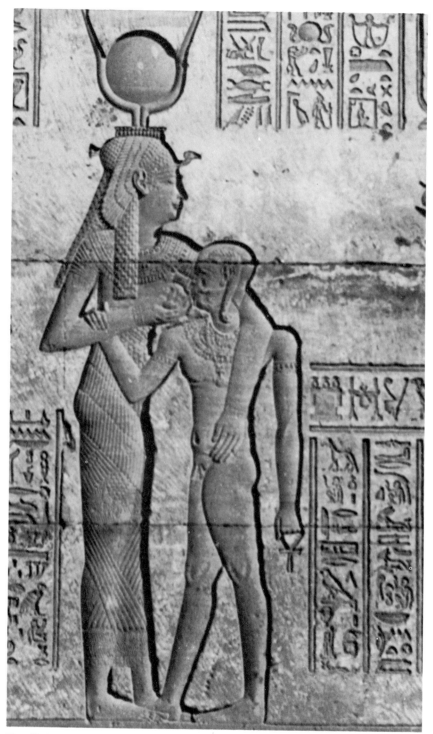

Fig. 19.1. Hathor feeding a young prince. Mammisi (House of Birth) of Dendera. Roman Period. Courtesy of Professor F. Daumas.

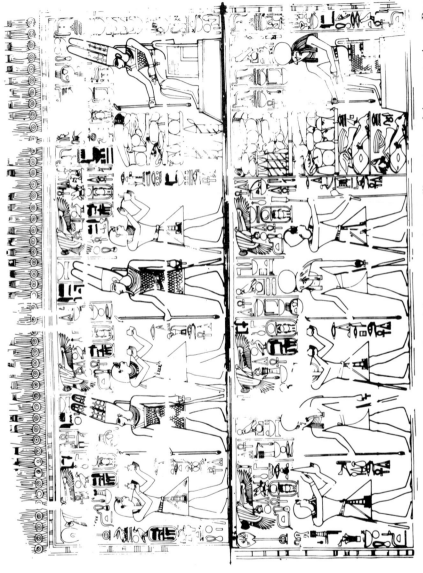

Fig. 19.2. Offerings of Amenhotep II. Left to right, upper register: milk, water, and incense to Amon-Ra; lower register: white bread, and victuals to Re-Harakhte. Temple of Amada, Nubia. New Kingdom. Centre of Documentation, Cairo.

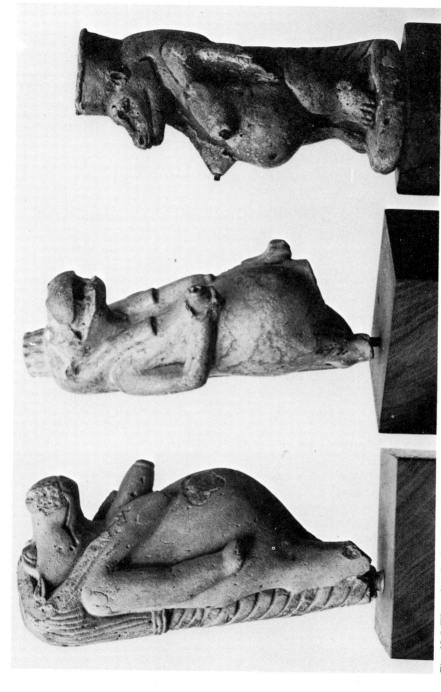

Fig. 19.3. Three jars in the shape of the hippopotamus goddess Ta-urt, with perforated nipples. The Louvre Museum. Courtesy of Mme Desroches-Noblecourt.

(*A.R.*, III, 17); and in his coronation inscription, Tutmose III declared that, in compliance with Amon's command, he had filled with milk the vessels of silver, gold and bronze that he had made for the god, and that he had instructed the priests to fill his altar with milk (*A.R.*, II, 571).

Milk in Infant Feeding

Milk was freely given to children. In a tomb of the eighteenth dynasty at El-Kab it is recorded that 60 children consumed the milk of 3 cows, 52 goats, and 9 she-asses (Ruffer, 1929, p. 25); and drugs destined for infants were given mixed with milk. The milk was probably spoon-fed, but three types of contrivance might have been used in feeding babies.

The first was a hollow statuette of the hippopotamus-cow goddess Ta-urt (Thueris), the protector deity of birth and childhood. The large hanging breasts, shaped like multiparous human breasts, are bored at the nipple with small perforations fitted with removable opercula. It has been conjectured by Borchardt (1910) that these were used as milk bottles, making believe that the sucklings were fed by the goddess herself. But Desroches-Noblecourt (personal communication, 1974) expressed the belief that these jars were water bottles used in the special Ta-urt rites. She very kindly gave us in December, 1974, pictures of three of these bottles, now kept in the Louvre Museum (Fig. 19.3), with the comment that one is of the usual type of heavy breasted hippopotamus; the second holds her right breast in her right hand; while the third, one of whose breasts is standing higher than the other, suggests that she dispenses her provend without restricting its aim.

The second type was a small vessel made in the shape of a woman carrying in her lap a child which, in some examples, is a weakly creature, in others, a vigorous infant. Desroches-Noblecourt (1952) suggested that the group represented Isis and the child that she had conceived from the dead Osiris; and she further made the brilliant suggestion that these jars were made to consecrate and keep a remedy that was held in highest regard, namely, the milk of a woman who had a male child (Fig. 19.4). For this substance, by being placed into these jars, probably to the accompaniment of some incantations, was thereby identified with the milk that Isis fed her child; hence its miraculous virtues (see also p. 771).

The third type was a hollow horn fitted at the tip with a Hathor head or with a spoon (Fig. 19.5). Mme Desroches-Noblecourt, who noticed the existence of similar horns on the lap of the woman of the above-mentioned jars, contended that they served to administer rectal or vaginal douches. We would rather look at them as containers for oil or scent, or possibly as milk bottles from which consecrated, or even ordinary, milk was fed (Ghalioungui, 1963, p. 120).

Our speculation is supported by the knowledge that various devices, such as jars with nipples or spouts, spoons and horns have been utilized throughout history as substitutes for the breast. An ovoid flask of polished burnt clay in The Cairo Museum with a nipple-shaped mouth-piece has been described as a milk bottle (Garrison, 1923, p. 16) although it could well have been simply a water drinking jar. Sucking horns are mentioned in early Mediaeval and in Renaissance literature (Garrison, 1923, p. 66) and a horn similar to the Ancient Egyptian one we have just described is illustrated in a small Meissen porcelain group, now in the Wellcome Historical Museum, of a fawn feeding an infant fawn by means of a cow's horn.

Still, in *The History of Paediatrics* (1931), has examined the evolution of infant feeding apparatus. Although he does not discuss its use in Ancient Egypt, he notes a curious lack of reference to any form of baby feeding device by Greek and Roman writers. He states

"... but such certainly existed, at least as early as the latter part of the first century (A.D.)"

and depicts a more or less globular terracotta Roman specimen with a small nipple-like spout dated about A.D. 200. (This specimen is in the Wellcome Historical Medical Museum.) He further notes that similar vessels are known from the periods of Domitian and of Constantine the Great. Still also reproduced a thirteenth century illustration (from the Wellcome Museum) of the horn in use as a baby feeder and states that during mediaeval and later times its use was common. He cites Simon de Vallambert as first giving mention of such an apparatus in his first French treatise on diseases of children (1565), translated as

"... a horn with an opening at both ends, one end being made into the shape of a teat, through which the infant sucks the pap just as it sucks breast milk by the nipple ..."

The feeding horn, likewise, was referred to by Rosen von Rosenstein

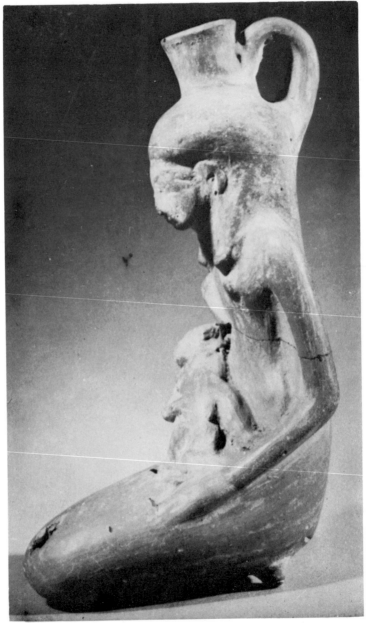

Fig. 19.4. Jar supposed to have contained, either the milk of a woman who had a male child, or milk consecrated to the treatment of burns (see text). Leiden: Rijksmuseum van Oudheden. Courtesy of W. D. van Wijngaarden.

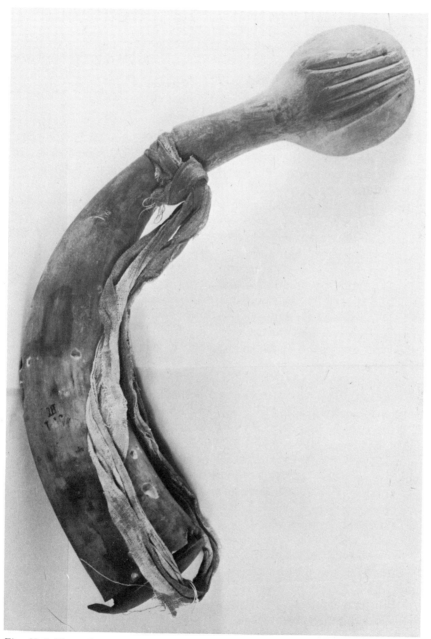

Fig. 19.5. Horn shaped container fitted with a spoon. Said to have been a clyster; more likely, it was used to dispense oil, scent or milk. Cairo Museum. Used with permission.

during the eighteenth century, and discussed in detail by George Armstrong of London. Armstrong, who in 1769 established the first free dispensary to help children of the poor, described according to Still

> ". . . two ways of feeding children who are bred up by the hand: the one is by means of a horn, and the other is with a boat or spoon . . ."

He described a kind of artificial nipple made of parchment for the horn.

The striking similarities of these vessels to those of Ancient Egypt and their documented use over several centuries make most plausible our interpretation given here.

Nevertheless, the possibility of direct feeding at animals' udders cannot be entirely excluded. In the charming fantasy of misty archetypal thought, animals and men were but separated by most tenuous barriers that artists, poets, and philosophers glibly crossed. Throughout Volume 1, we have seen numerous examples of this kind of assimilation. In classical mythology, Zeus changed into a bull, a swan, or any other animal to seduce the girls he coveted; Dionysus could transform himself into a lion and the sailors who captured him into dolphins; Apollo in a glance gave Midas the ears of an ass. Such transformations make it difficult to distinguish between zoomorphic gods and deified animals; they provided Ovid with the fifteen books of his *Metamorphoses*.

Numerous stories also tell of animals suckling children (McCartney, 1924; Rose, 1953). The best known is that of the founders of Rome, Romulus and Remus, fed by a she-wolf, but we read also of Pelias fed by a mare, of Neleus by a bitch, of Asklepios and Aigisthos (the goatman?) by a goat, of Aiolos and Biotos by a cow, of Telephos by a doe, of Atalanta by a she-bear. The list is endless. No animal is missing, even panthers were said to have fed Kybele.

The tales are not restricted to mythological figures for they relate, as an instance, that Cyrus the Great was fostered by a bitch,[1] and that the founder of the Ptolemaic Dynasty was fed by an eagle that gave him its blood.

Such legends may not be, however, entirely mythical. They are supported by the perennial reports in the press of wolf-children discovered in wild areas. Even if fabricated, they reveal a deep-rooted belief in their truth. It may not be irrelevant, therefore, to point here to a statuary group showing a cow suckling both a child and a calf, none of the three having any divine attributes (Fig. 2.1).

At least in the Greek Period, goddesses not only nurtured humans, but they also suckled animals which were, thereby, deified (Fig. 19.6).

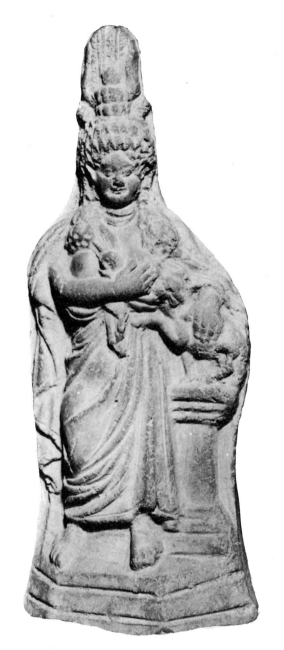

Fig. 19.6. Statuette of a woman, fitted with all the attributes of Isis, feeding a young animal, probably a young Apis bull. Personal collection of the authors. Ptolemaic/Roman Period.

Milk in Adult Nutrition

In many countries of the Far East and Central Africa adults manifest a profound dislike of milk and consider it a child's food. This may or may not be related to the milk intolerance known to result from intestinal lactase deficiency developing after weaning. This deficiency is said to be rare in Caucasians of Northern and Western Europe, of the United States, and of Australia, regardless of whether they persevere in drinking milk. By contrast, it is stated to be common in Blacks, Orientals, Jews, Arabs, Eskimos and American Indians, and it may occur as a transitory phenomenon in febrile illnesses and malnutrition (Newcomer, 1973).

We have already mentioned one pattern of avoidance, current in the Middle East, which forbids the consumption of milk or its products together with fish (See Chapter 7). Another is the Biblical prohibition of cooking meats in dairy products (Deuteronomy, 14, 21).

None of these restrictions seemed to have existed in Ancient Egypt, and milk must have been as freely consumed as it is today in all Arab countries, especially among the Bedouins for whom it is a staple food. We read in the *Tale of Two Brothers* that the younger brother came back every evening with the products of the field of which milk was one (Lefebvre, 1949, p. 142), although there were no children in the household. In another popular tale of the period, Sinouhe, dying with thirst, was happy to be offered cooked milk by a Bedu chief. As noted, when later he was covered with honours in Retenu (Syria), he boasted that there was milk in everything cooked (Lefebvre, 1949, p. 12), a favourite way of preparing meats and vegetables in the Near East. There is no evidence, however, that Egyptians were given to anything like the modern addiction to milk, widely advocated by health authorities and the media (Snapper, 1967).

Unfortunately, Egyptians had no gossipist like Pliny to tell us whether their "belles" preserved the beauty of their complexions in the same way as Nero's wife Poppaea, who used to drag five hundred she-asses with foals about with her everywhere, and actually soaked her whole body in a bath tub with ass's milk, believing that it smoothed her wrinkles (*N.H.*, XI, XCVI, 238).

Medical Uses of Milk

Medically, both human and animal milk were utilized, in some cases without addition; in others as a base or vehicle.

Human milk could be from any woman; and it was given by mouth (*Eb.*, X, 30); in enemata, alone or with other drugs (*Ber.*, 163, h); or in external applications.

In one case, nurse's milk was specified as a vehicle for a paediatric medicine

"if he is a big child, he shall swallow it down, if he is in swaddle, it shall be rubbed out for him by his nurse in milk which will come out for four days." (*Eb.*, L, 273)

Much more valuable, however, was the

"milk of a woman who had a male child"

one of the preferred drugs for eye diseases (*Eb.*, LIX, 368; LX, 384; LXII, 408; LXII, 414, etc.). Hippocrates (*Historia Animalia*, 7, 4) also recommended it (*On Sterile Women*, No. 214), and Aristotle gave a ready explanation for its value by stating that, in general, women bearing a male child are in better health and keep a better complexion; unlike those who bear girls as their pregnancies are difficult. The milk of the latter is therefore less recommendable. After them, Dioscorides (V, 99), Pliny (*N.H.*, XX, LI, 4) and the Copts (Chassinat, 1921, p. 301, no. 206) followed suit. Its supreme value made it an ideal magic medium: the incantation of the burning Horus (*Eb.*, LXIX, 499, see Vol. 1, Ch. 9) was to be recited over a mixture of this precious liquid with gum and ram's hair. Over a similar mixture the following spell, giving a striking description of an influenzal syndrome, had to be uttered to clear a fetid nose (*Eb.*, XCI, 763)

"Another, incantation of fetid nose: flow out, fetid nose! Flow out, son of fetid nose [polypus?]! Flow out, thou who breakest bones, destroyest the skull, diggest in the bone-marrow and makest the seven holes in the head ill! Re's servants, praise Thoth! Behold, I have brought thy remedy against thee, thy protecting drink against thee: milk of [a woman] who has borne a male [child] and fragrant gum; it expels thee, it removes thee. Is repeated backwards. Go out to the ground, thou fetid, thou fetid one!

four times. Is recited over milk of [a woman] who has borne a male [child], and fragrant gum; is placed in the nose."

In a third charm, it was mixed with papyrus stems, dry carob, and given to a child to cure a disease called *baa* (*Zaub.*, 1, 7, 3–5).

Its most marvellous use, however, was a fertility test. The propositus had to swallow, or to have a vaginal injection of, water-melon and sycamore mixed in this wonderful product. If she vomited, she could conceive. If she passed flatus, she could not (*Ber.*, 193). And yet, strange as this test appears, it bears a great resemblance to one of the Aphorisms of Hippocrates (V, 41)

"If you wish to know whether a woman is with child, give her hydromel to drink . . . if she has colic . . . she is with child; otherwise she is not."

One cannot refrain from thinking that the great Greek physician borrowed the idea (Ghalioungui, 1960).

The milk from asses and small cattle (goats) was, on the other hand, prescribed for more prosaic purposes, in mixtures (*Eb.*, XXXIX, 127), vaginal injections (*Ber.*, 179), mouth rinses (*Eb.*, LXXXVI, 698), or ointments (*Eb.*, LXIX, 512). In some of these, milk of a milch cow was specified (*Eb.*, LXXV, 585; von Deines *et al.*, IV, Vol. 1, p. 109).

Butter and Cheese

Cream rises only after churning
(Popular saying)

She serves cheese on paper, and bread from the market
(Of a bad housewife)

From the Pharaonic Period, no word designating butter or cheese has been identified with certainty, but this *argumentum a silentio* is, of course, of poor value, since many food articles, known from other evidence to have been consumed, are not mentioned in food lists. The word *srw* has indeed been proposed for butter on the strength of its similarity to Coptic *sir*; but in the opinion of Kuentz (personal communication), neither the context of the Pyramid Text where it is found, nor the use after this word in writing of the signs for granules or powder as a determinative, admit of such a hypothesis.

In 1942, Zaky and Iskandar, having examined the contents of two jars of the first dynasty, came to the conclusion that these were cheese. They based their opinion on the facts that the jars contained fatty matter in proper proportion; that they contained nitrogenous matter which they thought was most probably casein because it contained calcium in organic combination; and that the residues contained calcium in combination with higher fatty acids, as well as phosphate and sulphur.

The jars bore on the outer, some words that read as: "ʿ*rwt* of the North" and "ʿ*rwt* of the South", and they boldly identified ʿ*rwt* with *srw* which, as we have seen, is thought by some authors to mean cheese.

This identification is questionable, however, for the following reasons: the sound sign *s* is absent from ʿ*rwt*; ʿ*rwt* is feminine whereas *srw* is masculine; and the animal sign read *r* is written in such a way that the word could equally be read *iwt*, *zwt* or *wnt*, neither of which is identifiable with any known word (Kuentz, personal communication).

Some scholars have explained a scene in a Ramessid tomb at Thebes (Fig. 19.7) as illustrating the preparation, transport and bartering of butter. They based this on the proximity of goats being led to pasture; on the illustration of implements, looking like churn bags, being carried by arm, on poles, and on donkeys; and on two spherical objects that are the object of a deal (balls of butter?). This interpretation has not met, however, with general acceptance.

Knowledge of cheese is attested in late epochs by many Greek documents. About 245 B.C., a certain Demeter wrote to Ptolemaeus

". . . Send me also as many cheeses as you can." (*S.P.*, I, 95)

Later, Athenaeus saw fresh cheese served at Naucratis (*Deipnos.*, 4, 149, F). Diodorus gave indirect proof by recording the avoidance of cheese by certain sectors of the population (1, 89, 4); while his statement that sheep and cows were sacred because

"by their milk and cheese they furnish food that is both appetizing and abundant" (1, 87, 2)

intimates that cheese had an antique history, since hallowing animals always goes back to the beginnings of history.

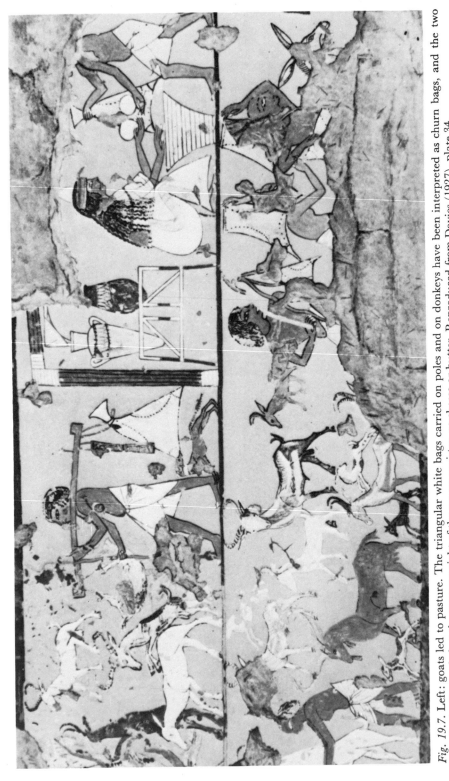

Fig. 19.7. Left: goats led to pasture. The triangular white bags carried on poles and on donkeys have been interpreted as churn bags, and the two globular bodies traded at the extreme right of the upper register, as cheese or butter. Reproduced from Davies (1927), plate 34.

In Saidic Coptic, butter was known as *sir*, a word that, though attested in Demotic, does not seem to have any antecedent in Ancient Egyptian. In Bohairic Coptic, it was called *seli* and *halom*, the latter cognate with modern Egyptian *haloum*, a variety of white cheese. As this word is unknown in any other Arabic dialect, it may well be a descendent of Coptic.

Pliny, in his long list of cheeses, did not mention Egyptian cheese. He added the curious remark that

> ". . . the foreign races, that live on milk for so many centuries, have not known or have despised the blessing of cheese, at most condensing their milk into agreeable sour curds and fat butter (*N.H.*, XI, XCVI, 237; XI, XCVII, 242)

Other Milk Preparations

Smy, or thickened milk, both human and animal, is often mentioned in medical prescriptions. This has usually been translated as "cream" (e.g. Ebbell in *Eb.*, LIII, 310; LIV, 315, 317). Von Deines and Grapow, however, pointed to the difficulty of producing cream from woman's milk, and were more inclined to interpret it as milk thickened after being kept standing, i.e. curdled (*Wb. Dr.*, 439). They found support in *Eb.*, LXXX, 642, H, 111.

> ". . . the milk of a woman who has born a male child, will be left overnight in a new vessel until its *smy* is formed."

Salt was added to this preparation to quicken the process. This thickened milk was specially recommended against cough. In a few instances, *white smy* was prescribed, the meaning of which is obscure since milk, curdled milk and cream, are all white; unless "fresh" curdled milk was meant by this expression (*Wb. Dr.*, 440).

In addition, the word *ḏśrt* (*Eb.*, LV, 335; XCIV, 802, 805, 807) has been interpreted by Lefebvre (1956, p. 106, n.9) as a special preparation of milk, while Von Deines and Grapow translate it as a variety of beer (*Wb. Dr.*, 604). The latter authors point out, however, that *ḏśrt* is enumerated alongside beer and wine in one and the same prescription (*Eb.*, LV, 335), which would throw some doubt on their interpretation.

Oils

"Then Samuel took a vial of oil, and poured it upon his head, and kissed him." (I, Samuel, 10, 1)

". . . and Samuel said to all the people, See ye him whom the Lord hath chosen . . . And all the people shouted and said God save the King." (I, Samuel, 10, 24)

There is no example in history of any product that has received as much regard, with as persistent a continuity, as has oil. In religious symbolism, to anoint with oil is to consecrate the anointed to God

"Then Samuel took the horn of oil and anointed him in the midst of his brethren: and the spirit of the Lord came upon David from that day forward." (I, Samuel, 16, 13)

Similary, no other word has ever attained the glorious fortune of *mashiah*, the Biblical word for "anointed": this became "Messiah", the name of the long-awaited Redeemer and, translated into Greek, gave their names to Christ (the Anointed, from *chrio*, anoint), Christianity, and Christendom.

Western kings followed the examples of Biblical kings; ever since the Middle Ages, a strict ritual regulated the anointment which was the central event of their coronation, and which was purported to impart to them their divine rights, even before their investment with the royal insignia.

The oils utilized in this and other ceremonies were very special, holy substances. The French invented the legend that a "Sainte Ampoule" filled with the Coronation oil had come down from heaven, borne by the Holy Spirit; and the English did not lag in asserting that Thomas Becket received the Holy oil from the Holy Virgin.

Nowadays, the traditional regard of oil as a vehicle of supernatural power is perpetuated in many Churches which confer the sacraments of Baptism, Confirmation and Extreme-Unction through the medium of the "Holy Chrism", a mixture of olive oil and balsam ceremonially consecrated on Maundy Thursday; and the same oil is used to consecrate churches, altars, chalices, pattens and church bells.

This is but a persistence of Egyptian traditions. Under the fifth dynasty, *sft*-oil, from the income of the King's Mother, coming from the temple of Ptah, was brought as a mortuary offering to Persen's tomb (*A.R.*, I, 241); and later, under Pepi-II (sixth dynasty), it was brought by a pious son to the tomb of his father, "Keeper of the Door of the South", an office traditionally belonging to the southern frontier nobles of Elephantine (*A.R.*, I, 382). At about the same period, Sebni, the Count, the Wearer of the Royal Seal, etc., equally manifested his filial feelings by bringing, to embalm his father, "festival oil from the Double White House" together with "secret things" from the Double Pure House (*A.R.*, I, 370).

Later, under the Middle Kingdom, it happened once that the god's statue was temporarily removed from the temple of Abydos while the temple was cleaned. Its return was recorded in the following terms:

"Then came the protector of the oil tree [the god] to assume his place in the temple . . ." (*A.R.*, I, 785)

thus stressing the appurtenance of oil to Gods.

As with wine, there is no temple in which kings do not offer some kind of oil or ointment (Fig. 19.8). Rameses III's gifts of the holy liquid were, as was his wont, on a munificent scale. In the inscriptions published by Breasted, a list of gifts to Amon records

". . . 2,743 *mn*-jars of oil of Egypt, 53 *mshy* jars and 1,757 jars of oil of Syria." (*A.R.*, IV, 233)

Another donation is on a still grander scale

". . . 513 *mn*-jars of oil of Egypt, 543 *mn*-jars of oil of Syria, one *mn*-jar of *bk* oil, one of red *bk* oil, and one of *sft* oil." (*A.R.*, IV, 376)

Twenty-three similar donations were made by the same king on other occasions (*A.R.*, IV, 1–456).

To satisfy these huge requirements, Rameses III established "oil-lands", in one of which, in Kanekem, oil was said to be

". . . more abundant than the sand of the shore." (*A.R.*, IV, 216)

Another oil-land, in Heliopolis, was equipped with gardeners to make pure oil, the best of Egypt

". . . to light the flame of the august house of the gods." (*A.R.*, IV, 263)

Oil Impositions, Imports and Taxes

To serve the huge lighting and ritual requirements of temples, oil had to be levied

". . . from the people and the serf-labourers as yearly dues to the estates of Amon at Thebes." (*A.R.*, IV, 228)

and the same impositions were current in Ra's domains at Heliopolis (*A.R.*, IV, 283).

The local production, however, could not meet the needs of the country. Oil was, therefore, exacted as tribute from Asia (*A.R.*, II, 462, 750, 771, etc.), where sesame and olives were plentiful. At least at late epochs, foreign oils were also bought. It is even related that Plato could defray the expenses of his sojourn in Egypt only by trading in this commodity (*Plutarch's Lives*, Vol. 1; *Solon*, II, 4, p. 409).

The intricate system of laws, whereby Ptolemy II Philadelphus (*Revenue Laws*, Grenfell, 1896) exerted a strict State monopoly on all aspects of the oil economy, provides an early example of rigid control of agricultural production. Mahaffy (1895, pp. 145–147) contended that this minute and complicated legislation was adopted from that of the pharaohs, because it was unlike anything that would be tolerated by either Greeks or Macedonians. In that system monopolies were farmed to contractors who bought the right of selling the oil to retailers, and so make their profit. The seed was distributed by the State; the acreage to be planted in every nome was determined; the retail price was fixed; a list of the retailers and of the amount of which each could dispose was fixed by the State. Import of Syrian oil beyond the requisite for three days' use was prohibited, and cooks were forbidden to melt suet and pass it off for oil

"The butchers shall use up the lard every day and in the presence of the oil contractor, and shall not sell it separately to any person on any pretext or melt it down nor store it up." (*S.P.*, II, 203)

Only the royal factories could process the seeds.

Excepted were the temples, whose freedom in that respect was, however, very strictly limited. Their authorities had to declare the number

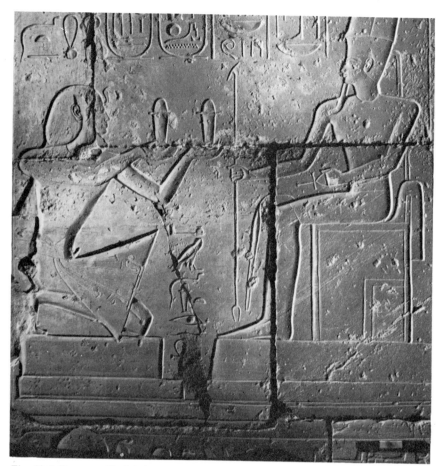

Fig. 19.8. Rameses II and Amon-Ra. The vertical inscription below the king's hands reads: An offering of *mdt* (ointment). Ramesseum. Thebes. Documentation Centre Cairo.

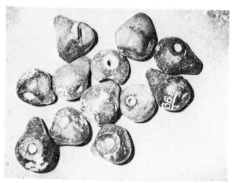

Fig. 19.9. Fruits of *Balanites aegyptiaca*. Saqqara. Third dynasty. Dokki Agricultural Museum. Note the holes through which the fat-containing nut was extracted. Photographed 1969.

of their oil factories and presses. Production was restricted to certain parts of the year, and carried out under the surveillance of a State official. They could sell no oil to the public.

Even the manufacture of oil mortars and presses was strictly controlled, and extensive powers of search were given to government contractors (see also Bouché-Leclercq, 1963, Vol. III, p. 253).

Varieties of Oil

The oils mentioned in the above laws were those of sesame, ricinus, carthamum, colocynth and linseed. This makes it clear that olive oil was not produced in important quantities at the time, that is before Greek veterans established themselves and planted the olive tree in the Arsinoite nome, which was the only region where Strabo found it planted (Strabo, 17, 1, 35).

On the other hand, Erman and Grapow, in their encyclopaedic dictionary of the Egyptian language, mention 28 terms for oil (*Wb.*, Belegstellen, 6). Of these, five are general terms for oils, two are "fine oils", and 21 are listed as varieties of oil (Table 1). From the resemblance between some of these terms, one may surmise that these were synonyms. On the other hand, a few terms probably designated oily preparations rather than unblended oils.

We shall limit our discussion to oils on which literary or factual information is available. Further discussion and information will be found in the sections on the individual sources of oil, almonds, sesame, etc.

Almond Oil

Almonds were known to Egyptians (Chapter 18), but they were mostly, or totally, imported and, if grown, were never produced in quantities sufficient to serve as a source of oil or of revenue. This is why they were not mentioned in the *Revenue Laws* (Grenfell, 1896). The only literary

Table 1

Oils mentioned in the Wörterbuch (Wb)

Type of oil	Documented date	Reference in the Wörterbuch
General oils		
$^c\underline{d}$	Old Kingdom	*Wb.*, I, 239
$b\,\underline{3}\underline{k}$	Middle Kingdom	*Wb.*, I, 424
mrḥ . t	Old Kingdom	*Wb.*, II, 111
nḥḥ	New Kingdom	*Wb.*, II, 302
śgnn	Nineteenth dynasty	*Wb.*, IV, 322
Fine oils		
tpy-ḥ 3 . t	Old Kingdom	*Wb.*, V, 290
ḥ 3 . t-mrḥt	Old Kingdom	*Wb.*, II, 111
Varieties of oil		
3ib 3. t	Eighteenth dynasty	*Wb.*, I, 62
3bs	Old Kingdom	*Wb.*, I, 64
^{c}ḥ3-t	Old Kingdom	*Wb.*, I, 217
ḥm-śbḳt	Greek	*Wb.*, I, 224
d^c. t	Old Kingdom	*Wb.*, I, 240
^{c}dr . t	Old Kingdom	*Wb.*, I, 242
ft	New Kingdom	*Wb.*, I, 581
nḥnm	Pyramids	*Wb.*, II, 319
nkftr	New Kingdom	*Wb.*, II, 346
ḥknw	Pyramids	*Wb.*, III, 180
ḥs3j . t	Middle Kingdom	*Wb.*, III, 400
śwr	Old Kingdom	*Wb.*, IV, 70
śfṯ	Pyramids	*Wb.*, IV, 118
śty-ḥb	Pyramids	*Wb.*, IV, 350
šš 3 . t	Old Kingdom	*Wb.*, IV, 543
šs . t	Old Kingdom	*Wb.*, IV, 543
ḳnny	New Kingdom	*Wb.*, V, 54
Ḳḏwr	New Kingdom	*Wb.*, V, 82
gt	New Kingdom	*Wb.*, V, 208
ty-š ps'	Middle Kingdom	*Wb.*, V, 243
dšr . t	Middle Kingdom	*Wb.*, V, 493

mention of almond oil concerns its inclusion in a scent described by
Pliny (XIII, 11, 8)

".. . Metopium . . . an oil made in Egypt, pressed out of bitter almonds
with the addition of omphacium [oil or juice of unripe olives or grapes],
cardamon, rush, reed, honey, wine, myrrh, seed of balsam, galbanum, and
terebinth resin . . ."

As it was well established in the time of Pliny, one may reasonably infer,
owing to the normal time lag between introduction and establishment,
that the almond tree was introduced long before the Roman Period.

Balanites Oil

Other names: thorn tree, Egyptian balsam, Zachum oil tree
Arabic: *haglig, hegelig*

The fruit of *Balanites aegyptiaca* (Fig. 19.9) has been found in many
Egyptian tombs (*Fl.*, 102), e.g. under the Step Pyramid at Saqqara
(Lauer *et al.*, 1951; Schweinfurth, 1885–1886). Nowadays, the tree is very
rare in Egypt, but it is widely grown in the Sudan and Ethiopia. Pliny
(*N.H.*, XIII, II, 8) stated its oil was part of the Mendesian scent that was
made of Balanites (*behen*) oil, resin, and myrrh; and he described an
unguent of cinnamon that included it and that fetched enormous prices
(*N.H.*, XIII, II, 15). Theophrastus referred to it also but, according to
him, the husks of the fruit were used by perfumers for its fragrancy (IV, I,
5) (see also Chapter 18).

Castor Oil

This oil has been a traditional food article in China and in some parts of
Central Africa. Its flavour, however, is most repulsive to Near Eastern
and Western palates. Its oil was well-known in Egypt, where Herodotus
(II, 94), Strabo (17, 2, 5) and others, reported its use in lighting and,

according to Strabo (*loc. cit.*), as a body inunction as well. The latter practice was still observed among the Bisharin and Ababda of the southeastern Egyptian deserts, by Ruffer in the early twentieth century (Ruffer, 1919, p. 82). Its medical uses are discussed on p. 788.

Cnecus Oil

There has been a good deal of argument about the plant *cnecus*, which has wrongly been identified as an artichoke, or even sunflower (Lucas, 1962, p. 336). Pliny (*N.H.*, XV, VII, 31) mentioned an oil from the nettle called *cnidium*, and this may be the reason for the confusion, as he elsewhere wrote

> "they [the Egyptians] hold in highest esteem one [a plant] called cnecos; . . . and the Egyptians . . . value it not as a food but for its oil . . ." (*N.H.*, XXI, LIII, 90)

It is now admitted that this plant is *Carthamus tinctorius*. Although it was not edible, it was of sufficient economic importance to be included in the taxable oils (see p. 780).

Colocynth Oil

This was also subject to the State Monopoly. According to Ruffer (1919, p. 83), its pulp contained about 3%, and its seeds about 15% of oil; and he added that it was used only by the poorer people. It is not now utilized in Egypt, where people say

> "Don't be a sugar; people would eat you; nor a [bitter] colocynth, they would pound you and throw you away."

Linseed Oil

Likewise included in the *Revenue Laws*, this was used only for lighting. It is nowadays called *zeit harr* "hot oil", and on account of its slight pungency, is considered to be the ideal seasoning of stewed horse-beans, *foul medammes*, the popular common dish. It is, otherwise, never used as a dressing.

Moringa Aptera (Ben) Oil

Ben oil, extracted from *Moringa aptera* (ben-oil tree, horse-radish tree; Arabic: *al Bán*) is an odourless, sweet oil, that keeps well and is, therefore, highly esteemed as an extracting oil in perfumery. The fruits of the tree have been found in many tombs (e.g. Newberry, 1890; Schweinfurth, 1886). It is frequently mentioned in ancient texts under the name of $b\mathsf{3}k$. Medicinally, it had wide applications (see later). At present, it forms part of a complicated polypharmacal preparation designed for the rapidly diminishing population of women who wish to grow fat (Ducros, 1930, pp. 39, 40).

Olive Oil

The history of the olive tree in Egypt was discussed in Chapter 18. According to Breasted's translations, olive oil (*djedet*, cognate with Semitic *zeit*, and Coptic *djoit*), was known in the time of Rameses II. The Greek authors did not think highly of the Egyptian olive oil. Strabo (17, 1, 35) wrote of the Arsinoite nome (in Fayoum) that

> ". . . it alone is planted with olive trees that are large and full-grown and bear fine fruit, and it would also produce good olive oil if the olives were carefully gathered. But since they neglect this matter, although they make much oil, it has a bad smell. The rest of Aegypt has no olive trees, except the gardens near Alexandria, which are sufficient for supplying olives, but furnish no oil."

He thus intimated that in Alexandria, either the quality of the fruit was not good enough to yield oil, or that its quantity barely met direct consumption. This, incidentally, could explain its non-inclusion in the *Revenue Laws*. Theophrastus also stated that its smell was less pleasant than in Greece; this he attributed to the unfavourable quality of the soil (IV, 2, 9); and Pliny asserted that the Egyptian olives, although very fleshy, yielded only scant oil (*N.H.*, XV, IV, 15).

The only references of the Dynastic Period to olive oil are to be found in the oft-quoted ration of Seti I's Messenger and Standard-Bearer (*A.R.*, III, 208), and in the donations of Rameses III, one of which records the creation of great olive-lands in *Kanemeke*, where oil was more abundant than the sand of the shore (*A.R.*, IV, 216). In addition, the gifts of olives to temples were of such magnitude that one may safely assume that they could not all have been eaten and that, at least partly, they were pressed (*A.R.*, IV, 239, 241, 379, 393, etc.). Nevertheless, olive oil was never as important to Egyptians as it was and still is to Greeks, Lebanese and Syrians.

Radish Oil

This was made in large quantities, according to Pliny (*N.H.*, XV, VII, 30), and he commented

". . . in Egypt, the radish is held in remarkable esteem because it produces oil which they make from its seed. The people are very fond of sowing radish if opportunity offers, because they make more profit from it than from corn [wheat] and have a smaller duty to pay on it, and because no plant there yields a larger supply of oil." (*N.H.*, XIX, XXVI, 79, 80)

Dioscorides (1, 45) reported the occasional use of this oil in medicine and Herodotus informs us that a method of embalming for the poorer classes utilized it as an enema to clear out the intestines (II, 86).

Sesame Oil

Sesame seeds (Sesamum orientale or *S. indicum)* yield on extraction about 50% of a peculiarly scented oil. The evidence for its use in Ancient Egypt rests on the presumed existence of this plant in Egypt since the beginnings of its history (see p. 489), on records of the use of sesame paste and oil dating to the third century B.C. and on reports of Theophrastus and other Greek authors.

As the production of olives in Egypt far from covers the needs of the country, sesame oil was used before the introduction of arachis, cotton seed, maize and lettuce seed oils; and until recently whenever animal fat could not be used, either because of its cost or because of the Coptic religious prohibition of animal products during fasts. The traditional (although now waning) popularity of this oil, called *sireg*, gave its name to oil-lamps, *mesraga*, and to the oil-presses, *serga*. The latter are thriving enterprises that produce, in addition, a sesame butter or paste called *taheena* (from *tahana*, to grind) which is a favourite dip and enters into a confectionery *halawa tahiniya*, and into many cooking recipes, especially in Syria and the Lebanon. *Taheena* is also often eaten with molasses. Its much appreciated smooth taste gave rise to the saying

"to change the rough sea into taheena"

meaning to smooth out all difficulties.

A similar preparation, if not an identical one, was known in Egypt as early as the second century B.C. and possibly earlier, as evidenced by several papyri

"I sent him off telling him to come early next morning in order to get from me in Memphis a quarter of an artaba of sesame and pound me a paste as I wished to give it to someone to take to the city." (*S.P.*, I, 98, *c.* 160 B.C.)

". . . they shall sell the oil in the country at the rate of 48 drachmae in copper for a metret [es] of sesame oil . . . if any one is detected manufacturing oil from sesame or croton or cnecus in any manner whatsoever, or buying sesame oil or cnecus oil or castor oil from any quarter except from the contractors, the king shall decide his punishment." (*S.P.*, II, 203, *c.* 259 B.C.)

Other Oils

The records quoted at the beginning of this chapter, some jar labels, and medical papyri, enumerate other specifically named kinds of oils. These various appellations may designate

1. their grade: pure oil (*A.R.*, IV, 263), best oil (*A.R.*, IV, 394);

2. a specific quality: sweet oil (*A.R.*, II, 482; *A.R.*, III, 208); white oil (*Eb.*, XXIII, 84), green oil (*A.R.*, II, 509), red oil (*A.R.*, IV, 376), sweet oil of gums (*A.R.*, IV, 497);
3. the country of origin: oil of Syria (*A.R.*, IV, 233);
4. their use: Festival oil (*A.R.*, I, 382; IV, 376).

One variety, *sft*, is recorded among offerings (*A.R.*, I, 241), in medical recipes (*Eb.*, XCIV, 807), and on two jars found in the palace of Amenhotep III (Hayes, 1951). It is believed by Von Deines and Grapow (*Wb. Dr.*, 437) to be the oil of the fir, but Ebbell (*Eb.*, XCIV, 807) translated it as turpentine, and Hayes as resin.

Two jars, labelled *nḥḥ*, a word translated as sesame oil by Keimer (*Gpfl.*, 1, 18, 20), were also found in the palace of Amenhotep III, and the name is attested in lists of offerings (*A.R.*, IV, 234, 376). Two other jars from the same site bore on their labels, "oil of *tḥ(w)*", an aromatic plant of which the seeds were used in the manufacture of perfume. *Tḥnt* oil is listed among offerings (*A.R.*, I, 366). The three oils, *sft*, *ḥknw* and oil (*mrḥt*), were included among the seven so-called sacred oils which have been the subject of considerable discussion (*Wb.*, II, 111). But the exact nature of the oils designated by these names still escapes us.

In addition, lettuce was well known since the earliest times (see Chapter 17), and it is possible that the present day practice of extracting from its seeds a cooking and dressing oil, originated then, but there is nothing to prove this.

Uses of Oil

Oil can be drawn only with the press
(Popular saying)

Whereas the enormous quantities of oil given to the temples or presented as mortuary offerings were mainly used to light temples, to anoint priest and statues, or to extract perfumes, the very size of the gifts and their inclusion in men's rations prove that they were also utilized for culinary purposes. In the Silsileh quarry stele of Seti I (nineteenth dynasty) the ration of the King's Messenger and Standard Bearer, that we have often quoted, comprised a daily provision of "sweet oil", "olive oil" and fat (*A.R.*, III, 208). In addition, the very large quantities of olives apportioned to the temples (*A.R.*, 239, 241, etc.) could not all have served for food, and a significant proportion must have gone to the oil press.

Medically, oil (*mrḥt*) is recorded in 30 recipes prescribed *per os*. In fifteen of these the medicine had to be swallowed (eaten); in eleven it had to be drunk, some other liquid like beer, water, or milk, being included; and in four it was drunk without any other added liquid. In three of the last group, cooking (frying) was understood. In one prescription, oil had to be swallowed after an inhalation, presumably to soothe the irritated mucosa. Moreover, as an aid in dispensing, *mrḥt* (oil) is mentioned about seventy times.

Two examples of healing by "transfer" and by "sympathy" used oil. The first prescribed for hemicrania the skull of a silurus fish, boiled with oil, to be rubbed on the side of the head (*Eb.*, XLVII, 250). The second, possibly capitalizing on the resemblance between a bald head and the glabrous smooth skin of worms, introduces us right into harem intrigue

> ". . . to cause the hair to fall out: burnt chaenopod worm, boiled with oil and balanites oil, applied to the head of a hated woman [a rival in the husband's affection]." (*Eb.*, LXVII, 474)

Specific types of oil had particular indications.

Castor oil was the subject of a long paragraph in the Ebers papyrus (*Eb.*, XLVII, 251).

> "To know what is made with the *dgm* (ricinus) plant . . . if its roots [according to Loret, 1902] are crushed in water and applied to a head which is ill, then he will get well immediately, like one who is not ill. But if a little of its seeds is chewed with beer by a man with looseness in his excrements, then it expels the disease in the belly of the man. Further, the hair of a woman is made to grow by means of its seed: it is ground, mixed together and put into oil by the woman who shall rub her head herewith. Further its oil in its seed is used to annoint one who [suffers] from the nose with bad putrid [. . .]. Really excellent, [proved] many times." (see Loret, 1902)

Moringa oil was very often included in enemas to treat anal conditions (*Ber.*, 165–171). It was cooked with a chaenopod worm and applied to the scalp of a hated rival to bring down her hair (*Eb.*, LXVII, 474, see above) and it was applied to ears to improve hearing (*Eb.*, XCI, 764).

Sft oil (fir-oil? turpentine?) had special indications. With copper flakes, malachite, scent and spices, it was applied to putrefying burns (*Eb.*, LXVIII, 491) and to purulent toe and finger infections to kill the *sp* worm (*Eb.*, LXXVIII, 617). It entered also in emmenagogue applications to the hypogastrium (*S.*, Verso 13–21, 3), and in remedies to ease delivery (*Eb.*, XCIV, 807).

Notes: Chapter 19

1. According to Herodotus (I, 122), Cyrus, exposed at his birth in the wilderness to be killed by wild beasts, was adopted by a cowherd's wife named Spaca, Mede for bitch. When, later, he was reclaimed, his parents, wishing to persuade the Persians that there was a special providence in his preservation, spread the report that Cyrus, when he was exposed, was suckled by a bitch. This, according to Herodotus, was the sole origin of the rumour.

Chapter 20   Spices and Herbs

"A garden locked is my bride,
my sister . . . Your shoots are an
orchard of pomegranates . . . henna
with nard, nard and saffron,
calamus and cinnamon, with all
trees of frank-incense, myrrh,
and aloes . . ."

(Song of Solomon, 4, 12–14)

Taste and smell, the only two senses based on chemical perception, are the oldest and most fundamental of the five. The magic spell of fragrance, the subtle charm of a recalled taste may evoke the past and recreate experience as can no other sense. Marcel Proust's *Remembrance of Things Past* finally revolved around the retrieval of memories confusedly aroused by the taste of a "madeleine" dipped in sweet tea, that, like the thread of Ariadne, slowly led the author through the labyrinth of his past.

If food were a mere mixture of essential nutrients, a synthetic diet including these in optimal proportions and quantities might be theoretically perfect, but would be devoid of any pleasurable associations and quickly lead to disinterest. Man has always embellished his food with seasoning to whet his appetite, contribute to his enjoyment and aid his digestion. Unfortunately, these advantages were often more than offset by the toll his gluttony paid to disease.

Nevertheless, skilfully used, these relishes enhance secretion of digestive juices and act as carminatives. They satisfy the gourmet *joie de vivre* for "smell explores and taste decides", said the supreme connoisseur, Brillat-Savarin (1884, p. 49); so much so that the word spice, like salt, has come to be applied to anything giving piquancy to character, speech or life.

In the past, however, spices played a more functional role. In the absence of refrigeration, meats, dried or salted in autumn, had to be kept and eaten through the long winter and, in time, turned bad. Even if spices could not prevent decomposition, just as "all the perfumes of Arabia" could not sweeten the little hand of Macbeth (V, I), they could, at least, hide the smell of spoilage. In some countries and at certain periods in history, before bathing became habitual, they were used also to mask personal odours, and were incorporated into fragrant mixtures and ointments. Their use in cosmetics stems from antiquity, as does their role today in medicinal preparations.

The demand for these correctives was enormous; prices soared and brought incalculable profits to those merchants who dared to speculate on their transport or trade, or to sail the high seas and affront piracy to obtain them.

It is, indeed, difficult to realize the full impact of spices on life and politics throughout history; of this, there are many historical or semi-historical records. In the fifteenth century B.C. Queen Hatshepsut thought it worthwhile to record on her temple at Deir el-Bahari the details of the expedition she launched to the distant land of Punt on the Red Sea to fetch the myrrh and spices demanded by Amon's cult; it was a group of spice-trading Ishmaelites who bought Joseph from his brothers; and it is related that King Nero burnt a year's supply of Rome's cinnamon at the funeral of Poppaea.

In more modern times, kings, governments, and powerful trading companies vied in armed expeditions to the sources of spices to by-pass the middlemen, usually Arab sailors and merchants, and the trading countries which hid the secret of their routes and weaved fantastic legends around them to discourage competitors.

When the sources were finally discovered, Portuguese, Dutch, French, British and other colonizers enslaved and killed aborigines to exact increasing supplies, and fought fierce wars to maintain their monopolies. In short, the traders in spices wrote as horrid a page of war and slavery in history as did the traffic in sugar; spices being then, like oil nowadays, behind many significant political moves.

In Egypt, the spice traffic was especially prosperous during the Mameluke period (A.D. 1250–1517), when its profits just from re-sale to Europeans, especially to Venetians, played a dominant role in the prosperity of Cairo.

This manna seemed so providential that fabulous tales circulated around its origin, and spices were said to fall from Eden into certain trees, then carried by the Nile to Egypt (cf. Genesis, 2, 13)

> "The name of the second river [that flows from Eden] is Gihon; it is the one which flows around the whole land of Cush."

In fact, apart from a few spices like anis, cumin and mint, that were local products, spices were imported. Cinnamon came from Ceylon, India and China by way of the Red Sea, or from the Levant; cloves from the Mollucas Islands, Malacca and Amboina (Indonesia), by way of Java and Aden; nutmeg from the Mollucas, Amboina and Banda; pepper from Ceylon, Malabar and Ethiopia, the last source being particularly appreciated; pepper from Cochin, Sumatra and Java; saffron from Persia, Cilicia and Spain; cardamom from Malabar by way of Aden; various kinds of ginger from India, Arabia, Zanzibar, Madagascar and Turkey.

Many of these products were heavily adulterated, and there are records of protests from German traders who bought them in Venice, to which the Venetian Consul answered that they, themselves, had to buy them without previous examination.

The trade became more difficult in the beginning of the sixteenth century when, with the rise of Portuguese sea-power, communications with India became insecure. In 1501, many spice-laden boats were sunk by the Portuguese in Calcutta. In 1503, a boat carrying to Cairo cinnamon and ginger was destroyed by Vasco de Gama. Merchants began to desert the Venetian market and go to Lisbon. Thereupon, the Venetian Senate sent an ambassador to Cairo to study measures against the Portuguese. Sultan al-Ghoury sent a monk as an emissary to the Pope, and Julius II gave a letter addressed to the kings of Portugal and Spain. This being of no avail, al-Ghoury took reprisals against Italian merchants in Cairo. The situation was extremely critical, and a Spices Commission was set up in Venice, while the European diplomacy entered into feverish action. Venetian Ambassadors to Cairo Domenico Trevisiano (cf. Fig. 5.17) and Benedetto Sanuto; the Embassy of Jean Thénaud, delegated by Louis XII of France to the Sultan; and the mission of Sagadino, sent by al-Ghoury to Venice, were particularly concerned with the re-establishment of the spice traffic; but they were ineffective and the source of wealth partially drifted to Damascus, Baghdad, and other routes (Clerget, 1934, Vol. II, pp. 344–346).

The continuing importance of that trade is illustrated by two examples. Until 1813, the Cairo merchants of coffee and spices accepted only French currency for their wares, and it was Mohamed Aly who compelled them to accept only Egyptian currency. Two years later, the monopoly on Upper Egyptian fennel, cumin, anise and caraway, was granted to an Armenian for a large sum. Previously, the proceeds of this trade were a mortmain in favour of the two Holy cities of Islam (Al-Djabarti, 1896, Vol. IX, pp. 77, 186).

Today, owing to a wide local consumption, both in food and in herbalist medicine, the spice trade still occupies in Egypt a multitude of merchants centering their activities mainly in very picturesque markets [*Taht el-Rab*ʿ in Cairo, and *Attarine* (the grocers) in Alexandria] where the surrounding air is heavily fragrant with their exotic wares.

The present size of the world spice market may be gauged from the following figures. According to the Foreign Agricultural Circulars of the US Department of Agriculture (FTEA 1–72 and 1–73), the US in 1971 imported condiments and flavouring materials totalling $80,847,000; in 1972, the figure rose to approximately $86,058,000. On an international scale, world trade in the nine principal spices, covering two-thirds of the world trade, averaged a yearly 113 million dollars in the 1959–1968 period (Rosengarten, 1969, pp. 5, 468).

"The number of savours", as Brillat-Savarin also said, "is, however, infinite" (1884, p. 58), and individual tastes differ, at different longitudes and latitudes. The differences do not depend entirely on availability, since most spices are imported, a feature that gave to groceries their German name "Kolonialwaren"; but they are, by and large, a matter of associations, habits, childhood conditioning, past experience and other factors that are sweepingly included under the general term "personal taste".

Particular flavours are preferred by particular social groups or environments. It is easy to distinguish by sight, smell, or taste between American, French, Spanish, Swedish, Arabic, Chinese and African cooking. Within each of these, subtler distinctions can be made today between the south and the north of, say, France, the United States, or Egypt; and this must have always been the case. These distinctions are largely a reflection of the spices used.

In the Mediterranean and Near Eastern countries, sweetening agents, jams, sweet jellies, or fruits, are not generally eaten with meats or cooked dishes, as they are in northern Europe or America. But spices are used more freely. Speaking in a rather schematic way, mint, oregano, thyme and laurel prevail in Greece; fennel, laurel, tarragon in Southern France; coriander, cumin and black pepper in Egypt; hot peppers in the Sudan and Congo; cardamon and saffron in the Arabian Peninsula; while pine seeds, raisins, pistaccio nuts and almonds are often added to rice or to stuffing in Syria and the Lebanon.

One relish that is specific to the Near East is *doqqa*, a varying mixture of thyme, marjoram and other herbs, made into a powder and eaten with bread. It is remarkable, moreover, that the nearer one approaches the Equator, the sharper the flavour of the food, which may be an instinctive response to the inhibition of appetite by excessive heat and humidity, or a precaution against spoilage.

The distinction between herbs and spices is artificial and often arbitrary. Rosengarten (1969, p. 3) defines herbs as aromatic products from temperate regions, and spices as the exotic products of tropical lands. Others differ only slightly and would call spices the aromatic natural products which are the seeds, buds, fruit or flower parts, bark or root of plants, usually of tropical origin, and herbs the aromatic leaves or flowers of plants, usually of temperate origin (R. Hall, personal communication).

These plants have a long history in the Near East. In Chapter 17, the use in Egypt of several fragrant plants, like onion, garlic, parsley, etc., to enrich the flavour of food, has been discussed along with vegetables, but much remains to be learned on culinary methods and seasoning in Ancient Egypt. The main writer on the subject, Apicius, lived in Alexandria, but he could hardly be considered an authority on Pharaonic cooking, although he might have inherited some of his recipes from Ramessid or Thutmoside "Chefs".

The discussion here is limited to those individual spices that have a documented record in Ancient Egypt, thus leaving aside coffee, tea, and cocoa which were introduced much later. The reservation must be made that specific identification is usually at best an informed guess because of the uncertain classification of many current spices, of changes with shifting supplies and commercial considerations, and of widespread adulteration throughout history.

Ami (Carum copticum)

Synonyms: Ethiopian cumin, Royal cumin, Bishop's weed

The use of ami is not documented by any Ancient Egyptian evidence. But it was mentioned by Pliny

". . . its use is similar to that of cumin, for it is put under loaves of bread at Alexandria and included among the ingredients of Alexandrian sauces. It dispels flatulence, promotes urine and menstruation, relieves bruises and fluxes of the eyes and, taken in wine with linseed in doses of two drach-mae, it is good for the wounds of scorpions, and with an equal proportion of myrrh it is especially good for the bite of the cerastes [horned viper]. Like cumin, it produces pallor in the complexion of those who drink it. A fumigation of it with raisins or resin acts as a purge upon the womb. It is believed that those women more easily conceive who smell the plant during sexual intercourse . . . " (*N.H.*, XX, LVIII, 163–164)

Anise (Pimpinella anisum)

Ancient Egyptian: *inst* (*Wb. Dr.*, 44)
Greek: *anison*
Arabic: *yansoon*

There is still some debate about the meaning of *inst*, which was stated to designate anise, by analogy with its Greek and Arabic names. Lefebvre (1956, p. 61) assessed it as a very likely correct translation, but Loret (*Fl.*, 51) translated it as "sage" (*Salvia aegyptiaca*).

Pliny, however, expressly mentions anise as an Egyptian plant

". . . the most esteemed variety is the Cretan; next comes the Egyptian." (*N.H.*, XX, LXXIII, 187)

The same with Dioscorides (III, 56) who gave a lengthy list of its indications.

Inst, untranslated by Ebbell, was used medicinally in abdominal and dental diseases (*Eb.*, XLIII, 210; XLIV, 219; XLV, 226, etc.).

Caper (Capparis spinosa)

The earliest reference that has come to our attention concerning capers in Egypt dates to the first century A.D. by Pliny

". . . in Egypt also grows the caper tree, a shrub with a rather hard wood; also its seed is well known as an article of food." (*N.H.*, XIII, XLIV, 127)

In the sixteenth century A.D., Pierre Belon du Mans found it growing abundantly in the regions of Alexandria, Suez and Sinai. He found the trees to be different from the Greek and European varieties, being thornless, as large as fig trees, keeping their leaves in winter, and bearing fruits the size of walnuts. The seeds, he said, tasted like pepper and were added to wine to keep it sweet (Sauneron, 1970, 94a, 97b, 125a, b, 129b).

Later, in the nineteenth century, Alfred Kaiser collected in Sinai specimens of *C. cartilaginea Decne*. He noted that the plant is called there *lassaf;* the fruit, *girru* or *agra*; and the bud, *kabr*. The plant was used there as fodder; its fruits were eaten raw or were used in preparing a refreshing drink; and its buds and seeds, that taste like pepper, were utilized as condiments.

He also found there another variety, *C. spinosa v. aegyptiaca*, now called *C. aegyptia*, used in the same way, in addition to being prescribed for chest diseases (Täckholm, 1969).

Cinnamon (Cinnamomum zeylanicum)

Ancient Egyptian: *ty-šps* (*Wb. Dr.*, 549)
Arabic: *gerfa*

Ty-šps was used medicinally in suppositories, ointments, and dressings (*Eb.*, XXXI, 140; XLVIII, 255; LXVIII, 491; *H.*, 108; *Ber.*, 51).

Rameses III, on many occasions, presented the gods with gifts of this plant

"246 measures and 82 bundles" (*A.R.*, IV, 235)
"17 measures of sticks" (*A.R.*, IV, 287)
"and 3036 logs" (*A.R.*, IV, 300)

It was one of the Oriental aromatic plants mentioned by Theophrastus (4, 4, 14; 9, 4, 2, etc.), and it figured among the precious spices carried in the Dionysiac processions described by Athenaeus

". . . then came camels some of which carried three hundred pounds of frankincense, three hundred of myrrh, and two hundred of saffron, cassia, cinnamon . . . " (*Deipnos.*, 5, 201, A)

If *malobathrum*, that was said by Jones (Vol. 7, p. 519) perhaps to be *Cinnamomum tamala*, could be identified with this plant with certainty, it must have been imported from Syria or from India. Pliny wrote

"Syria also supplies the malobathrum . . . from it oil is pressed to use for unguents, Egypt also producing it in still greater quantity. But the kind that comes from India is valued more highly" (*N.H.*, XII, LIX, 129)

According to Jones (Vol. IV, p. 88, n.c.), its attribution to Syria instead of India (since in Sanskrit this word is derived from *tamalapatra*, cinnamon-leaf) only reflected the trade routes through which it transited.

Coriander (Coriandrum sativum)

Ancient Egyptian: *š3w, pr . t š3w* (*prt shaw*, grains of *shaw*)
Arabic: *kuzbara*

"And the House of Israel called the name thereof Manna: and it was like coriander seed, white; and the taste of it was like wafers made with honey." (Exodus, 16, 31)

The identification by Loret of coriander with *wnšy* (*Fl.*, 72) is considered now erroneous, especially by Keimer (*Gpfl.*, 159) who points to the accepted translation of this word as one of the names of grapes (see Chapter 18).

Another word *š3w* or *prt . š3w* (*F.*, 261; *Wb. Dr.*, 47) seems more appropriate in view of its resemblance to the Coptic name of the plant *bershyw. š3w* is mentioned in the Ebers papyrus, especially as a treatment of *áaá* (*Eb.*, XXXV, 174; XLV, 226) and of diseases of the limbs (*Eb.*, VI, 19; XXXII, 145; *Ber.*, 188).

Remains of coriander found in Tut-ankh-Amon's tomb are now kept at lhe Dokki museum (Cat. no. 4206); Schweinfurth found coriander in material from a twenty-first dynasty tomb at Deir el-Bahari (1885); and Newberry, in the Graeco-Roman necropolis of Hawara (1889); two packets of coriander grains are also said to be in the Leyden Egyptian Museum (*Fl.*, 72).

The plant was mentioned by Apicius as a condiment for marrows

(3, 4, 3) and fish (10, 1, 7–8), and Pliny commended it in different passages

"... the best, as is generally agreed, is the Egyptian. It is an antidote for the poison of one kind of serpent the amphisbaena, both taken in drink and applied ... spreading sores also are healed by coriander with honey or raisins, likewise diseased testes, burns, carbuncles, and sore ears, fluxes of the eyes too if woman's milk be added, it is also taken in drink with rue for cholera. Intestinal parasites are expelled by coriander seed ..." (*N.H.*, XX, LXXXII, 216, 18 select)

Cumin (Cuminum cyminum)

Ancient Egyptian: *tpnn* (*Fl.*, 144; *Wb. Dr.*, 557)
Coptic: *tapen*
Hebrew: *kammou*
Arabic: *kammoun*
Roman: *cuminum*

According to Keimer, Egyptian cumin (*Cuminum cyminum*) is different from the European cumin, *Carum carvi* (*Gpfl.*, 41). From the fact that the Egyptian name *tpnn*, preserved in Coptic *tapen*, is different from the Semitic names of the plant, one could conclude that the Arabs introduced the Semitic appellation *kammoun* when they invaded Egypt.

Of this plant a gift of 5 *heket* from Rameses III to Ra at Heliopolis is on record (*A.R.*, IV, 287). A few grains coming from Deir el Medineh, during the New Kingdom are on view in the Agricultural Museum, Dokki, Cairo, and in the museum of Florence (*Fl.*, 72; Bonnet 1900).

From a later period, Apicius (3, 4, 3; 10, 1, 6) mentioned it as an ingredient used by Egyptians in cooking marrows and grilled fish, and Pliny commended it highly

"Yet of all the seasonings which gratify a fastidious taste cumin is the most agreeable ... Another kind of cumin is the wild variety called country cumin or by other people Thebaic cumin. For pounding up in water and using it as a draught in case of stomach ache the most highly esteemed kind in our continent is that grown at Carpetania, though elsewhere the prize is awarded to Ethiopian and African cumin; however some prefer the Egyptian to the African." (*N.H.*, XIX, XLVII, 161)

This practice is quite in accord with the present day household treatment of colic and indigestion with cumin tea.

Today, similarly, cumin is added to drinks served to women recently delivered of a child—a custom that lead to the saying (of some one taking premature decisions)

> "She has prepared cumin before being with child, and she called the child Ma'mun [a boy's name—assuming a male child] before its birth."

If *tpnn* is identified with cumin, then this plant was prescribed by Egyptian physicians internally in gastro-intestinal disease (*Eb.*, V, 17; LII, 299), to expel worms (*Eb.*, XXII, 79), and to treat various other disorders. It was also included in mouth rinses (*Eb.*, LXXXV, 700), suppositories (*Eb.*, IX, 26), external applications (*Eb.*, XXVI, 111; *H.*, 125), powders (*Eb.*, LXV, 446), and ear instillations (*Eb.*, XCII, 770).

Dill (Anethum graveolens)

Ancient Egyptian: *imst* (*Fl.*, 137; *Gpfl.*, 37, 147; *Wb. Dr.*, 34). Arabic: *shabath*

Loret (1886) in his introductory remarks on dill wrote that since it is a common observation that the Egyptian flora has hardly changed since antiquity, nowadays finding dill growing wild in Egypt is practically sufficient to prove its existence in Ancient Egypt as well. This was later proved true by Schweinfurth who found in the tomb of Amonophis II eight twigs of this plant (personal communication to Keimer, quoted in *Gpfl.*, 37 and 99).

As the plant *imst* is homonymous with Amsety, one of the four sons of Horus to protect the Canopic jars, and the only one with a human head, Kees (1961, p. 77) could write of it

> ". . . a medicinal herb called *amsety*, elevated to become one of the four divinities of the Canopic jars who protected the stomach and entrails of the dead so that they could not suffer hunger or want. In this way it personified certain vital characteristics of man in divine form."[1]

Imst was believed to relieve headache and to soften the vessels (or limbs, *mtw*) (*Eb.*, XLVII, 249; *Eb.*, LXXXI, 650; *Ber.*, 163e).

Fennel (Foeniculum vulgare, Anethum foeniculum)

Ancient Egyptian: *shamari*? (*Fl.*, 143)
Arabic: *shamar*

Loret points to several words that could have designated fennel. One is *shamari*, mentioned in the Leyden Gnostic Papyrus (according to Keimer: *Gpfl.*, p. 150), a misspelling of the scribe. This word is close to *shamarin* of the Great Harris Papyrus, and to Coptic *shamar hout*, that is translated into Arabic *shamar barri* (wild fennel) in a Scala (*Fl.*, 143).

Another suggested name is *besbes*, cognate with Arabic *bisbas*, that Loret translated fennel (*Fl.*, 71), but that was more correctly translated as "myristica" by Schweinfurth (1912, p. 55). Dioscorides called it *sampsoth* (III, 70, 71)

In a personal communication, R. Hall commented that there are two kinds of myrrh, one of which is *bisabol* myrrh (*Commiphora erythraea*), and he made the interesting suggestion that the closeness of *bisabol* to *bisbas*, and of *myrrh* to *myristica* could have misled some authors.

Bsbs is known from the medical papyri to have been used internally in the treatment of a disease called *nsyt* (*Eb.*, LXXXIX, 751), and externally against some skin diseases (*Eb.*, XXIII, 90); it was also included in suppositories (*Eb.*, XCIV, 802), mouth rinses (*Eb.*, LXXII, 554), fumigations (*Ber.*, 58) and vaginal injections (*Eb.*, XCVI, 830). But it was left untranslated by Ebbell, and was said to be an unknown plant by V. Deines and Grapow (*Wb. Dr.*, 180).

Fenugreek (Trigonella foenum grecum)

Ancient Egyptian: $hm \cdot y \cdot t$ (*S.*, 21, 9–10)
Arabic: *helba*

Loret (1935–1938) identified fenugreek with $hm \cdot y \cdot t$ on the basis of the resemblance of the latter word with Arabic *helba*. On the other hand, Dawson (1926) was of the opinion that fenugreek bore the name *šny . t*ʒ, which is now identified with *Cyperus esculentus* (see *Wb. Dr.*, 496 and Chapter 16, p. 649).

Hm yt was subjected to a lengthy preparation to extract its oil which was used as a medium of rejuvenation (*S.*, 21, 9–10). Seeds of this plant have been recovered from a Maadi site dating to 3000 B.C. (quoted by Renfrew, 1973, p. 188).

Nowadays, germinated *helba* is eaten usually with lupine. It is added to bread for its flavour, and the powdered grains, or an oil extracted from it are taken as galactagogues. Its presumed innumerable virtues are proclaimed in a street cry

"Healing from God, Helba!"

Laurel (Laurus nobilis)

Arabic: *ghar*

The only finds of this plant, now widely used in cooking in Greece and the Near East, are twigs found around garlands of the Graeco-Roman period (Newberry, 1889; Pleyte, 1882).

Marjoram (Origanum majorana)

Arabic: *samsaq, mardaqush, bardaqush*

Marjoram was a favourite component of the wreathes with which mummies were decorated (Newberry, 1889; Bonnet, 1900; *T.*, II, 96). Of this plant Dioscorides said that it grew in Egypt where it was called *sofo* (III, 39); and Pliny (*N.H.*, XIX, L, 165) reckoned Egyptian marjoram to be superior to *cunila* [according to Jones (Vol. VII, 503) summer savory or sweet winter marjoram], adding that

"Diocles the physician and the people of Sicily have called sweet marjoram the plant known in Egypt as *sampsucum*." (*N.H.*, XXI, XXXV, 61)

The Egyptian name of the plant is, however, unknown, unless it be permissible to see a relationship between *sofo*, the *sampsucum* of the Greeks, *smsq*, one of the Arabic names of the plant, and *šft*, a plant that appears in the Ebers papyrus

"To expel burning in the lower part of the belly: figs, cinnamon, manna, honey, *šft*, the lower part of the belly is bandaged therewith." (*Eb.*, XXXV, 176)

Mint (Mentha spicata, M. sativa)

Arabic: *na ʿna ʿ*

Schweinfurth (1881, p. 666) described twigs of this plant in a wreath found in a tomb at Sheikh-Abdel Gournah. Loret (*Fl.*, 53) thought that its Egyptian name was *agai* though, at times, it was abusively called *napkata*, this latter word being in his opinion the name of rosemary. Keimer (*Gpfl.*, 138), however, rejected these two interpretations. In some Scalae, *amisi*, elsewhere translated dill, is given as the name of mint, so that this word, too, could be one of the names for mint. Apicius mentioned the plant among cooking ingredients (3, 4, 3).

Mustard (Sinapis alba)

Arabic: *khardal*

This plant now grows wild in Egyptian fields. Parts of it have been found in large quantities in a twelfth dynasty tomb by Schweinfurth (1885). It is mentioned by Newberry (1889) among plants authenticated in Egypt, though he did not find any sample of it in Hawara. New Kingdom specimens are kept at the Dokki Agricultural Museum,

Cairo. Pliny (*N.H.*, XII, XIV, 28) incidentally recorded its existence in Egypt

> ". . . there are three kinds of mustard plant . . . The best seed comes from Egypt."

Pepper (Piper nigrum)

Arabic: *felfel*

At least in the Graeco-Roman Period, pepper (probably *Piper nigrum*) was utilized in Egypt. It was discussed by several Graeco-Roman authors (Theophrastus, 9, 20, 2; Dioscorides, II, 198, 199; Apicius, 3, 4, 3; 10, 1, 6–8). About A.D. 54–80 it was imported into Red Sea ports from India (Schoff, 1912). Later, in Byzantine times, its price and distribution were under Government control (Crum, 1925).

Rosemary (Rosmarinus officinalis L.)

Arabic: *hasalban*

Rosemary naturally grows in Egypt, but the only specimen reported to date to Ancient Egypt was found by Prosper Alpino (1735, Vol. I, VII, 36) in a garland adorning an Egyptian body. Loret (*Fl.*, 54), who recognized Alpino's experience, commented, however, that as the sample consisted of green leaves (*folia viridia*), the distinguished visitor might have been fooled by guides in playful mood. Nevertheless, Breasted recorded that 125 measures of the plant were offered to Amon at Thebes by Rameses III (*A.R.*, IV, 234).

Its Ancient Egyptian name was tentatively said by Loret (*Fl.*, 54, 141) to be *nkpty*.

Safflower (Carthamus tinctorius)

Arabic: *gortom,* ʿ*osfor*

Safflower was well known to Egyptians who used it, with other flowers, to make the garlands that adorned their mummies and that were possibly worn in religious and profane festivities (Schweinfurth, 1886; *Gpfl.*, 7). Samples from Kom Ouchim, dating to the Roman Period are found at the Dokki Agricultural Museum, Cairo (G.C. 4177). Moreover, chemical analysis of textiles from the twelfth dynasty showed it to be one of the dyes used (Huebner, quoted by Harris, 1962, p. 153).

Several names have been advanced for this plant, but none is as yet certain (see *Gpfl.*, 128, 154; *Wb. Dr.*, 316). Its Greek name was *cnecos* (Jones, Vol. 7, p. 500); this was said to be an Egyptian plant, by Pliny who went on to record the lore with which it was associated

". . . Nor would it be right to describe fully the *onecos*, otherwise *atractylis*, an Egyptian plant, were it not for the great help it affords against venomous creatures as well as against poisonous fungi. It is a well-known fact that as long as they hold this plant, those stung by scorpions feel no sharp pain." (*N.H.*, XXI, CVII, 184)

Elsewhere, he seemed to confuse the safflower with the nettle from which he said that an oil, *cnidium* (from *cnicos*, a nettle, but more correctly called *cnecicum* in another manuscript) was obtained (*N.H.*, XV, VII, 30).

The suggestion that *cnecos* oil was made from the thistle is, according to Harris (1962, p. 336) unsupported by any evidence.

Saffron (Crocus sativus)

Arabic: *zaafarân*

Saffron was widely used in antiquity as a perfume, but it is not known to have been cultivated in Egypt before recent times (*T.*, III, 511).

Athenaeus mentions it among the perfumes carried in Dionysiac processions in Alexandria

> ". . . then came camels, some of which carried three hundred pounds of frankincense, three hundred of myrrh, and two hundred of saffron, cassia, cinnamon, orris, and all other spices . . ." (5, 201, A)

A certain plant *sn-wt . t* was identified by Ebbell as *Crocus sativus* (*Eb.*, LI, 294), but Dawson (1934b) translated it *Convolvulus*. It was prescribed both internally and externally (*Eb.*, LI, 294; *Eb.*, XC, 759).

Another drug, *matet*, repeatedly mentioned in the Ebers papyrus, was translated *Chelidonium majus* by Ebers (*T.*, III, 515), *Apium graveolens* by Keimer (*Gpfl.*, 40) and Loret (1894) (see Lefebvre, 1956, p. 149), and *mandrake* by Dawson (1933). Täckholm and Drar, however, believe it to be *Crocus* (*T.*, III, 515).

Though saffron is now widely used in the Arab world as a seasoning to rice and fish, this seems to be an influence of Persian or Indian usage, and there is no indication that it was utilized in cooking in Ancient Egypt.

Thyme (Thymus acinos)

Ancient Egyptian: *innk*

> *Like thyme, it is full of virtues*
> (Popular saying)

Innk is a still undefined plant that Loret thought to be either conyza or thyme (*Fl.*, 67), and Ebbell accepted the latter interpretation in his translation of the Ebers papyrus. *Innk* was used internally against worms (roundworms) (*Eb.*, XXI, 69; XXXII, 81) and the disease conditions *whdw* and *áaá*, as well as various abdominal complaints (*Eb.*, XXXV, 173) (see also *Wb. Dr.*, 39–41). If *innk* is to be identified with the *acinos* of Pliny which, according to Jones (Vol. 7, p. 487), is possibly *Thymus acinos*, the only indication as to its dietary use in Ancient Egypt is the following remark by Pliny

> ". . . the Egyptians sow acinos both for chaplets and for food . . ."
> (*N.H.*, XXI, XCIX, 174)

Other Spices and Flavouring Agents

In addition to the more familiar spices and herbs already discussed in this chapter, many others were undoubtedly used.

Specimens of black cumin, *Nigella sativa L.*, nowadays called in Arabic *habbet el baraka* (grain of blessing), were recognized by Braun, mixed with linseed grains, in the Berlin museum (1879). They are at present sprinkled over bread before baking

"Like black cumin, a thousand on a morsel of bread."

Grains of sage (*Salvia aegyptiaca*) were found by Unger in a brick at El-Kab (quoted in *Fl.*, 54); the stem of a *clove* tree is kept in the Historical Section of the Dokki Agricultural Museum, Cairo (G.C. 293), and Apicius (10, 1, 6–8) mentioned water plantain (*Alisma plantago*) and *asafetida* as ingredients of Alexandrian sauces to complement grilled fish.

These are the flavouring herbs and spices of which we have records. It should be stressed again, however, that most of our information on these come from Greek authors or from medical recipes. But from what is known of the thinking of Ancient Egyptians, or indeed of all the Ancients, no clear separation was made between the worlds of the living and of the dead, or between table, medicine and cult. We think it justifiable, therefore, to consider that herbs or spices, which were ritually or medicinally in use, had probable culinary applications or had originated therefrom.

Notes: Chapter 20

1. This was based on the oft-repeated attribution of the stomach and intestines to *imsety*, after, Pettigrew, who based his statement on the examination of a single mummy where carelessness on the part of the embalmer led to a wrong distribution of the viscera among the Canopic jars. Experience with large numbers of mummies has shown that *imsety* usually received the liver (Elliot-Smith and Dawson, 1924, p. 145).

Appendix

continued

Name; city (country) of origin	Range of known or estimated dates
Appuleius Barbarus (birthplace unknown)	fourth century A.D.
Archippus of Athens	416–403 B.C.
Aristobulus of Alexandria	second century B.C.
Aristobulus of Cassandreia	fourth century B.C.
Aristophanes of Athens	455–375 B.C.
Aristotle (Aristotles) of Stageira	384–322 B.C.
Arrian (Flavius Arrianus) of Nicomedia	A.D. 124–150
Asclepiades of Mendes	(before the Christian Era)
Athenaeus of Naucratis	A.D. 170–230
Augustine (Aurelius Augustinus or Saint Augustine) of Tagaste	A.D. 354–430
Callimachus of Cyrene	305–240 B.C.
Callixeinus of Rhodes	285–155 B.C.
Carneades of Cyrene	215–125 B.C.
Carystius of Pergamum	second century B.C.
Cato, Censorius Marcus Porcius of Tusculum	234–149 B.C.
Celsus, Aulus Cornelius of Verona	27 B.C.–A.D. 37
Censorinus of Rome	A.D. 238
Chaeremon of Alexandria	first century A.D.
Chaeremon of Athens	380 B.C.
Clearchus of Athens	third century B.C.

Name; city (country) of origin	Range of known or estimated dates
Clemens, Titus Flavius (Clement of Alexandria) of Athens	A.D. 150–220
Cocceianus (see Dio Chrysostomus)	
Columella, Lucius Junius Moderatus of Gades	A.D. 36–60
Damascenus (see Joannes)	
Deinon (Dinon) of Colophon	355–323 B.C.
Demetrius of Scepsis	(uncertain period before Athenaeus)
Democritus of Abdera	490–357 B.C.
Didymus of Alexandria	first century B.C.
Dinon (see Deinon)	
Dio Chrysostomus (Cocceianus or Dion) of Prusa	A.D. 40–117
Diodorus (Diodorus Siculus) of Agyrium	60–8 B.C.
Dion (see Dio Chrysostomus)	
Dioscorides Pedacius (Pedanius) of Anazarba	first to second centuries A.D.
Diphilus of Sinope	340–289 B.C.
Epaenetus of Syracuse	(uncertain period before Athenaeus)
Epicharmus of Cos	(uncertain period before Athenaeus)
Eubulus of Athens	375 B.C.
Eudoxus of Cnidus	408–352 B.C.
Eudoxus of Cyzicus	145–116 B.C.
Eudoxus of Rhodes	225–200 B.C.
Eusebius (Pamphili) of Caesaria	A.D. 260–340

continued

Name; city (country) of origin	Range of known or estimated dates
Galen (Galenus Cl. [Claudius or Clarissimus?]) of Pergamum	A.D. 129–210
George the Monk (see Syncellus)	
Hecataeus of Miletus	550–476 B.C.
Hecataeus of Teos	300 B.C.
Heliodorus of Emesa	third to fourth centuries A.D.
Hellanicus of Mytilene	500–405 B.C.
Heracleides (Heraclides) of Syracuse	(uncertain period before Athenaeus)
Hermeias of Methymne	third century B.C.
Herodotus of Halicarnassus	484–408 B.C.
Hipparchus (birthplace unknown)	(uncertain period before Athenaeus)
Hippocrates of Cos	460–352 B.C.
Homer (Homerus) of Chios	1184–684 B.C.
Horace (Horatius, Flaccus Quintius) of Venusia	65–8 B.C.
Ion of Chios	(uncertain period before Athenaeus)
Joannes (Damascenus or John of Damascus) of Damascus	A.D. 700–756
Julianus, Flavius Claudius (Julian the Apostate) of Constantinople	A.D. 332–363
Julius Pollux (see Pollux)	
Juvenal (Juvenalis, Decimusunius) of Agiunum	A.D. 40–140
Lucian (Lucianus or Lycinus) of Samosata	A.D. 90–180
Lucretius, Titus Carus of Rome	99–51 B.C.

Name; city (country) of origin	Range of known or estimated dates
Lyceus (birthplace unknown)	(uncertain period before Athenaeus)
Lycinus (see Lucian)	
Machon of Corinth	300–260 B.C.
Macrobius, Ambrosius Aurelius Theodosius of Parma	A.D. 400–415
Malchus (see Porphyry)	
Manetho of Sebennytus	300–250 B.C.
Martial (Martialis, Marcus Valerius) of Bilbilis	A.D. 40–104
Menander of Athens	342–291 B.C.
Mithaecus (birthplace unknown)	(uncertain period before Athenaeus)
Nicander of Colophon	185–135 B.C.
Nicator (see Seleucus)	
Oppian (Oppianus) of Anazarbos	second to third centuries A.D.
Oppian (Oppianus) of Apameia	A.D. 198–211
Ovid (Ovidius, Publius Naso) of Sulmo	43 B.C.–A.D. 18
Pamphili (see Eusebius)	
Panyassis of Halicarnassus	489–467 B.C.
Pausanias of Lydia	150–200 A.D.
Pedanius (see Dioscorides Pedacius)	
Phaedrus (Phaeder) of Thrace	15 B.C.–A.D. 50
Philochorus of Athens	306–261 B.C.
Philonides of Athens	414–410 B.C.

continued

Name; city (country) of origin	Range of known or estimated dates
Philoxenus of Cythera	(uncertain period before Athenaeus)
Phylarchus of Naucratis	221–210 B.C.
Plato of Athens	430–347 B.C.
Pliny (Plinius, Gaius Secundus) of Verona	A.D. 23–79
Plutarch (Plutarchus) of Chaeronea	A.D. 46–127
Pollux, Julius of Naucratis	A.D. 186
Polyaenus of Macedon	A.D. 163
Polybius of Megalopolis	206–120 B.C.
Porphyry (Porphyrius or Malchus) of Tyre	A.D. 232–306
Ptolemy of Ptolemais Hermiu	A.D. 90–168
Pythagoras of Samos	608–510 B.C.
Saint Augustine (see Augustine)	
Seleucus (Nicator) of Macedon	358–280 B.C.
Sextus Empiricus (birthplace unknown)	third century A.D.
Sextius Julius (see Africanus)	
Socrates of Athens	469–399 B.C.
Socrates of Cos	(uncertain period before Plutarch)
Solon of Salamis	640–560 B.C.
Strabo of Amasia (Amaseia)	66 B.C.–A.D. 25
Suetonus (Gaius Suetonus) Tranquillus of Rome	c. A.D. 75–160
Syncellus Georgius (George the Monk) of Constantinople	A.D. 800

Name; city (country) of origin	Range of known or estimated dates
Tacitus, Cornelius of Interamna	A.D. 55–117
Terence (Terentius, Publius Afer) of Carthage	195–159 B.C.
Theocritus of Syracuse	310–250 B.C.
Theogonis of Megara	570–490 B.C.
Theophrastus of Eresus	374–285 B.C.
Theopompus of Chios	404–305 B.C.
Thucydides of Athens	471–400 B.C.
Varro, Marcus Terentius of Reate	116–27 B.C.
Virgil (Vergilius, Publius Maro) of Andes	70–19 B.C.
Vopiscus, Flavius of Syracuse	A.D. 291–320
Xenocrates (birthplace unknown)	A.D. 60
Xenophon of Athens	430–354 B.C.

Table 2

Pre-Dynastic Egypt; major sites and technological development

Chronology	Upper Egypt	Lower Egypt	Classification by stone/metal	Associated technology
3,200 B.C.	(UNIFICATION OF UPPER AND LOWER EGYPT) Semainean (Naqada III)	Maadian	CHALCOLITHIC	Centralized Administration Metal tools
3,500 B.C.	Gerzian (Naqada II)	Omarian (B)		Painting
	Amratian (Naqada I)	Omarian (A) Fayoum (B)		Pottery Polished stone tools
	Badarian	Mermidian Fayoum (A)	NEOLITHIC	Community organization Agriculture

Date	Culture	Period	Technological/cultural development
		MESOLITHIC	Pressure-flaking of stone tools
5,000 B.C.			
	Sebilian (III)		
10,000 B.C.	Sebilian (II)	UPPER PALAEOLITHIC	Bow and arrow
	Sebilian (I)		
	Helwan		
30,000 B.C.	(SCATTERED FLINT TOOLS IN NILE VALLEY TERRACES)	MIDDLE PALAEOLITHIC	Cultural regionalization
187,000 B.C.	(SCATTERED FLINT TOOLS IN NILE VALLEY TERRACES)	LOWER PALAEOLITHIC	Diversification of stone tools
475,000 B.C.	(Present ?)		Stone tools of pre-determined shape
?			"Pebble-tools" Fire

Table 3

Egyptian chronology; Archaic Period and Old Kingdom king list and contemporary nobility

Dynasty	Date	Royal name	Contemporaries
First	3200 B.C.	Narmer (Menes?)	
		Aha	
		Djer	
		Djet	
		Udimu (Den)	
		Adjib	
		Smerkhet	
		Qa (Qa-ay)	
		Hetep-Sekhemui	
Second	?	Nebre	
		Neterimu	
		Peribsen	
		Sendji	
		Neterka	
		Neferkare	
		Kha-Sekhem	
		Kha-Sekhemui	
		Sa-Nakht	
	2778 B.C.	Zoser	Imhotep
		Nebkare	
		Sekhemkhet	

ARCHAIC PERIOD

Dynasty	Date	Kings	Officials/Tombs
Third		Hu-Djefa Kha-Djefa Kha-Bau Snefru (Soris)	Anubisemonekh, Itet, Methen, Nefermaat
	2723 B.C.		
Fourth		Khufu (Cheops) Djadef-Re (Ratoises) Khaf-Re (Cephren, Kephrem) Horedef Ba-ef-Re Men-Kau-Re (Mycerinus) Shepses-Kaf (Sebercheres) Khentkawes	
	2563 B.C.		
Fifth		User-Kaf (Usercheres) Sahu-Re (Sephres) Nefer-ir-ka-Re (Kakai) Ne-Woser-Re Men-Kew-Hor Djed-Ka-Re (Isesi)	Ti
	2423 B.C.		
Sixth		Unas (Onnos) Teti (Othoes)	Akhet-hotep, Ptah hetep, Ire-Nakhty Idut Ankh-ma-Hor, Ka-Gem-Ni, Mereruka
		Pepi I Mer-ne-Re Pepi II ———	Aba, Pepionkh (A2), Pepionkh (D2), Senbi
	2300 B.C.		

OLD KINGDOM

Table 4

Egyptian chronology; First Intermediate Period, Middle Kingdom, Second Intermediate Period with king list and contemporary nobility

Dynasty	Date	Royal name	Contemporaries
1st	2300 B.C.		
I N T E R M E D I A T E (Seventh)	?		
(Eighth)			
(Ninth)	2242 B.C.		
(Tenth)	2150 B.C.		(?) { Duaf, Merikere, Neferrohu
			(?) { Kawit, Amenemhat
M I D D L E K I N G D O M (Eleventh)	2143 B.C.	Intef I	(?) { Baqt I, Baqt III, Khety
	2140 B.C.	Intef II	Khnum-hotep
	2090 B.C.	Intef III	
	2088 B.C.	Mentuhotpe I	
	2070 B.C.	Mentuhotpe II	
	2019 B.C.	Mentuhotpe III	
	2007 B.C.	Mentuhotpe IV	
	2000 B.C.	Amenemhat I (Ammenemes I)	Senbi
(Twelfth)	1970 B.C.	Senusret I (Sesostris I)	Ukh-hotp
	1936 B.C.	Amenemhat II (Ammenemes II)	Menthuweser
	1906 B.C.	Senusret II (Sesostris II)	Antefoker
	1887 B.C.	Senusret III (Sesostris III)	(?) { Tehuti-Nekht, Thut-Hotpe
	1850 B.C.	Amenemhat III (Ammenemes III)	
	1800 B.C.	Hor	
	1800 B.C.	Amenemhat IV (Ammenemes IV)	
	1792 B.C.	Sebek-Nefru-Re	
	1785 B.C.	———	

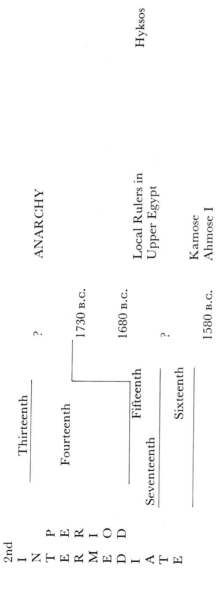

2nd
INTERMEDIATE PERIOD

Thirteenth

Fourteenth — ? — 1730 B.C.

Fifteenth — 1680 B.C.

ANARCHY

Hyksos

Seventeenth — ?

Sixteenth — 1580 B.C.

Local Rulers in Upper Egypt

Kamose
Ahmose I

Table 5

Egyptian chronology; New Kingdom (eighteenth to twentieth dynasties) king list and contemporary nobility

Dynasty	Date	Royal name	Contemporaries
	1580 B.C.	Ahmose I	Paheri, Reni
	1557 B.C.	Amenhotep I	Senmut, Nebamun,
	1530 B.C.	Thutmose I	Amenemhat, Amenhab,
	1520 B.C.	Thutmose II	Horemheb, Ineni,
		Hatshepsut	Menkheperrasonb,
		Thutmose III	Minnakht, Neb-Amon,
			Rekhmire, Menkheper
			(?) Inena
Eighteenth	1450 B.C.	Amenhotep II	Meryet-Amun, Suemmut
	1425 B.C.	Thutmose IV	Mena, Nakht, Nebamun, Thanunu
	1405 B.C.	Amenhotep III	Amenmose, Tiy
	1370 B.C.	Amenhotep IV (Akhenaten)	Mery-Ra, Nefertiti
	1352 B.C.	Smenkhkare	
		Tut-ankh-Amon	Huy
		Eye (Ai)	

R A M E S S I D P E R I O D	Nineteenth	1341 B.C.	Horemheb (Harmais)	Roy
		1320 B.C.		Ipy, Nefertari, Nekhtamun, Penehsi, Tjunersy, Nebunenef
		1318 B.C.	Seti I (Sethos)	
		1298 B.C.		
		1232 B.C.	Meneptah (Menephthes)	
			Amenmesses	
			Siptah-Meneptah	
			Seti II	
		1200 B.C.	Setnakht	(?) Sennutem
		1198 B.C.	Rameses III	
		1166 B.C.	Rameses IV	
			Rameses V	
			Rameses VI	
			Rameses VII	
	Twentieth		Rameses VIII	
			Rameses IX	
			Rameses X	
			Rameses XI	
			Rameses XII	
		1085 B.C.	Nesbanebdedi (Smendes)	Wenamon

Table 6

Egyptian chronology; New Kingdom (Late Dynastic Period), Second Persian Occupation, king list and contemporary nobility

Dynasty	Date	Royal name	Contemporaries
Twenty-first	1085 B.C.	Nesbanebdedi (Smendes)	
	1054 B.C.	Psusennes I	
	1009 B.C.	Amenemopet (Amenophthis)	
	1000 B.C.	Siamun	
	984 B.C.	Psusennes II	
	950 B.C.	Sheshonq I	
Twenty-second	929 B.C.	Osorkon I	
	893 B.C.	Takelot I	
	870 B.C.	Osorkon II	
	847 B.C.	(Beginning Rule of 5 Minor Kings)	
Twenty-third	817 B.C.	Petubastis	
	763 B.C.	(Beginning Rule of 5 Minor Kings)	
	730 B.C.	Tafnakht	
Twenty-fourth	720 B.C.	Bekenranef (Bochchoris)	
	716 B.C.	Pi'Ankhi	Nemlot
Twenty-fifth	716 B.C.	Shabaka (Sabacon)	
	701 B.C.	Shabatoka	
	690 B.C.	Taharqa (Taracos)	
	664 B.C.	Tanutamun	

L
I
B
Y
A
N

E
T
H
I
O
P
I
A
N

Period	Dynasty	Date	Ruler	
S A I T E	Twenty-sixth	663 B.C.	Psammetik I	Ibi
		609 B.C.	Nekaw (Necho)	
		594 B.C.	Psammetik II	(?) Pbes
		588 B.C.	Apries (Hophra)	
		568 B.C.	Amasis (Ahmose II)	
		525 B.C.	Psammetik III	
1st		525 B.C.	Cambyses	
P E R S I A N	Twenty-seventh	522 B.C.	Darius I	
		485 B.C.	Xerxes	
		464 B.C.	Artaxerxes I	
		424 B.C.	Darius II	
	Twenty-eighth	404 B.C.	Amyrtaeos	
		398 B.C.	Nepherites I	
	Twenty-ninth	392 B.C.	Achoris (Hagar)	
		380 B.C.	Psammuthis	
	Thirtieth	379 B.C.	Nepherites II	
		378 B.C.	Nectanebo I	
		361 B.C.	Teos (Djed-Hor)	
		359 B.C.	Nectanebo II	(?) Petosiris
2nd Persian Occupation		341 B.C.	Artaxerxes II (Ochus)	
		338 B.C.	Arses	
		335 B.C.	Darius III	
		332 B.C.	Alexander the Great	

Table 7

Egyptian chronology; Ptolemaic (Greek) Period, king list and contemporary nobility

Name and Titles	Dates of rule	Contemporaries
Alexander the Great	332–323 B.C.	
Ptolemy I		Archephon
(Soter I, Lagides)	323–285 B.C.	
Ptolemy II		
(Philadelphus I)	285–247 B.C.	Cydippus, Manetho, Zenon
Ptolemy III		
(Euergetes I)	247–221 B.C.	
Ptolemy IV		
(Philopator)	221–205 B.C.	
Ptolemy V		
(Epiphanes)	205–181 B.C.	
Ptolemy VI		
(Philometor)	181–145 B.C.	
Ptolemy VII		
(Eupator)	(never ruled)	
Ptolemy VIII		
(Neos Philopator)	(never ruled)	
Ptolemy IX		
(Euergetes II, Physcon)	169–116 B.C.	
Cleopatra II	130–101 B.C.	
Ptolemy X		
(Soter II, Lathyros)	116–80 B.C.	
Ptolemy XI		
(Alexander I)	108–88 B.C.	
Ptolemy XII		
(Alexander II)	80 B.C.	
Ptolemy XIII		
(Neos Dionysos, Auletes)	80–51 B.C.	
Ptolemy XIV	51–48 B.C.	
Ptolemy XV	48–44 B.C.	
Cleopatra VII	51–30 B.C.	Antony, Julius Caesar

ROMAN CONQUEST–30 B.C.

Table 8

Egyptian chronology; Roman Period, king list and contemporary nobility

Ruler	Dates	Contemporaries
Augustus (Octavianus)	30 B.C.–A.D. 14	
Tiberius	A.D. 14–37	
Caligula (Caius)	A.D. 37–41	
Claudius	A.D. 41–54	
Nero	A.D. 54–68	
Galba, Otho, Vitellius	A.D. 68–69	
Vespasian	A.D. 69–79	
Titus	A.D. 79–81	
Domitian	A.D. 81–96	
Nerva	A.D. 96–98	
Trajan	A.D. 98–117	
Hadrian	A.D. 117–138	
Antonius Pius	A.D. 138–161	
Marcus Aurelius, Lucius Verus	A.D. 161–169	
Marcus Aurelius	A.D. 161–180	
Commodus	A.D. 180–192	
Pertinax, Pescinius Niger, Septimus Severus	A.D. 193–194	
Septimus Severus	A.D. 193–211	
Caracalla, Geta	A.D. 211–212	
Caracalla	A.D. 211–217	
Macrinus	A.D. 217–218	
Eliagabalus	A.D. 218–222	
Alexander Severus	A.D. 222–235	
Maximinus	A.D. 235–238	
Gordianus I, Gordianus II, Balbinus Pupienus	A.D. 238	
Gordianus III	A.D. 238–244	
Philippus	A.D. 244–249	Aurelius Besarion
Decius	A.D. 249–251	
Gallus	A.D. 251–254	
Gallus, Aemilianus	A.D. 252	
Gallus, Aemilianus, Valerianus	A.D. 253–254	
Valerianus	A.D. 253–260	
Gallienus	A.D. 260–268	
Claudius II	A.D. 268–270	
Aurelianus	A.D. 270–275	

continued

Ruler	Dates	Contemporaries
Tacitus	A.D. 275–276	
Probus	A.D. 276–282	
Carus	A.D. 282–283	
Carinus, Diocletian	A.D. 283–285	
Diocletian	A.D. 284–305	

LATE ROMAN/BYZANTINE PERIOD

Table 9

Egyptian chronology; Arabic, Turkish, Modern Periods

		LATE ROMAN/BYZANTINE PERIOD (A.D. 305–642)	
A		Orthodox Khalifs	A.D. 642
R		Umayyad Governors	A.D. 661
A		Abbasid Governors (I)	A.D. 750
B		Tulunids	A.D. 868
I	P	Abbasid Governors (II)	A.D. 905
C	E	Ikhshidits	A.D. 934
	R	Fatimids	A.D. 969
	I	Ayoubids	A.D. 1171
	O	Bahrite Mamlukes	A.D. 1252
	D	Circassian Mamlukes	A.D. 1382
			A.D. 1517
TURKISH PERIOD			
			A.D. 1804
M O D E R N	P E R I O D	ERA OF MOHAMED ALY DYNASTY	
		REPUBLICAN EGYPT	A.D. 1952
			(Present)

Maps Section

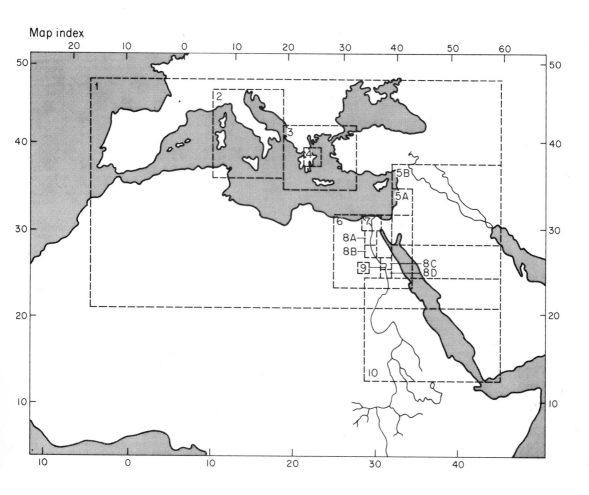

The numbered areas 1–10 refer to Maps 1–10 on the following pages.

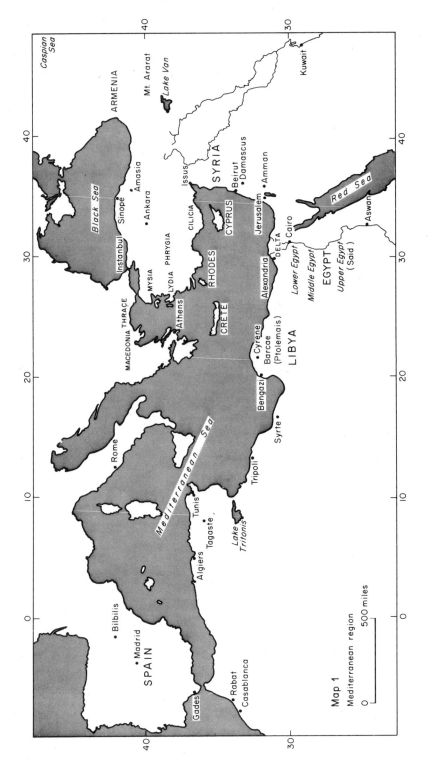

Map. 1. Mediterranean region.

Caspian Sea

ARMENIA
Mt. Ararat
Lake Van

Black Sea
• Amasia
• Ankara
Sinope
Instanbul
SYRIA
• Beirut
• Damascus
• Amman
CILICIA
CYPRUS
Jerusalem
Red Sea
• Cairo
• Aswan
MYSIA
LYDIA PHRYGIA
MACEDONIA THRACE
RHODES
Athens
CRETE
Alexandria
DELTA
Lower Egypt
Middle Egypt
Upper Egypt
(Said)
EGYPT
Cyrene
Barcae
(Ptolemais)
LIBYA
Bengazi
Syrte •
• Rome
Mediterranean Sea
Tunis
Tagaste •
Lake
Tritonis
Tripoli
Algiers
• Bilbilis
• Madrid
SPAIN
Rabat
Casablanca
Gades

Map 1
Mediterranean region

0   500 miles

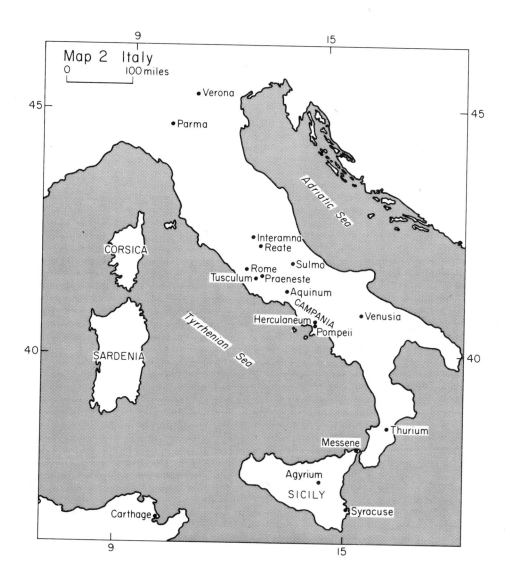

Map 2 Italy

0 _____ 100 miles

Verona

Parma

CORSICA

Adriatic Sea

Interamna
Reate

Sulmo

Rome
Tusculum • Praeneste

Aquinum

CAMPANIA

Herculaneum
Pompeii

Venusia

Tyrrhenian Sea

SARDENIA

Thurium

Messene

Agyrium

SICILY

Syracuse

Carthage

Map 2. Italy.

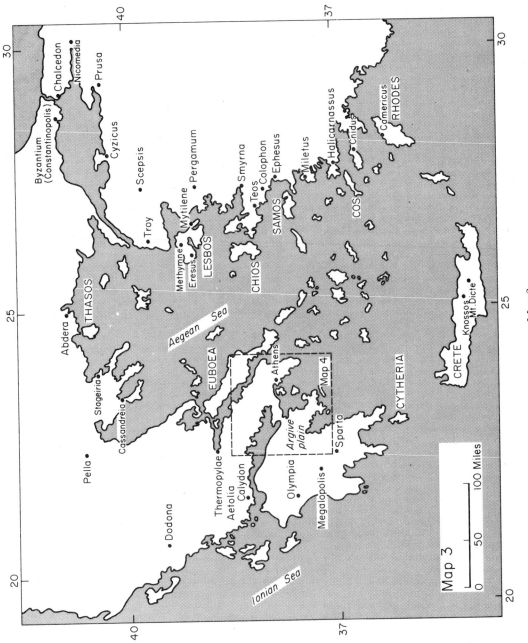

Map 3.

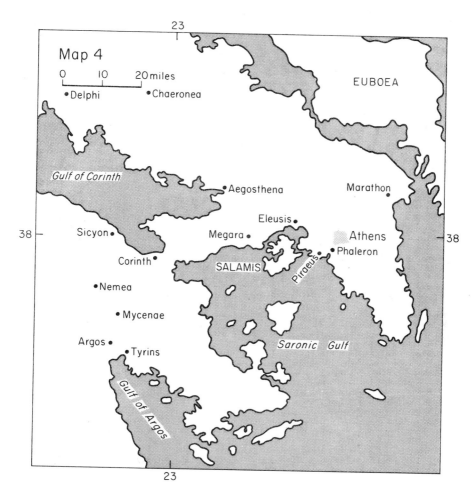

Map 4. Athens and vicinity.

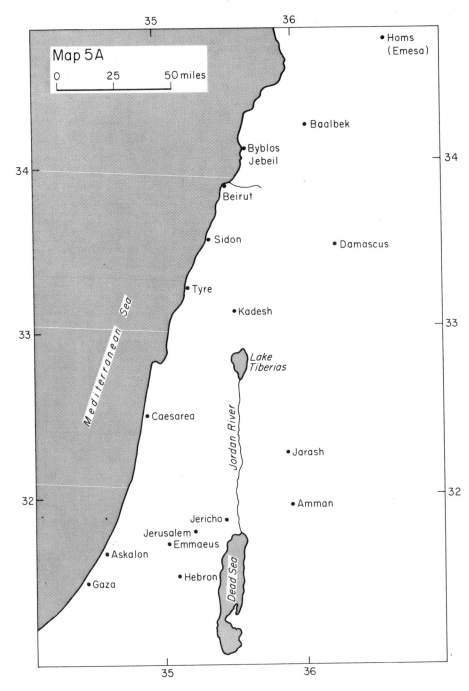

35

36

• Homs
(Emesa)

Map 5A

0   25   50 miles

• Baalbek

• Byblos
Jebeil

34

34

Beirut

• Sidon

• Damascus

Mediterranean Sea

• Tyre

• Kadesh

33

33

Lake Tiberias

• Caesarea

Jordan River

• Jarash

32

• Amman

Jericho •

Jerusalem •

• Emmaeus

Dead Sea

• Askalon

• Hebron

• Gaza

32

35

36

Map 5A. The Levant.

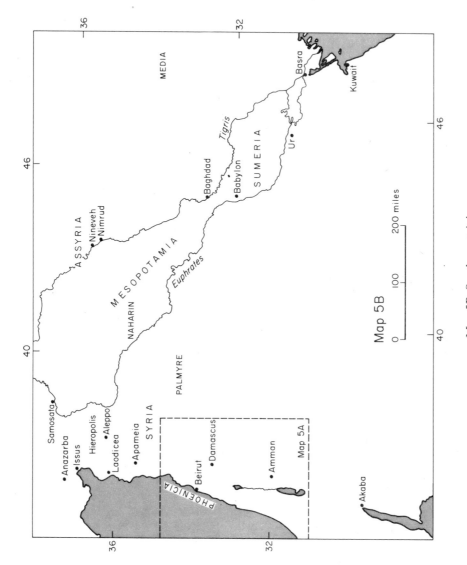

Map 5B. South-west Asia.

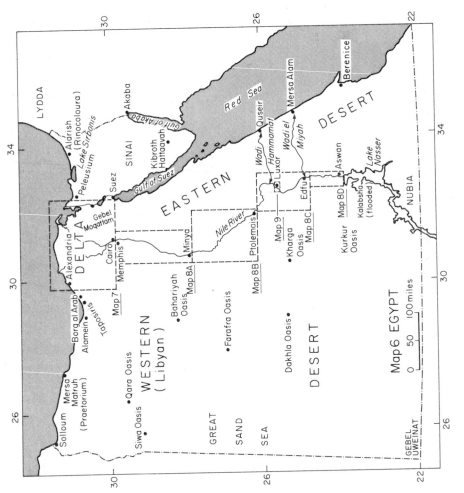

Map 6. Egypt.

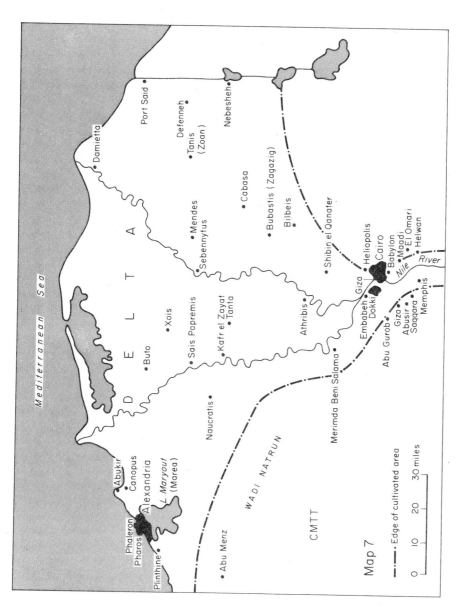

Map 7. Lower Egypt.

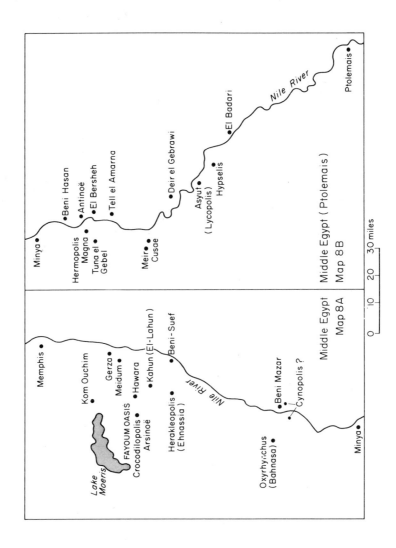

Maps 8A, 8B. Middle Egypt: Memphis-Ptolemais.

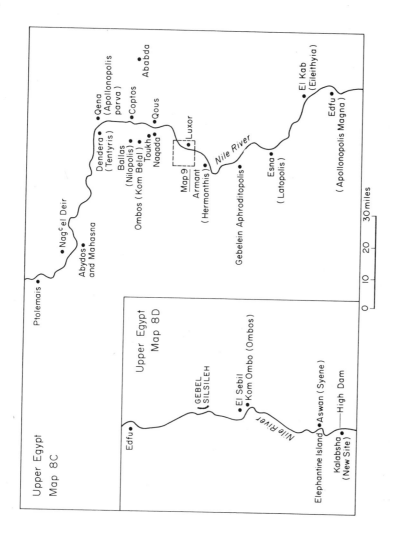

Maps 8C, 8D. Upper Egypt: Ptolemais-Aswan.

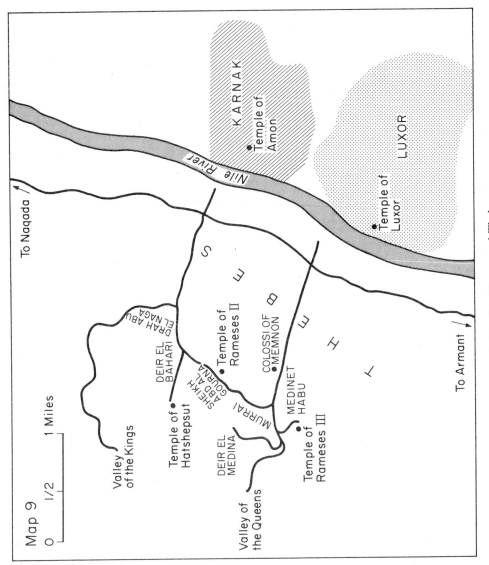

Map 9. Details of Luxor and Thebes.

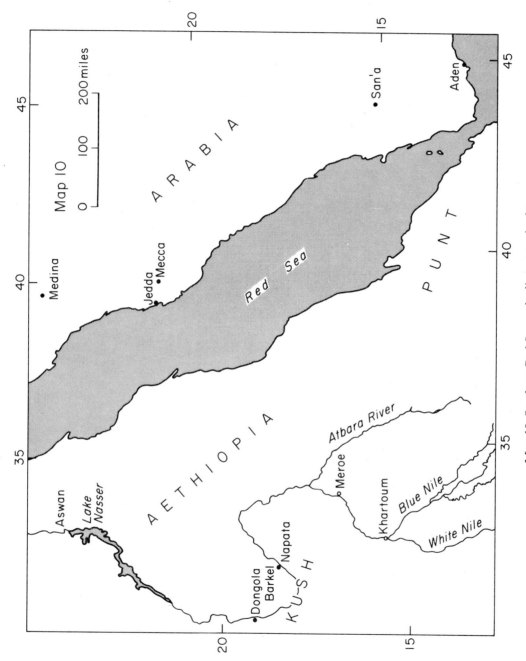

Map 10. Southern Red Sea and adjacent territories.

Abdal Latif al-Baghdadi (1965), *Kitab al Ifadah wa'l I'tibar* (The Eastern Key). Translated by Kamal Hafuth Zand, J.A. Videan, and I.E. Videan. London: George Allen and Unwin.

Abdou, I.A. (1965). A study of pellagra in the Egyptian region, U.A.R. *Bulletin of the Nutrition Institute, U.A.R.*, **1**, 61.

Abu-Bakr, A.M. and A. Badawy (1953). *Excavations at Giza*. 1949–50. University of Alexandria. Faculty of Arts. Cairo: Government Press.

Achilles Tatius (1918). *Adventures of Leucippe and Clitophon*. Translated by S. Gaselee. New York: G.P. Putnam's Sons.

Adams, A.L. (1870). *Notes of a Naturalist on the Nile Valley and Malta*. Edinburgh: Edmonston and Douglas.

Aelian (1958–59). *On the Characteristics of Animals*. Translated by A.F. Scholfield. 3 Vols. Cambridge: Harvard University Press.

Aeschylus (1889). *The Supplices of Aeschylus*. Translated by T.G. Tucker. London: Macmillan.

Al-Demiri, Kamal el Dine Mohammed ibn Musa al (1956). *Hayat al Hayawan al Kubra*, 3rd edition. Cairo: Mustafa al-Baby al-Halaby (in Arabic).

Al-Djabarti, el Cheikh Abdel Rahman (1896). *Merveilles Biographiques et Historiques*. 9 Vols (French translation). Cairo: Imprimerie Nationale.

Alevi, S.M.B. (1924). *Arabian Poetry and Poets*. Aligarh: Jami Millia Press.

Al-Hussaini, A.H. (1938). Short notes: The avifauna of the Bahariya Oasis in winter. *Ibis*. Series 14, 2, 544–547.

Al-Hussaini, A.H. (1959). The avifauna of Al-Wadi al-Gadid in the Libyan Desert. *Zoological Society of Egypt*, **14**, 1–14.

Alpinus, Prosper (1640). *De Plantis Aegypti Liber*. Patavii: Typus Pauli Frambotti Bibliopolae.

Alpino Prosper (1735). *Historia Naturalis Aegypti*. Lugduni Batavorum.

Amenemope (1925). *Das Weisheitsbuch des Amenemope*. Translated by H.O. Lange. Det Kgl. Danske Videnskabernes Selskab. Historisk-filologisk Meddelelser. **XI**, 2.

Ames, D. (Tr.) (1965). *Egyptian Mythology*. New York: Tudor.

Anabasis, *See under* Arrian, Xenophon.

Andersson, E. (1912). Dénomination égyptienne des boeufs sans cornes. *Sphinx*, **16**, 145–164.

Apicius (1958). *The Roman Cookery Book. A Critical Translation of the Art of Cooking, for Use in the Study and the Kitchen*. Translated by Barbara Flower and Elisabeth Rosenbaum. London: George G. Harrap.

Apollodorus (1921). *The Library*. Translated by James George Frazer. 2 Vols. New York: G.P. Putnam's Sons.

Aristophanes (1930). *The Frogs* in Vol. 2 of Aristophanes. Translated by Benjamin B. Rogers. New York: G.P. Putnam's Sons.

Aristotle (1910). *Historia Animalium* (History of Animals). Translated by D'Arcy.Wentworth Thompson. Vol. 4 of *The Works of Aristotle*. Edited by J.A. Smith and W.D. Ross. Oxford: Clarendon Press.

Aristotle (1936). On plants in *Aristotle: Minor Works*. Translated by W.S. Hett. London: William Heinemann.

Aristotle (1937). *Problems*. Translated by W.S. Hett. London: William Heinemann.

Armstrong, E.A. (1958). *The Folklore of Birds. An Enquiry into the Origin and Distribution of Some Magico-Religious Traditions*. London: Collins.

Arrian (1929). *Anabasis Alexandri*. Translated by E.I. Robson. London: William Heinemann.

Athenaeus (1927–41). *The Deipnosophists*. Translated by Charles Burton Gulick. 7 Vols. New York: G.P. Putnam's Sons.

Avicenna *See* O.C. Gruner (1930).

Avicenna, *The Canon*, (*Al-Qanun fil-Tibb*), 3 volumes, no date. Baghdad: Al-Muthanna Library (in Arabic).

Aykroyd, W.R. (1967). *The Story of Sugar*. Chicago: Quadrangle Books.

Aykroyd, W.R. and J. Doughty (1970). *Wheat in Human Nutrition*. Rome: Food and Agriculture Organisation of the United Nations.

Ayrton, E.R. and W.L.S. Loat (1908). *Pre-Dynastic Cemetery of El Mahasna*. Egypt Exploration Fund. 31st. Memoir. London: Egypt Exploration Society.

Badawi, A and M.S. Khafaga (1966). *Herodotus Talks of Egypt*. Cairo: Dar el Qalam (in Arabic).

Baer, K. (1962). The low cost of land in Ancient Egypt, *Journal of the American Research Center in Egypt*, **I,** 25–45.

Ball, J. (1942). *Egypt in the Classical Geographers*. Ministry of Finance. Survey of Egypt. Bulaq: Government Press.

Barguet, P. (1964). *See* Herodotus.

Barguet, P. (1967). *Le Livre des Morts des Anciens Egyptians*. Paris: Les Editions du Cerf.

Baron, S. (1962). *Brewed in America. The History of Beer and Ale in the United States*. Boston: Little, Brown and Co.

Bates, O. (1917). Ancient Egyptian fishing. *Harvard African Studies*. **1,** 199–271.

Beadnell, H.J.Ll. (1909). *An Egyptian Oasis. An account of the Oasis of Kharga in the Libyan Desert with reference to its history, physical geography and water supply*. London: G. Murray.

Beauverie, M.A. (1930). Sur quelques fruits de l'Ancienne Egypte exposés au musée de Grenoble. *Bulletin de l'Institut Français d'Archéologie Orientale*, **28,** 393–405.

Belgrave, C. Dalrymple (1923). *Siwa. The Oasis of Jupiter Ammon.* London: John Lane the Bodley Head.

Benedite, G. (1918). The Carnarvon Ivory. *Journal of Egyptian Archaeology,* **5,** 1–15, 225–241.

Bevan, E. (1927). *A Study of Egypt Under the Ptolemaic Dynasty.* London: Methuen.

Bible, The Holy (1953). King James Edition. London: Collin's Clear Type Press.

Bible, The Holy (1956). Douay Version, translated from the Latin Vulgate (Douay, A.D. 1609, Rheims, A.D. 1582). London: Catholic Truth Society.

Biggs, E.J. (1969). Molluscs from human habitation sites and the problem of ethnological interpretation, in *Science in Archeology.* Edited by D. Brothwell, and E. Higgs. pp. 423–428. London: Thames and Hudson.

Bissing, F.W. von (1896). *Die sogenannte statistische Tafel Thutmosis III von Aegypten,* Neue Herausgebung uebersetzt und erlautert von F.W. Bissing, Teil I, Einleitung. Leipzig: August Pries.

Bissing, F.W. von (1905). *Das Re-Heiligtum des Königs Ne-Wser-Re.* Vol. III, p. 55, plate 28, No. 432, plate 30, No. 459. Berlin: Alexander Duncker.

Bissing, F.W. von (1904–1906). *Denkmaeler Aegyptische Skulptur,* herausg. und mit erlauternden Texten versehen, 13 parts. Munich: F. Bruckman.

Bissing, F.W. von, A.E.P. Weigall, and M. Bollacher (1905–1911). *Die Mastaba des Gem-ni-kai.* 2 Vols. Berlin: Alexander Duncke.

Blackman, Aylward M. (1914). *The Rock Tombs of Meir: Vol. 1 The Tomb-Chapel of Ukh-Hotp's Son Senbi.* Archaeological Survey of Egypt. Memoir 22. London: Egypt Exploration Fund.

Blackman, Aylward M. (1915a). *The Rock Tombs of Meir: Vol. 2 The Tomb-Chapel of Senbi's Son Ukh-Hotp.* Archaeological Survey of Egypt. Memoir 23. London: Egypt Exploration Fund.

Blackman, Aylward M. (1915b). *The Rock Tombs of Meir: Vol. 3 The Tomb Chapel of Ukh-Hotp Son of Ukh-Hotp and Mersi.* Archaeological Survey of Egypt. Memoir 24. London: Egypt Exploration Fund.

Blackman, Aylward M. (1924). *The Rock Tombs of Meir: Vol. 4 The Tomb Chapel of Pepi'onkh the Middle Son of Sebkhotpe and Pekhernefert.* Archaeological Survey of Egypt. Memoir 25. London: Egypt Exploration Fund.

Bodenheimer, F.S. (1951). *Insects as Human Food: A Chapter of the Ecology of Man.* The Hague: W. Junk.

Bonnet, E. (1900). Végétaux antiques du Musée Egyptien de Florence. *Comptes-Rendus de l'Association Française pour l'Avancement des Sciences. Congrès de Paris.*

Bonnet, E. (1902). Plantes aquatiques des Nécropoles d'Antinöe. *Annales du Musee Guimet,* **30,** 153–159.

Bonnet, H. (1952). *Reallexikon der Aegyptischen Religionsgeschichte.* Berlin: Walter de Gruyter.

Borchardt, L. (1910). *Das Grabdenkmal des Königs Sahure.* Leipzig: Hinrichs.

Borchardt, L. (1932). Ein Brot, *Zeitschrift für Aegyptische Sprache und Alter-tumskunde*, **68**, 73–79.

Bouché-Leclercq, A. (1963). *Histoire des Lagides*, 4 Vols. Bruxelles: Culture et Civilisation.

Boulenger, F.R.S. (1907). *Zoology of Egypt: The Fishes of the Nile*. London: Hugh Rees.

Boussac, H. (1896). Le Tombeau d'Anna. *Mémoires de la Mission Archéologique Française au Caire*. Paris: Leroux.

Bradford, E.W. (1958). Food and the Peridontal Diseases. *Proceedings of the Nutrition Society*, **18**, 75–78.

Braun, A. (1879). On the vegetable remains in the Egyptian museum at Berlin. Edited from the author's manuscript by P. Ascherson and P. Magnus. *Journal of Botany, London*, New Series **8**, 19–23; 48–62, 91–92.

Breasted, J.H. (1906). *Ancient Records of Egypt*, 5 Vols. Chicago: University of Chicago Press.

Breasted, J.H. (1909). *A History of Egypt*. Reprinted in 1959. London: Hodder and Stoughton.

Brehant, J. (1966). A propos d'une Intoxication collective par le miel. Celle des Hébreux au Désert par les Cailles. *La Presse Médicale*, **74**, 1157–1158.

Brillat-Savarin, A. (1884). *A Handbook of Gastronomy. Brillat-Savarin's "Physiologie du Goût"*. Translated by A. Lalauze. London: Nimo and Bain.

Brockedon, W. (1846–49). *Egypt and Nubia from Drawings Made on the Spot, by David Roberts*. 3 Vols. London: F.G.Moon.

Brodrick, M. and A.A. Morton (1945). *A Concise Dictionary of Egyptian Archaeology*. London: Methuen.

Brodrick, A.H. (1948). *Early Man*. London: Hutchinson.

Brothwell, D.R. (1958). Teeth in Earlier Human Populations. *Proceedings of the Nutrition Society* **18**, 59–64.

Brothwell, D.R. (1967). *Diseases in Antiquity*, Springfield, Illinois: Thomas and Co.

Brothwell, D.R. and Higgs, E. (1969). *Science in Archaeology*. London: Thames and Hudson.

Brown, E. (1739). *The Travels and Adventures of Edward Brown Esq*. London. (n.p.)

Browne, W.G. (1806). *Travels in Africa, Egypt and Syria from the Year 1927 to 1798*. Second Edition. London: T. Cadell and W. Davies.

Browning, D.C. (1960). *Everyman's Dictionary*. London: J.M. Dent and Sons.

Brugsch, H. (1878). *Reise nach der Grossen Oase el Khargeh in der Libyschen Wuste*. Leipzig: Hinrichs.

Brunner, H. (1954). Die theologische Bedeutung der Trunkenheit. *Zeitzchrift für Aegyptische Sprache und Altertumskunde*. **79**: 81–83.

Brunton, G. (1937). *Mostagedda and the Tasian Culture*. British Museum Exped. to Middle Egypt, First and Second Years 1928–1929, London: Bernard Quaritch.

Brunton, G. (1948). *Matmar.* London: Bernard Quaritch.

Brunton, G. and G. Caton-Thompson (1928). *The Badarian Civilisation and Predynastic Remains near Badari.* British School of Archaeology in Egypt. Publication no. 46. London: Bernard Quaritch.

Bruyère B. (1937). *Deir el Medineh.* II. La Nécropole de l'Est. Cairo: Fouilles de l'Institut Français d'Archéologie Orient. Années 1934–1935.

Bryan, C.P. (1930). *The Papyrus Ebers.* London: Geoffrey Bles.

Buchheim, L. (1956). Die Arteriosklerose der alten Aegypten. *Therapeutiche Berichte,* **28,** 108.

Budge, E.A.T.W. (1895). *First Steps in Egyptian. A Book for Beginners.* London: Kegan Paul, Trench, Trübner, and Co.

Budge, E.A.T.W. (1928). *The Book of the Dead. Three Volumes Combined.* Second edition. London: Kegan Paul, Trench, Tübner, and Co.

Budge, E.A.T.W. (1949). *The Book of the Dead.* Second edition. London: Routledge and Kegan Paul.

Budge, E.A.T.W. (1959). *Egyptian Ideas of the Future Life: Egyptian Religion.* New York: University Books.

Budge, E.A.T.W. (1960). *The Book of the Dead.* New York: University Books.

Budge, E.A.T.W. (1967). *The Book of the Dead. The Papyrus of Ani in the British Museum. The Egyptian Text with Interlinear Transliteration and Translation. a Running Translation. Introduction, etc.* New York: Dover.

Budge, E.A.T.W. (1969). *The Gods of the Egyptians or Studies in Egyptian Mythology.* 2 Vols. New York: Dover.

Burckhardt, J.L. (1822). *Travel in Nubia.* 2nd edition. London: John Murray.

Bury, J.B. (1958). *The Ancient Greek Historians.* New York: Dover.

Butt, A. (1952). *The Nilotes of the Anglo-Egyptian Sudan and Uganda.* Ethnographic Survey of Africa. East Central Africa. Part 4. London: International Africa Institute.

Butzer, K.W. (1960). Archaeology and Geology in Ancient Egypt, *Science,* **132,** 3440: 1617–1624.

Caillaud, F. (1831). *Recherches sur les arts et métiers, les usage de la vie civile et domestique des anciens peuples de l'Egypte de la Nubie et de l'Ethiopie.* Paris. (n.p.)

Caminos, R.A. (1954). *Late Egyptian Miscellanies.* London: Oxford University Press.

Campbell-Thompson, R. (1949). *A Dictionary of Assyrian Botany.* London: Oxford University Press.

Candolle, A.L.P.P. de (1886). *Origin of Cultivated Plants.* Reproduction of 2nd edition, 1959. New York: Haffner.

Capart, J. (1941). Les poussins au tombeau de Ti. *Chronique d'Egypte,* **32,** 208–212.

Carson, R.A.G. (1963). *Coins of the World.* New York: Harper and Row.

Carter, H. (1923). An ostracon depicting a red jungle fowl. The earliest known drawings of the domestic cock. *Journal of Egyptian Archaeology,* **9,** 1–4.

Carter, H. (1923–1933). *The Tomb of Tut-Ankh-Amon.* 3 Vols. London: Cassel.
  Vol. 1 in collaboration with A.C. Mace (1923).
  Vol. 2 with appendices by D.E. Derry, A. Lucas, P.E. Newberry, A. Scott and H.J. Plenderleith (1927).
  Vol. 3 with appendices by D.E. Derry and A. Lucas (1933).
Caton-Thompson, G. and E.W. Gardner (1934). *The Desert Fayum.* London: Royal Anthropological Institute of Great Britain and Ireland.
Caton-Thompson, G. and E.W. Gardner (1952). *Kharga Oasis in Pre-history.* London: University of London Athlone Press.
Caylus, A.C. de (1752). *Recueil d'Antiquités Egyptiennes, Etrusques, Grecques et Romaines.* (7 Vols.) Vol. 1, p. 13, plate III: I and II. Paris: Chez Desaint et Saillant.
Celsus (1935–38). *On Medicine.* Translated by W.S. Spencer, 3 Vols. Cambridge: Harvard University Press.
Cerny, J. (1937). Deux noms de poisson du nouvel empire. *Bulletin de l'Institut Français d'Archéologie Orientale,* **37,** 35–40.
Chassinat, E. (1905). Note sur le titre . . ., *Bulletin de l'Institut Français d'Archéologie Orientale,* **IV,** 223.
Chassinat, E. (1921). Le papyrus Médical Copte. *Mémoire de l'Institut Français d'Archéologie Orientale no.* 32. Cairo: Institut Français d'Archéologie Orientale.
Childe, V.G. (1953). *New Light on the Most Ancient East.* Fourth edition. New York: F.A. Praeger.
Clark, G. (1948). Fowling in Prehistoric Europe, *Antiquity,* **22,** 116–130.
Clark, R.T.R. (1949). The Legend of the Phoenix. Part One. *University of Birmingham Historical Journal,* **2,** 1–29.
Clark, R.T.R. (1950). The Legend of the Phoenix. Part Two. *University of Birmingham Historical Journal,* **2,** 105–140.
Clark, R.T.R. (1959). *Myth and Symbol in Ancient Egypt.* London: Thames.
Clédat, J. (1901). Notes sur quelques figures égyptiennes. *Bulletin de l'Institut Français d'Archéologie Orientale,* **1,** 21–24.
Clemens, Titus Flavius Alexandrinus (Clement of Alexandria) (1953), Exhortation to the Greeks, in *Clement of Alexandria.* Translated by G.W. Butterworth. Cambridge: Harvard University Press.
Clerget, M. (1934). *Le Caire, Etude de Géographie Urbaine et d'Histoire Economique,* 2 Vols. Cairo: E. and R. Schindler.
Cobbold, T.S. (1866). On the discovery of Trichina. *The Lancet,* **I,** 224.
Codex Iustiniani (1870). *Digestia Iustiniani Augusti,* Vol. II. Berlin: Weidmann.
Coltherd, J.B. (1966). The Domestic Fowl in Ancient Egypt. *Ibis.* **108,** 217–223.
Columella, (1941–1955). *On Agriculture.* Translated by E.S. Forster, E.H. Heffner and H.B. Ash. 3 Vols. Cambridge: Harvard University Press.
Cosson, A.F.C. de (1935). *Mareotis, being a short account of the history and ancient*

monuments of the northwestern desert of Egypt and of lake Mareotis. London: Country Life Ltd.

Crum, W.E. (1925). Koptische Zünfte und das Pfeffermonopol. *Zeitschrift für aegyptische Sprache und Altertumskunde*, **60**, 103–111.

Crum, W.E. (1962). *A Coptic Dictionary*. Oxford: Clarendon Press.

Curto, S. *La Satira nell'Antico Egitto*. Torino: Fratelli Pozzo.

Danelius, E. and H. Steinitz (1967). The fishes and other aquatic animals on the Punt Reliefs at Deir el-Bahri. *Journal of Egyptian Archaeology*, **53**, 15–24.

Daressy, G. (1922). Le riz dans l'Egypte Antique, *Bulletin de l'Institut d'Egypte*, **4**, 35–37.

Daumas, F. (1957). Note sur la plante matjet, *Bulletin de l'Institut Français d'Archéologie Orientale*, **56**, 59–66.

Daumas, F. (1964). Quelques remarques sur les représentations de pêche à la ligne sous l'Ancien Empire. *Bulletin de l'Institut Français d'Archéologie Orientale*, **62**, 69–85.

Daumas, F. (1965). *La Civilisation de l'Egypte Pharaonique*. Paris: Arthaud.

Daumas, F. and Goyon, G. (1939). Le Tombeau de Ti. *Mémoire de l'Institut Français d'Archéologie Orientale* no. 65. Cairo: Institut Français d'Archéologie Orientale.

Davaine, C.J. (1860). *Traité des entozoaires et des maladies vermineuses de l'homme et des animaux domestiques*. Paris. (n.p.)

Davidson, B. (1965). *Old Africa Rediscovered*. London: V. Gollancz.

Davies, J.D. (1965). *Dictionary of the Bible*. Fourth edition. Westwood, N.Y.: Revell.

Davies, Nina de Garis (1936). *Ancient Egyptian Paintings*, 2 Vols. Chicago: Chicago University Press.

Davies, Nina de Garis (1949). Birds and Bats at Beni Hasan. *Journal of Egyptian Archaeology*, **35**, 13–20.

Davies, Norman de Garis (1900). *The Mastaba of Ptahhetep and Akhethetep at Saqqarah. Vol. 1*. Archaeological Survey of Egypt. 8th memoir. London: Egypt Exploration Fund.

Davies, Norman de G. (1901). *The Mastaba of Ptahhetep and Akhethetep at Saqqarah. Vol. 2*. Archaeological Survey of Egypt. 9th memoir. London: Egypt Exploration Fund.

Davies, Norman de G. (1902). *The Rock Tombs of Deir el Gebrawi Part I*. Archaeological Survey of Egypt. 11th memoir. London: Egypt Exploration Fund.

Davies, Norman de G. (1903). *The Rock Tombs of el Amarna. Part I*. Archaeological Survey of Egypt. 13th memoir. London: Egypt Exploration Fund.

Davies, Norman de G. (1913). *Five Theban Tombs*. Archaeological Survey of Egypt. XXI. London: Egypt Exploration Society.

Davies, Norman de G. (1927). *Two Ramesside Tombs at Thebes*, Robb de Peyster Tytus Memorial Series, Vol. 5. New York: Metropolitan Museum of Art.

Davies, Norman de G. (1930). *The Tomb of Ken-Amun at Thebes*, Vol. 1, Egyptian Expedition Publication No. 5. New York: Metropolitan Museum of Art.

Davies, Norman de G. (1943). *The Tomb of Rekh-mi-Re at Thebes*, 2 Vols. Metropolitan Museum of Art Egyptian Expedition. New York: The Plantin Press.

Davies, Norman de G. and A. H. Gardiner (1920). *The Tomb of Antefoker*. Egypt Exploration Society. London: George Allen and Unwin.

Dawson, W.R. (1926). The Plant called "Hairs of-the-Earth". *Journal of Egyptian Archaeology*, **12,** 240–241.

Dawson, W.R. (1928). The pig in ancient Egypt. A commentary on two passages of Herodotus. *Journal of the Royal Asiatic Society of Great Britain and Ireland*, 597–608.

Dawson, W.R. (1929). *Magician and Leech*. London: Methuen.

Dawson, W.R. (1930). *The Beginnings: Egypt and Assyria*. New York: Paul Huebner.

Dawson, W.R. (1932). Studies in the Egyptian medical texts. Part I. *Journal of Egyptian Archaeology*, **18,** 150–154.

Dawson, W.R. (1933). Studies in the Egyptian medical texts, Part II. *Journal of Egyptian Archaeology*, **19,** 133–137.

Dawson, W.R. (1934a). Studies in the Egyptian medical texts. Part III. *Journal of Egyptian Archaeology*, **20,** 41–46.

Dawson, W.R. (1934b). Studies in the Egyptian medical texts, Part IV. *Journal of Egyptian Archaeology*, **20,** 185–188.

Dawson, W.R. (1935). Studies in the Egyptian medical texts. Part V. *Journal of Egyptian Archaeology*, **21,** 37–40.

Debono, F. (1948). El Omari (près de Helouan), exposé sur les campagnes des fouilles 1943–1944 et 1948, *Annales du Service des Antiquités de l'Egypte*, **48,** 561–569.

De Buck, A. (1935–1961). *Coffin Texts*. 7 Vols. Chicago: University of Chicago Press.

De Buck, A. (1967). *Grammaire Elémentaire du Moyen Egyptian*. Leiden: Brill.

Deerr, N. (1949–1950). *The History of Sugar*. London: Chapman and Hall.

Deiber, A. (1904). Clément d'Alexandrie. *Mémoires publiés par les membres de l'Institut Français d'Archéologie Orientale du Caire. no. X.* Cairo.

Delile, A.R. (1813a). Florae Aegyptiacae Illustratio, in *Description de l'Egypte, Histoire Naturelle*. Volume 2. Part 1. pp. 49–82. Paris: Imprimerie Impériale.

Delile, A.R. (1813b). Flore d'Egypte. Explication des Planches, in *Description de l'Egypte, Histoire Naturelle*. Volume 2. Part 1. pp. 145–320. Paris: Imprimerie Impériale.

Delile, A.R. (1813c). Mémoire sur les Plantes qui croissent spontanément en Egypte, in *Description de l'Egypte. Histoire Naturelle*. Volume 2. Part 1. pp. 1–10. Paris: Imprimerie Impériale.

Delile, A.R. (1813d). *Histoire des Plantes cultivées en Egypte* in *Description de l'Egypte. Histoire Naturelle. Volume* 2. Part 1. pp. 11–24. Paris: Imprimerie Impériale.

Derchain, Ph. (1965). *Le Papyrus Salt* 825, Vol. II, 5–7, p. 137. Bruxelles: Académie Royale de Belgique. Mémoires. Classe des Lettres. Vol. 58.

De Ruiter, L. (1967). Critic's Comments, in *The Chemical Senses and Nutrition*. Edited by M.R. Kare and O. Maller, pp. 83–88. Baltimore: The Johns Hopkins Press.

Description de l'Egypte ou Recueil des Observations et des Recherches qui ont été faites en Egypte pendant l'Expédition Française (1813). Paris: Imprimerie Impériale.

Desroches-Noblecourt, Ch. (1952). Pots anthropomorphes et recettes magico-médicales dans l'Egypte Ancienne. *Revue d'Egyptologie*, **9**, 49–67.

Desroches-Noblecourt, Ch. (1963). *Tut-ankh-Amen*, New York: Graphic Society.

Desrousseaux, A.M. (1956). *Athénée de Naucratis. Les Deipnosophistes*. Paris: Les Belles Lettres.

Didymus *See* T. Owen (1805–1806).

Dimick, J. (1958). The Embalming House of the Apis Bulls. *Archaeology*, **II**, 183–189.

Dio Cocceianus, Chrysostomus (1932). Second Discourse on Kingship, in *Dio Chrysostom*. Translated by J.W. Cohoon. New York: G.P. Putnam's Sons.

Diodorus Siculus (1933–1967). *Library of History*, Translated by C.H. Oldfather, C. Sherman, C.B. Welles, R.M. Geer and F.R. Walton, 12 Vols. New York: G.P. Putnam's Sons.

Diogenes Laertes, *De Clarorum Philosoph*. London: Heinemann.

Dioscorides (1959). *The Greek Herbal of Dioscorides*. Translated by R.T. Gunther. New York: Hafner.

Dixon, D.M. (1969). A note on Cereals in Ancient Egypt, in *The Domestication and Exploitation of Plants and Animals*. Edited by P.J. Ucko and G.W. Dimbleby, pp. 131–142. London: Gerald Duckworth and Co.

Dolbey, R.V. and M. Omar (1924). A note concerning the incidence of goitre in Egypt. An analysis of 216 cases. *The Lancet*, **II**, 549–550.

Drioton, E. (1943a). Une représentation de la famine sur un bas- relief égyptien de la Ve Dynastie. *Bulletin de l'Institut d'Egypte*, **25**, 45–54.

Drioton, E. (1943b). Les Fêtes de Bouto. *Bulletin de l'Institut d'Egypte*, **25**, 1–19.

Drioton, E. (1952). Les origines pharaoniques du nilomètre de Rodah. *Bulletin de l'Institut d'Egypte*, **34**, 291–316.

Ducros, A.H. (1930). Essai sur le droguier populaire arabe de l'Inspectorat des Pharmacies du Caire. *Mémoire de l'Institut Français d'Archéologie. Orientale du Caire* no. XV. Cairo: Institut Français d'Archéologie Orientale du Caire.

Dümichen, J. (1865–1885). *Geographische Inschriften altaegyptischer*. Denkmäler, 4 Vols. Leipzig: Hinrichs.

Dumreicher, A. von. (1931). *Trackers and Smugglers in the Deserts of Egypt*. New York: The Dial Press.

Dunbar, J.H. (1941). *The Rock Pictures of Lower Nubia*. Service des Antiquités de l'Egypte. Cairo: Government Press.

Dunham, D. (1937). The Bird Trap. *Bulletin of the Museum of Fine Arts, Boston*, **35**, 52–54.

Ebbell, B. (1926). Die altaegyptischen Krankheitsnamen. *Zeitschrift für Aegyptischer Sprache und Altertumskunde*, **62**, 13–20.

Ebbell, B. (1937a). Altaegyptische anatomische Namen. *Acta Orient*, **15**, 293.

Ebbell, B. (1937b). *The Papyrus Ebers*. Oxford: Oxford University Press.

Edel, E. (1970). *Die Felsengräber der Qubbet el Hawa bei Assuan II Abteilung Die Althieratischen Topfaufschriften*. I Band. 2 Teil. pp. 24–27. Wiesbaden: Otto Harrassowitz.

Edgar, C.C. (1931). *Zenon Papyri in the University of Michigan Collection*. Ann Arbor: University of Michigan Press.

Edgerton, W.F. and J.A. Wilson (1936). *Historical Records of Ramses III: The Texts in Medinet-Habu*, vols 1 and 2 combined. Chicago: University of Chicago Press.

Egypte, L', Aperçu Historique et Géographique (1926). Cairo: Institut Français d'Archéologie Orientale.

Ehrich, R.W. (1965). *Chronologies in Old World Archaeology*. Chicago: University of Chicago Press.

Ellenbogen, M. (1962). *Foreign words in the Old Testament. Their Origin and Etymology*. London: Luzac and Co.

Elliot Smith, G. (1911). *The Ancient Egyptians and their Influence upon the Civilization of Europe*. New York: Harper.

Elliot Smith, G. and W.R. Dawson (1924). *Egyptian Mummies*. London: George Allen and Unwin.

Emery, W.B. (1958). *Great Tombs of the 1st Dynasty*. London: Egypt Exploration Fund.

Emery, W.B. (1961). *Archaic Egypt*. Baltimore: Penguin Books.

Emery, W.B. (1962). *A Funerary Repast in an Egyptian Tomb of the Archaic Period*. Leiden: Nederlands Institut voor het Nabije Osten.

Emery, W.B. (1966). Preliminary reports on the excavations at North Saqqara. *Journal of Egyptian Archaeology*, **52**, 3–8.

Emery, W.B. (1967). Preliminary reports on the excavations at North Saqqara. *Journal of Egyptian Archaeology*, **53**, 141–145.

Emery, W.B. (1970). Preliminary reports on the excavations at North Saqqara, *Journal of Egyptian Archaeology*, **56**, 5–11.

Emery, W.B. and Z.Y. Saad (1938). *The Tomb of Hemaka*. Cairo: Department of Antiquities.

Engelbach, R. (1924). Notes on the Fish of Mendes. *Annales du Service des Antiquités de l'Egypte*, **24**, 161–168.

Engelbach, R. (1961). *Introduction to Egyptian Archaeology with special reference* to the *Egyptian Museum*. 2nd edition. Cairo: General Organization for Government Printing Offices.

Erman, A. (1894). *Life in Ancient Egypt*, Translated by H.M. Tirard. London: Macmillan and Co.

Erman, A. (1927). *The Literature of the Ancient Egyptians*, Translated by A.M. Blackman. London: Methuen.

Erman, A. (1934). *Die Religion der Aegypter, ihr Werden und Vergehen in vier Jahrtausende*. Berlin: Walter de Gruyter.

Erman, A. (1966). *The Ancient Egyptians. A Sourcebook of their Writings*. Translated by A.M. Blackman. New York: Harper and Row.

Erman, A. and H. Grapow (1957). *Wörterbuch der aegyptischen Sprache*. Berlin: Akademie-Verlag.

Erman, A. and H. Grapow (1961). *Aegyptisches Handwörterbuch*. Darmstadt: Wissenschaftliches Buchgesellschaft.

Erman, A. and H. Ranke (1952). *La Civilisation Egyptienne*. French Translation by Charles Mathien. Paris: Payot.

Etchecopar, R.D. and F. Hüe (1967). *The Birds of North Africa from the Canary Islands to the Red Sea*. Translated by P.A.D. Hollum. London: Oliver and Boyde.

Fakhry, A. (1944). *Siwa Oasis. Its history and antiquities*. Cairo: Government Press.

Fakhry, A. (1973). *The Oases of Egypt. vol. 1 Siwa Oasis*. Cairo: American University in Cairo Press.

Faulkner, R.O. (1962). *A Concise Dictionary of Middle Egyptian*, Oxford: Oxford University Press.

Faulkner, R.O. (1968). The pregnancy of Isis. *Journal of Egyptian Archaeology*, **54**, 40–44.

Faulkner, R.O., E.F. Wente and W.K. Simpson (1972). *The Literature of Ancient Egyptians*. New Haven: Yale University Press.

Faust, E.C. (1949). *Human Helminthology*, 3rd edition. Philadelphia: Lea and Febiger.

Fustigière, A.J. (1945). *Hermes Trismegistus*, in *Asclepios*. Vol. 2. Paris: Les Belles Lettres.

Filce Leek, F. (1972). Teeth and bread in Ancient Egypt. *Journal of Egyptian Archaeology*, **58**, 126–132.

Filce Leek, F. (1973). Further studies concerning ancient Egyptian bread. *Journal of Egyptian Archaeology*, **59**, 199–204.

Firth, C.M. and B. Gunn (1926). *Teti Pyramid Cemeteries Excavations at Saqqara*. 2 Vols. Cairo: L'Institut Français d'Archéologie Orientale.

Flannery, K.V. (1965). The ecology of early food production in Mesopotamia. *Science*, **147**, 1247–1256.

Flower, S.S. (1932). Notes on the recent mammals of Egypt. *Proceedings of the Zoological Society*, London. 369–450.

Forbes, R.J. (1955). *Studies in ancient technology*, 9 Vols. Vol. V, pp. 79–81. Leiden: Brill.

Forde-Johnson, J.L. (1959). *Neolithic cultures of North Africa*. Liverpool: Liverpool University Press.

Foster, W.D. (1965). *A History of Parasitology*. London: E. and S. Livingstone.

Foucart, G. (1917). Sur quelques représentations des tombes thébaines découvertes cette année par l'Institut Français d'Archéologie Orientale. *Bulletin de l'Institut d'Egypte*, Serie V, **11**, 52.

Frazer, J.G. (1959). *The New Golden Bough*. Edited by Theodor H. Gaster. New York: New American Library.

Freeth, Z. (1956). *Kuwait Was My Home*. London: George Allen and Unwin.

Freud, S. (1947). *Leonardo da Vinci. A Study in Psychosexuality*. New York: Vintage Books.

Gabra, S., E.T. Drioton, P. Perdrizet and W.G. Waddell (1941). *Rapport sur les Fouilles d'Hermoupolis Ouest (Touna el Gebel)*. Université Fouad I. Cairo: l'Institut Français d'Archéologie Orientale.

Gaillard, Cl. (1912). Les tâtonnements des Egyptiens à la recherche des animaux à domestiquer. *Revue d'Ethnographie et de Sociologie*, 11–12, 19.

Gaillard, Cl. (1923). Recherches sur les poissons representés dans quelques tombeaux égyptiens de l'Ancien Empire. *Mémoire de l'Institut Français d'Archéologie Orientale* no. 51. Cairo: l'Institut Français d'Archéologie Orientale.

Gaillard, Cl. (1934). Contribution à l'étude de la faune préhistorique de l'Egypte. *Extrait des Archives du Museum d'Histoire Naturelle de Lyon*. Vol. 14.

Gaillard, Cl. and G. Daressy (1905). La faune momifiée de l'Antique Egypte. *Catalogue Général des Antiquités Egyptiennes du Musée du Caire*. Cairo: Institut Français d'Archéologie Orientale du Caire.

Gardiner, A.H. (1923). The eloquent peasant. *Journal of Egyptian Archaeology*, **9**, 5–25.

Gardiner, A.H. (1935). *Hieratic Papyri in the British Museum*. 3rd series, Vol. 1. London: British Museum.

Gardiner, A.H. (1947). *Ancient Egyptian Onomastica*, Vol. II, p. 222. Oxford: Oxford University Press.

Gardiner, A.H. (1950). *Egyptian Grammar*, 2nd edition. London: Oxford University Press.

Gardiner, A.H. (1961). *Egypt of the Pharaohs*. Oxford: Clarendon Press.

Garrison, F.H. (1923). History of Pediatrics, Vol. 1 of *Pediatrics*, Edited by I.A.Abt. Philadelphia and London: W.B. Saunders Company.

Gaster, T.H. (1959). Additional Notes, in *The New Golden Bough* by J.G. Frazer. Edited by T.H. Gaster. New York: New American Library.

Gauthier, H. (1911–1914). *Le Temple de Kalabchah. Les Temples immergés de la Nubie*. 2 Vols. Cairo: Service des Antiquités de l'Egypte.

Gauthier, H. (1931). *Les Fêtes du dieu Min*. Cairo: Institut Français d'Archéologie Orientale.

Geoffroy St-Hilaire, I. (1829). Des poissons du Nil, in *Description de l'Egypte. Histoire Naturelle*. Vol. 1. part 1. pp. 265–310.

Ghalioungui, P. (1960). Des papyrus égyptiens à la médecine grecque. *7th International Congress of the History of Medicine*, **I**, 296–307.

Ghalioungui, P. (1962). Some body swellings illustrated in two tombs of the Ancient Empire and their possible relation to *âaâ*. *Zeitschrift für Aegyptische Sprache und Altertumskunde*, **87, II**, 108–114.

Ghalioungui, P. (1963). *Magic and Medical Science in Ancient Egypt*. London: Hodder and Stoughton.

Ghalioungui, P. (1964a). Sur l'exophthalmie de quelques statuettes de l'Ancien Empire. *Bulletin de l'Institut Français d'Archéologie Orientale*, **62,** 63.

Ghalioungui, P. (1964b). *Thyroid enlargement in Africa with reference to the Nile basin*. Cairo: Institut d'Egypte.

Ghalioungui, P. and Z. Dawakhly (1965). *Health and Healing in Ancient Egypt*. Cairo: Egyptian Organization for Authorship and Translation.

Ghalioungui, P., Sh. Khalil and A.R. Ammar (1963). On an ancient method of diagnosing pregnancy and determining faetal sex. *Medical History*, **7, 3,** 241–246.

Ghandi, M.K. (1949). *Diet and Diet Reform*. Ahmedabad: Marajivan Publishing House.

Girard, M.P.S. (1813). Mémoire sur l'agriculture, l'industrie et le commerce de l'Egypte, in *Description de l'Egypte. Etat Moderne*. Vol. II, pp. 491–714.

Goodrich-Freer, A. (1924). *Arabs in Tent and Town*. London: Seeley, Service and Co.

Gould, S.E. (1945). *Trichinosis*. Springfield, Illinois: Charles C. Thomas.

Grapow, H. and W. Westendorf (1958). Uebersetzung der Medizischen Texte. Vol. IV of *Grundriss der Medizin der Alten Aegypter*. Berlin: Akademie Verlag.

Graves, R. (1955). *The Greek Myths*. 2 Vols. Baltimore: Penguin Books.

Gray, P.H.K., 1966. Radiological Aspects of the Mummies of Ancient Egyptians in the Rijksmuseum van Oudheden, Leiden. *Oudheidkidge Mededelungen*, **47,** 1–29.

Gray, P.H.K. (1967). Radiography of Ancient Egyptian Mummies. *Medical Radiography and Photography*, **43,** 34–44.

Greiss, E.A.M. (1955). Anatomical identification of plant remains and other materials from El-Omari excavations at Helwan neolithic period and the excavations at Helwan from the first Dynasty. *Bulletin de l'Institut d'Egypte*, **36,** 227–235.

Greiss, E.A.M. (1957). Anatomical identification of some ancient Egyptian plants and materials. *Mémoire de l'Institut d'Egypte*, n. 55. Cairo: Institut d'Egypte.

Grenfell, B.P. (1896). *The Revenue Laws of Ptolemy Philadelphus edited from a Greek Papyrus in the Bodleian Library*. 2 Vols. Re-edited by J. Bingen (1952). Oxford: Oxford University Press.

Griffith, F.Ll., P.E. Newberry and G.W. Fraser (1894). *El Bersheh*. Part 2. Special Publication no. 4. London: Egypt Exploration Fund.

Griffith, F.Ll. and H. Thompson (1904–1909). *The Demotic Medical Papyrus of London and Leyden*. London: H. Grevel and Co.

Griffiths, J. Gwyn (1948). Human sacrifices in Egypt: The Classical Evidence. *Annales du Service des Antiquités de l'Egypte*, **48**, 409–423.

Grivetti, L.E. (1971). *The European Migratory Quail (Coturnix coturnix L.): its role in culture-history and diet among peoples of the Eastern Mediterranean*. Unpublished manuscript in the Department of Geography Library, University of California, Davis.

Gruner, O.C. (1930). *A Treatise on the Canon of Medicine of Avicenna incorporating a translation of the first book*. London: Luzac and Co.

Grüss, J. (1932). Untersuchung von Broten aus der Aegyptischen Sammlung der Staatlichen Museen zu Berlin. *Zeitschrift für Aegyptische Sprache und Altertumskunde*, **68,** 79–80.

Guerini, V. (1909). *A History of Dentistry from the most distant times until the end of the 18th century*. New York: Milford Inc.

Gulick, C.B. (1927–1941). *See* Athenaeus *Deipnosophists*.

Gurney, J.H. (undated? 1875). *Rambles of a naturalist in Egypt and other countries*. London: Jarrold and Sons.

Hadjigeorge, E. (1952). Les cailles empoisonneuses. *La Presse Médicale*, **68,** 1469.

Hamlyn, P. (1965). *See* Ames *Egyptian Mythology*.

Harris, J.R. *See* Lucas, A. (1962).

Harris, J.E. and K.R. Weeks (1973). *X-Raying the Pharaohs*. New York: Scribner.

Hartmann, F. (1923). *L'agriculture dans l'Ancienne Egypt*. Paris: Imprimeries Réunies.

Hartmann, R. (1864). Versuch einer systematischen Aufzahlung der von alten Aegyptern bildlich dargestellten Thiere. *Zeitschrift für aegyptische Sprache und Altertumskunde*, **2,** 7.

Hayes, W.C. (1951). Inscriptions from the temple of Amenhotep III. *Journal of Near Eastern Studies*, **10,** 82–112.

Hayes, W.C. (1953–1959). *The Scepter of Egypt*, 2 Vols. Cambridge: Harvard University Press.

Hayes, W.C. (1964). *Most Ancient Egypt*. Edited by Keith C. Seele. Chicago: Chicago University Press.

Hefele, Ch. J. (1910). *Histoire des Conciles d'après les documents originaux*. French translation of 2nd German edition by Dom H. Leclercq. 11 Vols. Paris: Letouzy et Ané.

Helbaek, H. (1955). Ancient Egyptian Wheats. *Proceedings of the Prehistoric Society*, **21,** 94–95.

Helbaek, H. (1959). Domestication of Food Plants in the Old World. *Science*, **130,** 6, 8, n. 29.

Helbaek, H. (1966). Wheat Farming produced at Cypriote Kalopsidha, in Astrom, P., *Excavations at Kalopsidha and Ayios Iakovos in Cyprus.* **II.** Quoted by Renfrew (1973). p. 127.

Helck, W. (1971). *Das Bier im Alten Aegypten.* Berlin: Gesellschaft für die Geschichte und Bibliographie des Brauwesens. E.V. Institut für Garungsgewerbe und Biotechnologie.

Helck, H.W. and E. Otto (1956). *Kleines Wörterbuch der Aegyptologie.* Wiesbaden: Otto Harrassowitz.

Heliodorus (1587). *An Aethiopian Historie Written in Greeke by Heliodorus no less wittie than pleasaunt.* Translated by Thomas Underdowne. London: Francis Coldocke.

Henkin, R.I. (1967). Abnormalities of Taste and Olfaction in various disease states, in *The Chemical Senses and Nutrition,* Edited by M.R. Kare and O. Maller. Baltimore: The Johns Hopkins Press. pp. 95–114.

Herbst, G. (1851). Beobachtungen über Trichina spiralis in Betreff der Uebertragung der Eigeweidewürmer. *Nachrichten von der Gesellschaft der Wissenschaften, Göttingen,* pp. 200–264.

Hermes Trismegistus. *See:* Fustigière, A.J. (1945).

Herodotus (1885). Translated by George Rawlinson, 4 Vols. New York: D. Appleton and Co.

Herodotus (1920–30). Translated by A.D. Godley, 4 Vols. New York: G.P. Putnam's Sons.

Herodotus (1964). Translated by A. Barguet and D. Roussel (in French). Bibliothèque de la Pléiade. Paris: Editions Gallimard.

Herre, W. (1969). The Science and History of Domesticated Animals, in *Science in Archaeology.* Edited by Brothwell, D. and E. Higgs. London: Thames and Hudson, pp. 257–272.

Hilton, J. (1833). Notes on a Peculiar Appearance Observed in Human Muscle, Probably Depending Upon the Formation of Very Small Cysticerci. *London Medical Gazette,* **11,** 605.

Hilzheimer, M. (1936). Sheep. *Antiquity,* **10,** 195–206.

Hippocrates (1931a). Regimen, in Vol. 4 of *Hippocrates.* Translated by W.H.S. Jones. New York: G.P. Putnam's Sons.

Hippocrates (1931b). Regimen in Health, in Vol. 4 of *Hippocrates.* Translated by W.H.S. Jones. New York: G.P. Putnam's Sons.

Hippocrates (1945). *Les Aphorismes d'Hippocrate suivis des Aphorismes de l'Ecole de Salerne,* Translated from Greek by Ch. Daremberg. Paris: A l'enseigne du pot cassé.

Hippocrates (1952). *On Diet and Hygiene.* Collected Writings. Translated by J. Precope. London: Williams, Lee and Co.

Hirsch, A. (1885). *Handbook of Geographical and Historical Pathology.* Translated by Ch. Creighton. Vol. II. London: The New Sydenham Society.

Homer (1919). *The Odyssey*, Translated by A.T. Murray, 2 Vols. New York: C.P. Putnam's Sons.

Homer (1924–25). *The Iliad*. Translated by A.T. Murray, 2 Vols. New York: G.P. Putnam's Sons.

Homer (1967). The Odyssey, in *The Poems of Pope*. Vol. II. Yale: Methuen (*See* Pope).

Hoogstraal, H., W. Wassif and M. Kaiser (1955). Results of the NAMRU-3 Southeastern Egypt Expedition 1954. *Zoological Society of Egypt*, **13**, 52–75.

Horace (1947). *The Odes of Horace*. Translated by Lord Dunsany. London: Heinemann.

Horder, Lord, Sir Ch. Dodds and T. Moran (1954). *Bread. The Chemistry and Nutrition of Flour and Bread with an introduction to their history and technology*. London: Constable.

Hornblower, G.D. (1935). The barndoor fowl in Egyptian Art. *Ancient Egypt*, p. 82.

Hornell, J. (1947). Egyptian and medieval pigeon houses. *Antiquity*, **21**, 182–185.

Hort, Sir A. (1916). *See* Theophrastus.

Huffman, R. (1931). *Nuer Customs and Folk-lore*. International Institute of African Languages and Cultures. London: Oxford University Press.

Hugot, H.J. (1968). Origin of African agriculture. Part Two: the origins of agriculture, Sahara. *Current Anthropology*, **9**, 483–488.

Humbert, P. (1929). Recherches sur les sources égyptiennes de la littérature sapientiale d'Israël. *Mémoires de l'Université de Neuchâtel*, Vol. VII.

Hunt, A.S. and C.C. Edgar (1932–34). *Select Papyri*, 2 Vols. New York: G.P. Putnam's Sons.

Huzayyin, S.A. (1941). *The Place of Egypt in Prehistory. A Correlated Study of Climates and Cultures in the Old World*. Mémoires présentés à l'Institut Egyptien, Vol. 43. Cairo: l'Institut Egyptien.

Iason, A.F. (1946). *The Thyroid gland in Medical History*. New York: Froben.

Ibn Sina. (*See* O.C. Gruner (1930) and Avicenna).

Ibrahim, A. (1932). Endemic goitre in Dakhla Oasis of Egypt. *Journal of the Egyptian Medical Association*, **15**, 401–404.

Ingersoll, E. (1923). *Birds in Legend, Fable, and Folklore*. New York: Longmans, Green and Co.

Isfahany al, Abu Farag (1936). History of Imru' al Qeis, in *Kitab al Aghani*. Vol. 9, pp. 102–103. Cairo: Government Press (Arabic).

Issel, H. (1971). *Sacred Fish in the Ancient Near East and Nearby Areas and Avoidance of Fish as Food*. Unpublished manuscript in the Department of Geography Library, University of California, Davis.

Jackson, A. (1934). in Caton-Thompson, G. and E.W. Gardner, *The Desert Fayum*. The Royal Anthropological Institute of Great Britain and Ireland.

Jacobs, H.L. (1967). Taste and Role of Experience in the Regulation of

Food intake, in *The Chemical Senses and Nutrition.* Edited by M.R. Kare and O. Maller, pp. 187–200, Baltimore: The Johns Hopkins Press.

Jacquet-Gordon, H.K. (1962). *Les noms des domaines sous l'ancien Empire Egyptien.* Cairo: Institut Français d'Archéologie Orientale.

Jarvis, C.S. (1938). *Yesterday and Today in Sinai.* London: Blackwood and Sons.

Joachim, H. (1890). *Papyros Ebers. Das alteste Buch ueber Heilkunde.* Berlin: George Reimer.

Johnson, A.C. and L.C. West (1949). *Byzantine Egypt: Economic Studies.* Princeton, N.J.: Princeton University Press.

Joleaud, L. (1935). Les Ruminants Cervicornes d'Afrique. *Mémoire de l'Institut d'Egypte,* **27,** 1–85.

Jonckheere, F. (1944). *Une maladie égyptienne.* Bruxelles: Fondation Egyptologique Reine Elisabeth.

Jones, W.H.S. (1938–1956). *See* Pliny, *Natural History.*

Josephus, Flavius (1865). Antiquities of the Jews, in *The Works of Flavius.* Translated by William Whiston. Edinburgh: W.P. Nimmo.

Junker, H. (1906). Poesie aus der Spätzeit. *Zeitschrift für altegyptische Sprache und Altertumskunde,* **43,** 101–127.

Junker, H. (1929). Vorlaüfiger Bericht über die Grabungen der Akademie auf der neolithischen Siedelung von Merimde-Benisalâme. *Akademie der Wissenschaft. in Wien. Phil.-Hist. Klasse,* 16–18, 156–250.

Junker, H. and Winter, E. (1965). *Das Geburtshaus des Tempels der Isis in Philä.* Wien: Herman Böhlaus.

Juvenal (1957). The Satires of Juvenal, in *Juvenal and Persius.* Translated by G.G. Ramsay. **XV,** 10. London: Heinemann.

Kare, M.R. and O. Maller (1967). *The Chemical Senses and Nutrition.* Baltimore: The Johns Hopkins Press.

Kees, H. (1956). *Die Götterglaube im alten Aegypten.* Berlin: Akademie Verlag.

Kees, H. (1961). *Ancient Egypt. A Cultural Topography.* Translated by Ian F.E. Morrow. Edited by T.G.H. James. London: Faber and Faber.

Keimer, L. (1924a), *Die Gartenpflanzen im alten Aegypten.* Hamburg: Hoffmann and Campe.

Keimer, L. (1924b). Die Pflanze des Gottes Min. *Zeitschrift für altaegyptische Sprache und Altertumskunde,* **59,** 140–143.

Keimer, L. (1929a). Sur quelques petitis fruits en faïence émaillée datant du Moyen Empire. *Bulletin de l'Institut Français d'Archéologie Orientale,* **28,** 49–97.

Keimer, L. (1929b). Falcon Face, *Ancient Egypt,* **14,** 2, 47–48.

Keimer, L. (1929c). Bemerkungen und Lesefrüchte zur altaegyptischen Naturgeschichte. *Kemi,* **2,** 84–106.

Keimer, L. (1930). Quelques hiéroglyphes représentant des oiseaux. *Annales du Service des Antiquités de l'Egypte,* **30,** 1–26.

Keimer, L. (1931). L'arbre *Tr.t* est-il réellement le saule égyptien. *Bulletin de l'Institut Français d'Archéologie Orientale,* **30,** 177–235.

Keimer, L. (1932). Zu Appelts Aufsatz, Lotosfrucht als Ornament. *Mitteilungen des Deutschen Institutes für aegyptische Altertumskunde in Kairo*, **2**, 137–138.

Keimer, L. (1938). Remarques sur quelques représentations de divinités-béliers. *Annales du Service des Antiquités de l'Egypte*, **38**, 297–331.

Keimer, L. (1938–39). La boutargue dans l'Ancienne Egypte. *Bulletin de l'Institut d'Egypte*, **21**, 215–243.

Keimer, L. (1939). Pavian und Dum-Palme. *Mitteilungen des Deutschen Institutes für aegyptische Altertumskunde in Kairo*, **8**, 42–45.

Keimer, L. (1943a). L'identification de l'hiéroglyphe IW. *Annales du Service des Antiquités de L'Egypte*, **42**, 257–270.

Keimer, L. (1943b). Le chrisme sur une statuette de porc. Cairo: *Bulletin de la Société d'Archéologie Copte*, **IX**, 93–101.

Keimer, L. (1943c). Le représentation d'une antilope chevaline sur un bas-relief de Saqqarah. *Bulletin de l'Institut d'Egypte*, **25**, 101–128.

Keimer, L. (1943d). Note sur le nom égyptien du jujubier d'Egypte. *Annales du Service des Antiquités de l'Egypte*, **42**, 279–281.

Keimer, L. (1947). L'interprétation de quelques passages d'Horapollon. *Annales du Service des Antiquités de l'Egypte*. Supplément, no. 5.

Keimer, L. (1948). Quelques représentations rares de poissons égyptiens remontant à l'époque pharaonique. *Bulletin de l'Institut d'Egypte*, **29**, 263–274.

Keimer, L. (1951). Les oignons et les poissons de Cham en-Nessim. *Cahiers d'Histoire Egyptienne*, Serie 3, 352–356.

Keimer, L. (1953). La Musa Ensete. *Chronique d'Egypte*, **XXVIII**, 551, 107, 108.

Khalil, M. (1933). The life-history of the human trematode parasite Heterophyes heterophyes in Egypt. *The Lancet*, **2**, 573.

King, W.J.H. (1925). *Mysteries of the Libyan Desert*. London: Seeley, Service and Co.

Kloos, H. (1971). *Fish-avoidance in Sub-Saharan Africa*. Unpublished manuscript in the Department of Geography Library. University of California. Davis.

Koran, (1955). *The Koran Interpreted*. Translated by A.J. Arberry. London: George Allen and Unwin.

Kroeber, A.L. (1941–42). Culture element distributions. XV. Salt, Dogs, Tobacco. *Anthropological Records*, **VI**, 1–20.

Kueny, G. (1950). Scènes apicoles dans l'Ancienne Egypte. *Journal of Near Eastern Studies*, **9**, 84–93.

Langkavel, B. (1898–1900). Dogs and Savages. pp. 651–675. *Annual Report. Board of Regents of the Smithsonian Institutes*. Washington, D.C.

Lauer, J.P., V.L. Täckholm and A. Aberg (1951). Les plantes découvertes dans les souterrains de l'enceinte du roi Zoser à Saqqara (IIIe Dynastie). *Bulletin de l'Institut d'Egypte*, 1949–1950, **32**, 121–157.

Leclant, J. (1956). La mascarade des boeufs gras et le triomphe de l'Egypte.

Mitteilungen des Deutschen Institutes für aegyptische Altertumskunde in Kairo, **14,** 128–145.

Lefebvre, G. (1924). *Le Tombeau de Petosiris*. Vol. 3. Service des Antiquités de l'Egypte. Cairo: Institut Français d'Archéologie Orientale.

Lefebvre, G. (1949). *Romans et Contes Egyptiens de l'Epoque pharaonique*. Paris: Adrien-Maisonneuve.

Lefebvre, G. (1952). Tableau des parties du corps humain mentionnées par les Egyptiens. Supplement to: *Annales du Service des Antiquités de l'Egypte*. Vol. 17. Cairo.

Lefebvre, G. (1956). *Essai sur la médecine égyptienne de l'époque pharaonique*, Paris: Presses Universitaires de France.

Legge, F. (1900). The carved slates from Hieraconpolis and elsewhere. *Proceedings Society of Biblical Archaeology*, **22,** 125–139.

Leidy, J. (1846). Remarks on Trichina, *Proceedings of the Academy of Anatomical Sciences, Philadelphia*, **3,** 107–108.

Lemprière, J. (1963). *Classical Dictionary of Proper Names mentioned in Ancient Authors*. Revised by F.A. Wright. London: Routledge and Kegan Paul.

Lepsius, R. (1842). *Auswahl der wichtigsten Urkunden des aegyptischen Altertums*. Leipzig: G. Wigand.

Leuckhart, R. (1866). *Untersuchungen über Trichina spiralis zug ein Beitrag zur Kenntniss der Wurmkrankheiten*. Leipzig: C.F. Winter.

Lichtheim, M. (1957). *Demotic Ostraca from Medinet Habu*. Vol. 80. Chicago: University of Chicago Oriental Institute Publications.

Liddell, H.G. and R. Scott (1966). *Greek-English Lexicon*. Oxford: Oxford University Press.

Lindsay, J. (1966). *Leisure and Pleasure in Roman Egypt*. New York: Barnes and Noble.

Loat, W.L.S. (1904). *Gurab*. British School of Archaeology in Egypt. Vol. 10. London: Bernard Quaritch.

Long, A.R. (1931). Historical Review. Cardiovascular Renal Disease. Report of a case of three thousand years ago. *Archives of Pathology (Chicago)*, **12,** 92–94.

Lorenz, K.Z. (1952). *King Solomon's Ring*. London: Methuen.

Loret, V. (1886). Recherches sur plusieurs plantes connues des Anciens Egyptiens. *Recueil de travaux relatifs à la Philologie et à l'Archéologie égyptiennes et assyriennes*, **7,** 101–114.

Loret, V. (1892a). Note sur la faune pharaonique. *Zeitschrift für altaegyptische Sprache und Altertumskunde*, **30,** 24–30.

Loret, V. (1892b). *La Flore Pharaonique d'après les documents hiéroglyphiques et les spécimens découverts dans les tombes*. Paris: Ernest Leroux.

Loret, V. (1893). Recherches sur plusieurs plantes connues des anciens égyptiens. *Recueil de travaux relatifs à la Philologie et à l'Archéologie égyptiennes et assyriennes*, **15,** 105–130.

Loret, V. (1894). Recherches sur plusieurs plantes connues des Anciens égyptiens. *Recueil de travaux relatifs à la Philologie et à l'Archéologie égyptiennes et assyriennes*, **16**, 4–11.

Loret, V. (1900). Les livres III et IV (animaux et végétaux) de la Scala Magna de Schams-ar-Riâsah. *Annales du Service des Antiquités de l'Egypte*, **1**, 48–63. (1902).

Loret, V. (1902). Le ricin et ses emplois médicaux. *Revue de Médecine*, **22**, 696.

Loret, V. (1904). L'ail chez les anciens Egyptiens. *Sphinx*, **8**, 135–147.

Loret, V. (1935–38). Pour transformer un vieillard en jeune homme. *Mélanges Maspero*. Vol. 1, pp. 853–877. Cairo: L'Institut Français d'Archéologie Orientale.

Loret, V. and J. Poisson (1895). Etudes de Botanique Egyptienne. *Recueil de Travaux relatifs à la Philologie et à l'Archéologie égyptiennes et assyriennes*, **17**, 177–191.

Lortet, L.C. and C. Gaillard (1909). La faune momifiée de l'Ancienne Egypte. *Archives du Musée de Lyon*. Vol. X.

Lortet, L.C. and Hugounenq (1902). Recherches sur les momies d'animaux de l'Ancienne Egypte. *Annales du Service des Antiquités de l'Egypte*, **3**, 15–18.

Lucas, A. (1942). Notes on some of the objects from the tomb of Tutankamun. *Annales du Service des Antiquités de l'Egypte*, **41**, 135–147.

Lucas, A. (1962). *Ancient Egyptian Materials and Industries*. 4th edition. Edited by J.R. Harris. London: Edward Arnold.

Lucian (1921). On Sacrifices, in Vol. 3 of *Lucian*, Translated by A.M. Harman. New York: G.P. Putnam's Sons.

Lucian (1959). The Ship or the Wishes, in Vol. 6 of *Lucian*. Translated by K. Kilburn. London: William Heinemann.

Lucretius (1910). *De rerum natura* [On the nature of things]. Translated by C. Bailey, 3 Vols. Oxford: Clarendon Press.

Lutz, H.F. (1922). *Viticulture and Brewing*. Leipzig: Hinrichs.

Lynes, H. (1909–1910). Observations on the migration of birds in the Mediterranean. *British Birds*, **3**, 36–51 and 69–77.

Lynes, H. and H.F. Witherby (1912). Field Notes on a collection of birds from the Mediterranean. *Ibis*, Series 9, **6**, 121–187.

Mackworth-Praed, C.W. and C.H.B. Grant (1957). *Birds of Eastern and North Eastern Africa*. 2nd edition. London: Longmans, Green and Co.

MacPherson, H.A. (1897). *A History of Fowling*. Edinburgh: D. Douglas.

Macrobius, A.A.T. (1937). *Les Saturnales*. Translated by Henri Bornecque. 2 Vols. Paris: Garnier Frères.

Mahaffy, J.P. (1895). *The Empire of the Ptolemies*. London: Macmillan.

Maller, O. (1967). Specific appetite, in *The Chemical Senses and Nutrition*. Edited by Kare, M.R. and O. Maller. pp. 201–212. Baltimore: The Johns Hopkins Press.

Manetho (1940). *History of Egypt*. Translated by W.G. Waddell. Cambridge: Harvard University Press.

Maqrizi, Ahmed ibn Aly al (1958). *Kitab al-Solouk li-Marifat Dowal al-Muluk* (in Arabic). Cairo: Organization of Authorship and Translation.

Marco Polo (1929). *Travels.* New York: Everyman's Library.

Marie, A. (1910). *Transactions of the National Conference on Pellagra.* The South Carolina Board of Health (Nov. 3–4, 1909). Columbia S.C., The State Company.

Mariette, A.E. (1880). *Catalogue Général des Monuments d'Abydos.* No. 1464. Paris: Imprimerie Nationale.

Martial (1919–1920). *Epigrams.* Translated by Walter C.A. Ker. 2 Vols. New York: G.P. Putnam's Sons.

Maspero, G. (1883). *Guide to the Cairo Museum.* Fifth edition. Translated by J.E. Quibell. Bulak.

Maspero. G. (1885–86). Pots de miel, *Bibl. Egyptol. I*: Deuxième rapport à l'Institut Egyptien sur les fouilles et travaux éxécutés en Egypte. Cairo: Institut Egyptien.

Maspero, G. (1901). *The Dawn of Civilization. Egypt and Chaldaea.* Fourth edition. Translated by M.L. McClure. Edited by A.H. Sayce. London: Society for Promoting Christian Knowledge.

Mattirolo, O. (1926). I Vegetali scoperti nella Tomba dell'Architetto Kha e di sua moglia Mirit nella Necropoli di Tebe dalla Missione Archeologi Italiana diretta del Senatore E. Schiaparelli. *Atti della Reale Academia delle Scienze di Torino,* **61,** Disp. 13.

Maystre, C. (1941). Le Livre de la Vache di Ciel. *Bulletin de l'Institut Français d'Archéologie Orientale,* **40,** 53–115.

McCartney, E.S. (1924). Greek and Roman lore of animal-nursed infants. *Papers of the Michigan Academy of Sciences, Arts, and Letters,* **IV,** pp. 15–16.

Medinet Habu. (1930–1970). 8 Vols, by the Epigraphic Survey. Vol. 4 (1940), Vol. 5 (1957). Chicago: The University of Chicago Oriental Institute.

Megally, M. (1971). *Le Papyrus Comptable E 3226 du Louvre.* Vol. LIII. Bibliothèque d'Etude. Cairo: Institut Français d'Archéologie Orientale.

Meinertzhagen, R. (1922). Notes on Some Birds from the Near East and from Tropical East Africa. *Ibis* (Series 11) **4,** 1074.

Meinertzhagen, R. (1930). *Nicoll's Birds of Egypt.* 2 Vols. London: Hugh Rees.

Meinertzhagen, R. (1954). *Birds of Arabia.* London: Oliver and Boyd.

Meneely, G.R., C.O. Ball and J.B. Youmans (1957). Chronic sodium chloride toxicity. The protective effect of added potassium chloride. *Annals of Internal Medicine,* **II,** 263–273.

Menghin, O. and M. Amer (1932). The *Excavations of the Egyptian University in the Neolithic site of Maadi.* First Preliminary Report. 1930–1931. Cairo: Misr-Sokkar Press.

Menghin, O. and M. Amer (1936). *The Excavations of the Egyptian University in the Neolithic site of Maadi.* Second Preliminary Report. 1932. Cairo: Government Press.

Mercer, S.A.B. (1952). *The Pyramid Texts in Translation and Commentary.* 4 Vols. London: Longmans, Green and Co.

Meyerovitz, E.L.R., (1960). *The Divine Kingship in Ghana and Ancient Egypt.* London: Faber and Faber.

Michailidis, G. (1962). Nouvel Essai d'Interprétation d'une statuette de porc marquée du Chrisme. *Bulletin Société d'Archéologie Copte,* **16,** 253–260.

Michailidis, G. (1965). Moule illustrant un texte d'Hérodote relatif au bouc de Mendes. *Bulletin de l'Institut Français d'Archéologie Orientale,* **63,** 139–160.

Mond, R., O.H. Myers, T.J.C. Baly, J. Cameron, A.J.E. Cave, S. Huzayyin, J.W. Jackson and D. O'Leary (1937). *Cemeteries of Armant.* 42nd Memoir. London: Egypt Exploration Fund.

Mond, R., O.H. Myers, T.J.C. Baly, D.B. Harden and H.W. Fairman (1934). *Bucheum.* 41st Memoir. London: Egypt Exploration Fund.

Montet P. (1910). Les Scènes de boucherie dans les tombes de l'Ancien Empire. *Bulletin de l'Institut Français d'Archéologie Orientale,* **7,** 41–65.

Montet, P. (1913). Les Poissons Employés dans l'Ecriture Hiéroglyphique. *Bulletin de l'Institut Français d'Archéologie Orientale,* **11,** 39–48.

Montet, P. (1925). *Les scènes de la vie privée dans les tombeaux égyptiens de l'Ancien Empire.* Paris: Librairie Istra.

Montet, P. (1950). Etudes sur quelques prêtres et fonctionnaires du dieu Min. *Journal of Near Eastern Studies,* **9,** 18–27.

Montet, P. (1958). *Everyday life in Egypt in the days of Ramesses the Great.* Translated by A.R. Maxwell-Hyslop and M.S. Drower. London: Edward Arnold.

Moodie, R.L. (1931). Roentgen studies of Egyptian and Peruvian mummies. Chicago: *Field Museum Natural History,* Vol. III.

Moreau, R.E. (1927). Quail. *Zoological Society of Egypt,* **1,** 6–13.

Moreau, R.E. (1930). The Birds of Ancient Egypt, in *Nicoll's Birds of Egypt.* *See* Meinertzhagen (1930). Vol. 1, pp. 58–77.

Moreau, R.E. (1953). Migration in the Mediterranean area. *Ibis,* **95,** 329–364.

Moreau, R.E. (1966). *The Bird Faunas of Africa and Its Islands.* London: Academic Press.

Mosseri, V.M. (1922). Sur l'origine du Riz et l'Histoire de sa culture en Egypte. *Bulletin de l'Institut d'Egypte,* **4,** 25–34.

Mountfort, G. (1965). *Portrait of a Desert.* London: Collins.

Moussa, A.M. and H. Altenmüller (1971). *The Tomb of Nefer and Ka-Hay,* Mainz-am-Rhein: P. von Zabern.

Moustafa, Y.S. (1953a). A contribution to the knowledge of animal life in Predynastic Egypt. *Bulletin of the Faculty of Arts, Cairo University,* **15,** 207–211.

Moustafa, Y.S. (1953b). Preliminary notice on gazelles from Predynastic Wadi Digla. *Bulletin of the Faculty of Arts, Cairo University,* **15,** 213.

Moustafa, Y.S. (1955). *Canis familiaris aegyptiaca* from Predynastic Maadi, Egypt. *Bulletin de l'Institut d'Egypte,* **36,** 105–109.

Moustafa, Y.S. (1964). The domesticated animals of the Sekhemkhet Step Pyramid. *Annales du Service des Antiquités de l'Egypte,* **58,** 255–265.

Müller, W.M. (1893). *Asien und Europa nach altägyptischen Denkmälern.* Leipzig: Engelman.

Murdock, G.P. (1959). *Africa. Its Peoples and Their Culture History.* New York: McGraw-Hill.

Murray, M.A. (1905). *Saqqara Mastabas.* 2 Vols. London: Bernard Quaritch.

Murray, M.A. and K. Sethe (1937). *Saqqara Mastabas,* Vol. II, London: Bernard Quaritch.

Mustafa, M. (1969–1970). An illustrated manuscript of chivalry from the late Circassian Mameluke period. *Bulletin de l'Institut d'Egypte,* **51,** 1–14 and plate XVIII.

Nagaty, H.F., M.S. Gindy and M.A. Rifaat (1961). A parasitological survey of the school children of Kerdasa village in 1960. *Journal of Egyptian Medical Association,* **44,** 516–521.

Naville, E.H. (1894–1908). *The Temple of Deir el-Bahari.* 7 Vols. London: Kegan Paul.

Naville, E.H. (1907–1913). *The XIIth Dynasty Temple at Deir el-Bahari.* London: Kegan Paul.

Netolitzki, F. (1911). in *The Ancient Egyptians and their Influence upon the Civilization of Europe,* by G. Elliot-Smith, pp. 41–43. New York: Harper.

Newberry, P. (1889). On the vegetable remains discovered in the cemetery of Hawara, in *Hawara, Biahmu, and Arsinoe* by W.M.F. Petrie, pp. 46–53. London: Trubner and Co.

Newberry, P. (1890). The Ancient Botany, in W.M.F. Petrie, *Kahun Gurob and Hawara,* pp. 46–50. London: Kegan, Trench, Trubner and Co.

Newberry, P. (1928). The pig and the cult animal of Set. *Journal of Egyptian Archaeology,* **14,** 211–225.

Newberry, P.E. and G.W. Fraser (1893–1894). *Beni Hassan,* 2 Vols. London: Egypt Exploration Fund.

Newcomer, A.D. (1973). Disaccharidase deficiencies. *Mayo Clinic Proceedings,* **48,** 9, 648–652.

Nims, C.F. (1950). Egyptian Catalogue of Things. *Journal of Near Eastern Studies,* **9,** 253–262.

Nims, C.F. (1958). The beer and bread problems of the Moscow Mathematical Papyrus. *Journal of Egyptian Archaeology,* **44,** 56–65.

Northampton, W.G.S.S.C., W. Spiegelberg and P.E. Newberry (1908). *Theban Necropolis. Report on some excavations during the winter of 1898–1899.* London: Archibald Constable and Co.

Oakley, K.P. (1969). Analytical methods of dating bones, in *Science in Archaeology.* Edited by D. Brothwell and E. Higgs. pp. 35–45. London: Thames and Hudson.

Oliver, R. and J.D. Fage (1962). *A Short History of Africa.* London: Penguin Books.

Oppian (1928). *Halieutica-Cynegetica.* Translated by A. W. Mair. New York: G.P. Putnam's Sons.

Otto, E. (1964). Beitrage z. Geschichte der Stierkulte in Aegypten. Hildesheim, quoted from Ucko and Dimbleby, *The Domestication and Exploitation of Plants and Animals,* 1969, p. 314. Chicago: Aldine.

Ouzounellis, T.I. (1968). Myoglobinuries par ingestion de Cailles. *La Presse Médicale,* **76,** 1863–1864.

Ouzounellis, T.I. (1970). Some notes on quail poisoning. *Journal of the American Medical Association,* **211,** 1186–1187.

Ovid (1951–56). *Metamorphoses.* Translated by Frank Justus Miller. 2 Vols. London: William Heinemann.

Owen, R. (1835). Description of a microscopic entozoon infesting the muscles of the human body. *Transactions of the Zoological Society of London,* **1,** 315–324.

Owen, T. (1805–06). *Geoponics (Agricultural Pursuits).* 2 Vols. Combined edition. London: W. Spilsbury.

Owen, W.L. (1933). Production of industrial alcohol from grain by Amylo process. *Industrial and Chemical Engineering,* **25,** 87–89.

Paget, J. (1835). Oral communication. Minute-Book Abernethian Society. *Transactions of the Abernethian Society,* **2,** February 6th.

Paget, J. (1866). On the discovery of Trichina. *The Lancet,* **1,** 269–270.

Paget, R.F.E. and A.A. Pirie (1898). *The Tomb of Ptah-hetep,* London: Bernard Quaritch.

Parker, R.A. (1971). The calendars and chronology, pp. 23–24 in *The Legacy of Egypt,* Edited by J.R. Harris. Oxford: Clarendon Press.

Paton, D. (1925). *Animals of Ancient Egypt,* Princeton, N.J.: Princeton University Press.

Patwardhan, V.N. (1961). *Nutrition in India,* Bombay: Indian Journal of Medical Science Publications.

Patwardhan, V.N. and W.J. Darby (1972). *The State of Nutrition in the Arab Middle East.* Nashville, Tennessee: Vanderbilt University Press.

Pausanias (1918–35). *Description of Greece.* Translated by W.H.S. Jones. 5 Vols. New York: G.P. Putnam's Sons.

Peet, T.E. (1914). *The Cemeteries of Abydos. Vol. 2. 1911–12.* 34th Memoir. London: Egypt Exploration Fund.

Pendlebury, J.D.S. (1951). *The City of Akhenaten,* Part III, 2 Vols. London: Egypt Exploration Society. London: Oxford University Press.

Petrie, Hilda, F., M.A. Murray, F. Hansard, F. Kingsford, and L. Eckenstein (1952). *Seven Memphite Tomb Chapels.* British School of Archaeology in Egypt. Vol. 65. London: Bernard Quaritch.

Petrie, W.M.F. (1888). *Nebesheh (Am) and Defenneh (Tahpanhes),* Egypt Exploration Fund. London: Trübner.

Petrie, W.M.F. (1889). *Hawara, Biahmu and Arsinoe.* London: Trübner and Co.

Petrie, W.M.F. (1890). *Kahun, Gurob, and Hawara.* London: Kegan, Trench and Trübner.

Petrie, W.M.F. (1891). *Illahun, Kahun, and Gurob.* London: Trübner.

Petrie, W.M.F. (1892). *Medum.* London: David Nutt.

Petrie, W.M.F. (1894). *Tell el Amarna.* London: Methuen.

Petrie, W.M.F. (1896). *Koptos.* London: Bernard Quaritch.

Petrie, W.M.F. (1900). *Dendereh.* London: Egyptian Fund. Memoir no. 17.

Petrie, W.M.F. (1900). *I. The Royal Tombs of the First Dynasty.* London: Kegan Paul.

Petrie, W.M.F. (1901). *II. The Royal Tombs of the Earliest Dynasties.* London: Kegan Paul.

Petrie, W.M.F. (1914). *Amulets Illustrated by the Egyptian Collection in University College, London.* London: Constable and Co.

Petrie, W.M.F. (1920). *Prehistoric Egypt.* 2 Vols. London: Bernard Quaritch.

Petrie, W.M.F. (1925). The Cultivators and their Land. *Ancient Egypt*, **4**, 105–110.

Petrie, W.M.F., E. Mckay and G. Wainwright (1910). *Meydum and Memphis.* British School of Archaeology in Egypt. 16th Year. London: Bernard Quaritch.

Petrie, W.M.F., E. McKay and G. Wainwright (1912). *The Labyrinth, Gerzeh, and Mazghuneh.* British School of Archaeology in Egypt. Vol. 21. London: Bernard Quaritch.

Petrie, W.M.F., and J.E. Quibbel (1896). *Naqada and Ballas.* London: Bernard Quaritch.

Petrie, W.M.F., A.E. Weigall, and F.Ll. Griffith. (1903). *Abydos*, 2 vols. 24th Memoir. London: Egypt Exploration Fund.

Petronius (1965). *The Satyricon and the Fragments.* Translated by John Sullivan. Harmondsworth: Penguin Books.

Philo (1954). *The Special Laws*, in Vol. 8 of *Philo with an English Transl.* Translated by F.H. Colson. London: William Heinemann.

Piankoff, A. (1968). *The Pyramid Texts of Unas.* New York: Marchbanks Press.

Plato (1952). *Timaeus*, in Vol. 7 of *Plato*. Translated by R.G. Bury. London: William Heinemann.

Plato (1961). *Laws.* 2 Vols. Translated by R.G. Bury. London: William Heinemann.

Pleyte, W. (1882). Bloemen en Planten uit Oud-Egypte in het museum te Leiden. *Jaarvergad. d. Nederland. Botan. Vereenigung.* Leiden, nos. 46, 67, 82.

Plichet, A. (1952). Les Cailles Empoisonneuses. *La Presse Médicale*, **60**, 1189.

Pliny (1938–56). *Natural History.* Translated by H. Rackham and W.H.S. Jones. 8 Vols. Cambridge: Harvard University Press.

Plutarch (1920). in Vol. 9 of *Plutarch's Lives*. 11 Vols. Translated by Bernadotte Perrin. London: William Heinemann.

Plutarch (1924). *The Roman Questions of Plutarch*, Translated by H.J. Rose. Oxford: The Clarendon Press.

Plutarch (1936). Isis and Osiris in *Moralia*, Vol 5. Translated by F.C. Babbitt. Cambridge: Harvard University Press.

Plutarch (1959). Table Talk (Quaest. conv.) in *Moralia*, Vol. 9. Translated by E.L. Minar, F.H. Sandbach and W.C. Helmbold. Cambridge: Harvard University Press.

Polynaeus (1793). *Stratagems of War*. Translated by R. Shepherd, London.

Pope, A. (1967). *The Poems of Alexander Pope*. Yale: Methuen.

Porphyry (1965). *On Abstinence from Animal Food*. Translated by Thomas Taylor. London: Centaur Press.

Posener, G. (1962). *A Dictionary of Egyptian Civilisation*. New York: Tudor.

Pruner, F. (1847a). *Topographie médicale du Caire avec le plan de la ville et ses environs*. Munich: Author's edition.

Pruner, F. (1847b). *Die Krankheiton des Orients von Standpunkte der vergleichenden Nosologie*. Erlanger: J.J. Palm and E. Enke.

Quibbell, J.E. and F.W. Green (1900–02). *Hierakonpolis*. 2 Vols. London: Bernard Quaritch.

Radcliffe, W. (1926). *Fishing from the Earliest Times*. 2nd edition. London: John Murray.

Ragheb, F.H. (1939). *Hadiqat Al-Amthâl al 'ammiya*. Cairo: Amin Abdur-Rahman Press (in arabic).

Rawlinson, G. (1881). *History of Ancient Egypt*. 2 Vols. New York: J.B. Alden.

Rawlinson, G. (1885). (*See* Herodotus (1885).)

Reed, C.A. (1959). Animal domestication in the Prehistoric Near East. *Science*, **130**, 1629–1639.

Reekmans, T. (1966). *La sitométrie dans les archives de Zenon*. p. 108. Bruxelles: Fondation Egyptologique Reine Elisabeth.

Reisner, G.A. (1907). *Amulets*. Catalogue Général des Antiquités Egyptiennes au Musée du Caire. Vol. 35. Cairo: Institut Français d'Archéologie Orientale du Caire.

Reisner, G.A. (1931). *Mycerinus*. Cambridge: Harvard University Press.

Renfrew, J.M. (1973). *Palaeoethnobotany*. New York: Columbia University Press.

Ricci, C. (1924). *La cultura della vite e la fabricazione del vino nell' Egitto Greco-Romano*. Milano: Aegyptus.

Riddell, W.H. (1943). The domestic goose. *Antiquity*, **17**, 148–155.

Rifaat, M. and H.F. Nagaty (1961). The incidence of intestinal parasitic infection among the inhabitants of Cairo. *Journal of the Egyptian Medical Association*, **41**, 164–169.

Rifaud, M.J.J. (1830). *Voyage en Egypte, en Nubie et lieux circonvoisins depuis 1805 jusqu'à 1827*, Paris. (n.p.)

Roberts, D. *See* William Brockedon (1846–49).

Robinson, J.T. (1952). Teeth in earlier human populations. *Journal of Dental Association of South Africa*, **7**, 102.

Rohrbacher (1878). *Histoire Universelle de l'Eglise Catholique par Rohrbacher continuée jusqu'a nos jours par Mr. l'Abbé Guillaume*, 13 Vols. Paris: Société Générale de Librairie Catholique.

Rose, H.J. (1953). *A Handbook of Greek Mythology Including its Extension to Rome*, 5th edition. London: Methuen.

Rosellini, I. (1834). *I Monumenti dell Egitto e della Nubia*. Pisa: Nicolo Capurro.

Rosengarten, F. Jr. (1969). *The Book of Spices*, Philadelphia: Livingstone.

Rosner, F. (1970). The Biblical quail incident. *Journal of the American Medical Association*, **211**, 1544.

Rougé, J. de (1867). Textes géographiques du Temple d'Edfou. *Revue Archéologique*. (Nlle Serie), **XV**, 330–341.

Roushdy, M.E. (1911). The treading of sown seed by swine. *Annales du Service des Antiquités de l'Egypte*, **11**, 162–163, 281, 282.

Ruffer, M.A. (1919). *Food in Egypt*. Mémoire presenté à l'Institut Egyptien, **1**, 1–88.

Ruffer, M.A. (1921). *Studies in the Palaeopathology of Egypt*. Chicago: Chicago University Press.

Russell, A.S. (1974). Carbohydrates as a causative factor in dental caries: epidemiological evidence, in *Sugars in Nutrition*. Edited by H.L. Sipple and K.W. McNutt, pp. 635–645. New York: Academic Press.

Saad, Z. (1951). *Royal Excavations at Helwan, 1945–1947*. Cairo: Imprimerie de l'Institut Français d'Archéologie Orientale.

Saffirio, L. (1966). L'alimentazione umana nell'Egitto preistorico, III, *Aegyptus*, **46**, 26–59.

Salmon, G. (1901). Note sur la Flore du Fayoum d'après al-Naboulsii *Bulletin de l'Institut Français d'Archéologie Orientale*, pp. 25–72.

Sambon, L.W. (1905). The geographical distribution and etiology of pellagra: *Journal of Tropical Medicine*, **8**, 250–252.

Sandford, K.S. (1934). *Paleolithic Man and the Nile Valley in Upper and Middle Egypt. A Study of the Region During Pliocene and Pleistocene Times. Part 3*. University of Chicago, Oriental Institute Publication, Vol. 18. Chicago: University of Chicago Press.

Sandison, A.T. (1962). Degenerative vascular disease in an Egyptian mummy. *Medical History*, **6**, 77–81.

Sandwith, F.M. (1898). Pellagra in Egypt (Abstract). *British Medical Journal*, **11**, 881.

Sandwith, F.M. (1905). *The Medical Diseases of Egypt*, Vol. 1. London: Henry Kimpton.

Sandwith, F.M. (1913). Is Pellagra a disease due to deficiency of nutrition? *Transactions of the Royal Society of Medicine and Hygiene*, **6**, 143–148.

Sauer, C.O. (1969). *Agricultural Origins and Dispersals*. 2nd edition. Cambridge, Mass.: M.I.T. Press.

Sauneron, S. (1960). A propos d'un Pronostic de naissance. *Bulletin de l'Institut Français d'Archéologie Orientale*, **60**, 29–30.

Sauneron, S. (1959–69). *Le Temple d'Esna*. 4 Vols. Cairo: Institut Français d'Archéologie Orientale.

Sauneron, S. (1968). Les Inscriptions Ptolémaïques de Temple de Mout à Karnak. *Bulletin de l'Institut d'Egypte*, Session 1963–64. **45**, 45–52.

Sauneron, S. (1970). *Le Voyage en Egypte de Pierre Belon du Mans, 1547*. Cairo: Institut Français d'Archéologie Orientale.

Sauneron, S. (1971). *Le Voyage en Egypt de Jean Palerne Forésien, 1581*. Cairo: Institut Français d'Archéologie Orientale.

Säve-Söderbergh, T. (1957). *Four Eighteenth Dynasty Tombs*, plate XV, Oxford: Oxford University Press.

Scharff, A. (1957). *Die archaeologischen Ergebnisse des vorgeschichtlichen Grabenfelder von Abusir el Meleq, nach den Aufgezeichnungen*, G. Muller, Leipzig: Hinrichs.

Scheuthauer, G. (1881). Beiträge zur Erklärung Des Papyrus Ebers, Des Hermetischen Buches über die Arzneimittel der Alten Aegypter. *Virchow's Archiv*, **85**, 343–354.

Schleiden, M.I. (1875). *Das Salz*. Leipzig: Engelmann.

Schoff, W.H. (1912). *The Periplus of the Erythrean Sea, Travel and Trade in the Indian Ocean*. New York: Longmans, Green and Co.

Scholfield, A.F. *See* Aelian (1958–59).

Schulz, A. (1916). Die Getreide der alten Aegypter, *Abhandlungen d. Naturforschung Gesellschaft zu Halle*, Neue Folge, no. 5.

Schuz, E. (1966). Über Stelzvögel (Ciconiiformes und Gruidae) im Alten Aegypten. *Vogelwarte*, **23**, 264–283.

Schweinfurth, G. (1873a). *The Heart of Africa*. London: Sampson Low.

Schweinfurth, G. (1873b). Les végétaux cultivés en Egypte qui se trouvent à l'état spontané dans le Soudan et le Centre de l'Afrique. *Bulletin de l'Institut Egyptien*, **12**, 200–209.

Schweinfurth, G. (1883). De la flore pharaonique. *Bulletin de l'Institut Egyptien* (2nd series). Année 1882, **3**, 51–76.

Schweinfurth, G. (1885). Notice sur le restes de végétaux de l'ancienne Egypte contenus dans une armoire du musée de Boulaq. *Bulletin de l'Institut Egyptien* (2e serie). Année 1884. **5**, 3–10.

Schweinfurth, G. (1886). Les dernières découvertes botaniques dans les anciens tombeaux de l'Egypte. *Bulletin de l'Institut Egyptien* (2e série). Année 1885, 6, 256–283.

Schweinfurth, G. (1887). Sur les dernières trouvailles botaniques dan les tombeaux de l'Ancienne Egypte. *Bulletin de l'Institut Egyptien*, 1886 (2e. serie), **7**, 419–433.

Schweinfurth, G. (1888). Sur la flore des anciens jardins arabes d'Egypte. *Bulletin de l'Institut Egyptien*, 1887 (2e serie), **8**, 294–337.

Schweinfurth, G. (1891). Aegyptens auswärtige Beziehungen hinsichtlich der Kulturgewächse. *Verhandlungen der Berliner Gesellschaft für Anthropologie.* 656–669.

Schweinfurth, G. (1912). *Arabische Pflanzennnamen aus Aegypten Algerien und Jemen.* Berlin: Dietrich Reimer.

Sergent, E. (1941). Les cailles empoisonneuses dans la Bible et en Algérie de nos jours: aperçu historique et recherches expérimentales. *Archives de l'Institut Pasteur d'Algérie,* **19,** 161–192.

Sergent, E. (1948). Les cailles empoisonneuses en France. *Archives de l'Institut Pasteur d'Algérie,* **26,** 249–252.

Serjeant, R.B. (1968). Fish-folk and fish-traps in Al-Bahrain. *Bulletin of the School of Oriental and African Studies,* University of London, **31,** 487–514.

Sethe, K. (1906–09). *Urkunden der 18. Dynastie.* Leipzig: Hinrichs.

Sethe, K. (1916). Die älteste Erwähnung des Haushuhns in einem agyptischen Texte. *Festschrift Friedrich Carl Andreas,* 109–116. Leipzig: Hinrichs.

Sethe, K. (1932). *Urkunden des alten Reiches.* Vol. 1. Leipzig: Hinrichs.

Sextus Empiricus (1933). Outlines of Pyrrhonism, in Vol. 1 of *Sextus Empiricus.* Translated by R.G. Bury. New York: G.P. Putnam's Sons.

Shafei, A. (1939). Fayoum irrigation as described by Nabulsi in 1425 A.D. *Bulletin de la Société Royale de Géographie d'Egypte,* **20,** 285–314.

Shattock, S.G. (1909). A report upon the pathological condition of the aorta of King Meneptah, traditionally regarded as the Pharaoh of the Exodus. *Proceedings of the Royal Society of Medicine,* **2,** 122 (Pathological Section).

Sickenberger, E. (1901). Contribution a la Flore d'Egypte. *Memoire de l'Institut Egyptien,* **IV,** 167–335.

Simoons, F.J. (1961). *Eat Not this Flesh. Food Avoidance in the Old World.* Madison, Wisc.: The University of Wisconsin Press.

Sipple, H.L. and K.W. McNutt (1974. *Sugars in Nutrition.* New York: Academic Press.

Smith, H.S. (1969). Animal domestication and animal cult in dynastic Egypt, in *The domestication and exploitation of plants and animals,* Edited by P.J. Ucko and C.W. Dimbleby. London: Gerald Duckworth and Co.

Smith, S. (1928). Assryiological notes on a Babylonian fertility cult. *Journal of the Royal Asiatic Society of Great Britain and Ireland,* 848–875.

Smith, W.S. (1952). Inscriptional evidence for the history of the Fourth Dynasty. *Journal of Near Eastern Studies,* **II,** 113–128.

Snapper, I. (1967). The etiology of different forms of taste behaviour, in *The Chemical Senses and Nutrition.* Edited by M. R. Kare and O. Maller, pp. 337–346. Baltimore: Johns Hopkins Press.

Sobhy, G.P.G. (1921). Survival of Ancient Egyptian in modern dialect. *Ancient Egypt,* **3,** 70–75.

Sobhy, G.P. and M. Meyerhof (1937). *The Abridged Version of the Book of*

Simple Drugs of Ahmed Ibn Muhammad al-Ghafiki, 2 vols. Cario: Egyptian University, Faculty of Medicine Publication no. 4.

Sognnaes, R.F. (1956). Histologic evidence of developmental lesions in teeth originating from paleolithic, prehistoric, and ancient man. *American Journal of Physical Anthropology*, **32**, 547–577.

Sonnini, C.S. (1799). *Travels in Upper and Lower Egypt*. Translated by Henry Hunter. 3 Vols. London: John Stockdale.

Speleers, L. (1923–1924). *Les Textes des Pyramides Egyptiennes. Traduction et Vocabulaire*. 2 Vols. Ghent: Vanderpoorten.

St. John, J.A. (1834). *Egypt and Mohamed Ali or Travels in the Valley of the Nile*. 2 Vols. London: Longman.

Ste Fare-Garnot, J. (1949). Deux vases égyptiens représentant une femme tenant un enfant sur ses genoux. *Mélanges Ch. Picard*. Vol. II, p. 905. Paris: Presses Universitaires de France.

Steindorff, G. (1913). *Grab des Ti*. Leipzig: Hinrichs.

Still, G.F. (1931). *The History of Paediatrics. The Progress of the Study of Diseases of Children up to the End of the XVIIIth Century*. Oxford University Press. (Reprinted 1965, London: Dawsons of Pall Mall.)

Storcke, J. and W.D. Teague (1952). *A History of Milling. Flour for man's Bread*. Minneapolis: University of Minnesota Press.

Strabo (1917–1932). *Geography*. Translated by H.L. Jones. 8 Vols. New York: G.P. Putnam's Sons.

Strekalowski, N.W. (1949). *Shooting and Fishing in Egypt*. Egyptian State Tourist Department. Cairo: Schindler.

Struve, W.W. (1930). Mathematischer Papyrus des Staatlichen Museums der schonen Kunste in Moskau. *Quellen und Studien zur Geschichte der Mathematik*. Abt. A. 1 Band. Berlin: Julius Springer.

Suetonius, Gai Suetoni Tranquilli (1957). *De vita Caesarum: The Twelve Caesars*. Translated by Robert Graves. Baltimore: Penguin Books.

Tacitus (1931–7). *The Annals*. Translated by J. Jackson. 2 Vols. New York: G.P. Putnam's Sons.

Täckholm, V.L. (1941–1969). *The Flora of Egypt*.
    Vol. I. (1941). with G. Täckholm. Cairo: Bulletin of the Faculty of Science, Fouad I University.
    Vol. II. (1950). with M. Drar. Cairo: Bulletin of the Faculty of Science, Fouad I University.
    Vol. III. (1954). with M. Drar, Cairo: Cairo University Press.
    Vol. IV. (1969). with M. Drar, Cairo: The Public Organization for Books and Scientific Appliances.

Täckholm, V.L. (1961). *Le Monastère de Phoebammon dans la Thébaide*. Vol. III. *Botanical Identification of the Plants found at the Monastery of Phoebammon*. Cairo: Publications de la Société d'Archéologie Copte.

Täckholm, V. (1969). *Alfred Kaiser's Herbarium*. Cairo: Publication of the Cairo University Herbarium. No. 2, pp. 43–44.

Tannahill, R. (1973). *Food in History*. New York: Stein and Day.

Theognis (1962). *Poèmes élégiaques*. Translated into French by J. Carrière. 2nd Edition. Paris: Belles Lettres.

Theophrastus (1916). *Enquiry Into Plants:* Translated by Arthur Hort. 2 Vols. New York: G.P. Putnam's Sons.

Thesiger, W. (1964). *The Marsh Arabs*. London: Longmans.

Thompson, D'Arcy Wentworth (1928). On Egyptian fish names used by Greek writers. *Journal of Egyptian Archaeology*, **14**, 22–33.

Thompson, D'Arcy, W. (1966). *A Glossary of Greek Birds*. Hildersheim: George Olms.

Thucydides (1919–23). *History*. Translated by Charles Forester Smith, 4 Vols. Cambridge: Harvard University Press.

Tiedemann, F. (1821). Untitled. Under "Miscellany". *Notiz an der Gebiet der Natur und Heilkunde*, Weimar, 1, 64.

Tutuola, A. (1963). *The Palm-Wine Drinkard*. London: Faber and Faber.

Tylor, J.J. and Ll. Griffith (1895). *The Tomb of Paheri at El-Kab*, 11th Memoir. London: Egypt Exploration Society.

Tylor, J.J. and S. Clarke (1896). *Wall Drawings and Monuments of El-Kab. The Tomb of Sebeknekht*. London: Bernard Quaritch.

Ucko, P.J., and G.W. Dimbleby (1969). *The Domestication and Exploitation of Plants and Animals*. London: Gerald Duckworth and Co.

Underdowne, *See* Heliodorus (1587).

Unger, F (1860). Die Pflanzenresten des alten Aegyptens. *Sitzungberichte d. mathematische-naturwissenschaftliche Klasse der Akademie d. Wissenschaftlichen in Wien*, **38**, 68–140.

Unger, F. (1862). Botanische Streifzuge auf dem Gebiete der Kulturgeschichte. V. Inhalt eines alten aegyptisches Ziegels an organische Korpern. *Sitzungberichte der Kaiserichen Akademie der Wissenschaften in Wien. Mathem.-Naturwiss. Klasse*. **45,** 81.

Van de Walle, B. and J. Vergote (1943). Traduction des hieroglyphica d'Horapollon. *Chronique d'Egypte*, **35**, 39–89.

Vandier, J. (1936). *La Famine dans l'Egypte Ancienne*. Cairo: Institut Français d'Archéologie Orientale, Vol. 7.

Vandier, J. (1964). *Manuel d'Archéologie Egyptienne*. Vol. IV. Bas-reliefs et peintures. Scènes de la vie quotidienne (part 1). Paris: A. and J. Picard.

Vandier, J. (1969). *Manuel d'Archéologie Egyptienne*. Vol. V. Bas-reliefs et peintures. Scènes de la vie quotidienne (part 2). Paris: A. and J. Picard.

Van Veen, A.G. (1966). Toxic properties of some unusual foods, in *Toxicants Occurring Naturally in Foods*. Report of the Food Protection Committee, Food and Nutrition Board. National Research Council Publication no. 1345. Washington, D.C.: National Academy of Sciences.

Vilter, R.D., W.J. Darby and H.S. Glazer (1954). *A Survey of pellagra and nutritional anaemia in Egypt*. Geneva: W.H.O.

Virgil (1965). *Georgics*, with an English translation by H. Ruston Fairclough. London: William Heinemann.

Volten, A. (1942). *Demotische Traumdeutung*. Papyrus Carlsberg XIV Copenhagen: Levine and Munksgaard.

Von Deines H. and H. Grapow (1959). *Wörterbuch der aegyptischen Drogennamen*, Vol. 6 of *Grundriss der Medizin der Alten Aegypter*. Berlin: Akademie-Verlag.

Von Deines, H., H. Grapow and W. Westendorf (1958). *Uebersetzung der medizinischen Texte*, Vol. 4 of *Grundriss der Medizin der Altern Aegypter*. Berlin: Akademie-Verlag.

Waddell, W.G. (1940). *See Manetho.*

Wainwright, G.A. (1951). Egyptian origin of a ram-headed breast-plate from Lagos. *Man*, 231.

Walker, W. (1957). *All the plants of the Bible*. New York: Harper.

Wallert, I. (1962). *Die Palmen im Alten Aegypten*. Berlin: Bruno Hessling.

Waslien, C.I., Z. Farid and W.J. Darby (1973). The malnutrition of parasitism in Egypt. *Southern Medical Journal*, **66,** 47–50.

Weatherwax, P. (1954). *Indian Corn in Old America*, New York: Macmillan and Company.

Weill, R. (1908). *Des Monuments et de l'Histoire des IIe et IIIe dynasties egyptiennes*. pp. 240–251. Paris: Ernest Lebrun.

Weill, R. (1950). Les transmissions littéraires d'Egypte à Israel. *Revue d'Egyptologie*. Cahier Complémentaire.

Wendorf, F., R. Said, and R. Schild (1970). Egyptian prehistory: some new concepts. *Science*, **169,** 1161–1171.

White, R. C. (1910). *Transactions of the National Conference on Pellagra*, The South Carolina Board of Health. Nos. 3–4, 1909. Columbia, S.C.: The State Company.

Whymper, C. (1909). *Egyptian Birds for the Most Part Seen in the Nile Valley*. London: Adam and Charles Black.

Wiedemann, A. (1878). Die Phönix-Sage im alten Aegypten. *Zeitschrift für aegyptische Sprache und Altertumskunde*, **16,** 89–106.

Wiedemann, A. and B. Pörtner (1906). *Aegyptische Grabreliefs aus der Grossherzoglichen Altertumer-Sammlung zu Karlsruhe*. Strassburg: Schlesier und Schweikhardt.

Wild, H. (1966). Brasserie et Panification au tombeau de Ti. *Bulletin de l'Institut Français d'Archéologie Orientale*, **64,** 95–120.

Wilkinson, J.G. (1854). *A Popular Account of the Ancient Egyptians*. 2 Vols. New York: Harper.

Wilkinson, J.G. (1878). *The Manners and Customs of the Ancient Egyptians*. 3 Vols. London: John Murray.

Williams, J.G. (1967). *A Field Guide to the Birds of East and Central Africa*. 3rd edition. London: Collins.

Willis, E.H. (1969). Radiocarbon dating, in *Science in Archaeology*. Edited by D. Brothwell and E. Higgs, pp. 46–57. London: Thames and Hudson.

Wilson, W.H. (1921). The diet factor in pellagra. *Journal of Hygiene*, **20,** 1.

Winkler, H.A. (1938–1939). *Rock-drawings of Southern Upper Egypt.* 2 Vols. Vol. 1. Sir Robert Mond Desert Expedition. Season 1936–37. Preliminary Report. Egypt Exploration Fund. London: Oxford University Press.

Winlock, H.E. (1932). *The Tomb of Queen Meryet-Amun at Thebes.* Egyptian Expedition Publication. Vol. 6. New York: Metropolitan Museum of Art.

Winlock, H.E. (1942). *The Doorkeeper of the Temple of Amon-pe-khor-en-Khonsu.* Excavations at Deir el Bahari. 1911–1931. New York: MacMillan.

Winlock, H.E. (1955). *Models of Daily Life in Ancient Egypt.* Cambridge: Harvard University Press.

Winlock, H.E. and W.E. Crum (1926). *The Monastery of Epiphanus at Thebes.* part 1. New York: Metropolitan Museum of Art.

Winton, A.L. and K.B. Winton (1935). *Analysis of Foods.* New York: J. Wiley and Son.

Winton, A.L. and K.B. Winton (1945). *Analysis of Foods.* 2nd edition. London: Chapman.

Wissa Wassef, C. (1971). *Pratiques rituelles et alimentaires coptes.* Cairo: Institut Français d'Archéologie Orientale.

Wönig, F. (1886). *Die Pflanzen im alten Aegypten, ihre Heimat, Geschichte, Kultur, und ihre mannigfache Verwendung im soziale Leben, in Kultur, Sitten, Gebrauchen, Medizin, Kunst.* 2nd edition. Leipzig: Wilhelm Friedrich.

Wreszinski, W. (1909). *Der grosse medizinische Papyrus des Berliner Museums (pap. Berlin 3038) mit Uebersetzung, Kommentar und Glossar.* Leipzig: Hinrichs.

Wreszinski, W. (1912). *Der Londoner medizinische Papyrus (British Museum nr. 10059) und der Papyrus Hearst in Transkription, Uebersetzung und Kommentar.* Leipzig: Hinrichs.

Wreszinski, W. (1913). *Der Papyrus Ebers, Umschrift. Uebersetzung, und Kommentar.* Leipzig: Hinrichs.

Wreszinski, W. (1913–1942). *Atlas z. Altaegyptischen Kulturgeschichte.* Leipzig: Hinrichs.

Xenophon (1921–1922). *Anabasis*, in Vols 2 and 3 of *Works.* Translated by C.L. Brownson and O.J. Todd. London: William Heinemann.

Zaky, A. and Z. Iskandar (1932). Ancient Egyptian Cheese. *Annales du Service des Antiquités de l'Egypte*, **41,** 295–313.

Zander, E. (1941). *Beiträge zur Herkunfstbestimmung bei Hönig.* Vol. III, II Teil, Versuch der Pollenanalyse eines um 1350 v. Chr. einer aegyptische Mumie in der Nähe von Thebe beigegeben Honigs. Leipzig: Liedloff, Loth und Michaelis.

Zawzani, A.A.H. ibn A. El (1972). *Shark el-Moallaqat el Sab^c,* 2nd edition. Beirut: Dar el Gil (Arabic).

Zenker, F.A. (1860). Ueber die Trichinen-Krankheit des Menschen. *Virchows Archiv für pathologische Anatomie und Physiologie und fur klinische Medizin,* **18,** 561–572.

Index of Popular Sayings

Sayings are listed in the order in which they appear

I

Index to Volumes 1 and 2

The subentries have been arranged in order of reference, rather than in alphabetical order.

A

Âaâ
symptoms of, 74–76
suggested identification with occult poison, 75
incorrectly identified with *Schistosomum*, 76
suggested identification with Egyptian chlorosis or hypochromic anaemia, 76

Aardvark
sketch of dating to Pre-Dynastic period, 206

Ababdeh Desert, 737

Abesh wine, identification of, 608–609

Abortion wine, reference to during Roman Period, 614

Abu Gourob, mummified Latus fish found at, 392

Abu Mena, Christian archaeological site south of Borg el Arab, 607

Abu Simbel, temple of Rameses II at, 465

Abydos, bones of swine found at, 173
burial place of the heart of Osiris, 180

Abydos king list, 43

Acacia gum, 156

Achilles raised on intestines of lions and bear marrow, 90
raised on intestines of swine, 198
raised by Chiron the centaur, 198

Addax hunted as food, 103

Admonitions of a prophet, reports of swine kept by Ancient Egyptian nobility, 185

Adonis, followers of the Greek god rejected pork as food, 198

Aeson (father of Jason the Argonaut), suicide of by drinking bulls' blood, 167

Agrostis, rhizomes sold for treatment of urinary lithiasis, 667

Ahmed el Badawi, festival of, at Tanta, 165, 651

Ahura-Mazda, Persian god of light, 249

Akhmimic dialect (*see* Coptic language)

Alcohol, produced only through natural fermentation, 613

Alexander the Great
founded city of Alexandria, 10
visit of, to Siwa oasis, 218, 220
accused of being intoxicated, 584

Alexandria
general information, 11
data on Jewish community at, 201
foundations of laid out with barley, 482

Algeria, presence of toxic quail, 312

Almond
general, 751–752
associated with ease and pleasure, 752
consumption of thought to neutralize effects of alcohol, 752
medicinal uses of, 752
believed to induce sleep, 752
believed to increase appetite, 752

Almond oil
general, 752, 780–782

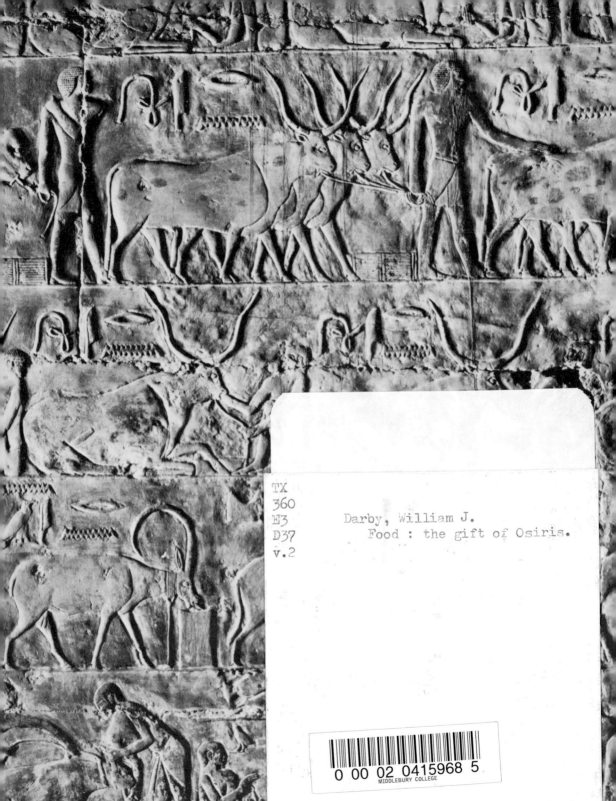